ATLANTIS STUDIES IN PROBABILITY AND STATISTICS

VOLUME 1

SERIES EDITOR: CHRIS P. TSOKOS

Atlantis Studies in Probability and Statistics

Series Editor:

Chris P. Tsokos, University of South Florida,
Tampa, USA

(ISSN: 1879-6893)

Aims and scope of the series

The Series 'Atlantis Studies in Probability and Statistics' publishes studies of high-quality throughout the areas of probability and statistics that have the potential to make a significant impact on the advancement in these fields. Emphasis is given to broad interdisciplinary areas at the following three levels:

(I) Advanced undergraduate textbooks, i.e., aimed at the 3rd and 4th years of undergraduate study, in probability, statistics, biostatistics, business statistics, engineering statistics, operations research, etc.;

(II) Graduate level books, and research monographs in the above areas, plus Bayesian, non-parametric, survival analysis, reliability analysis, etc.;

(III) Full Conference Proceedings, as well as Selected topics from Conference Proceedings, covering frontier areas of the field, together with invited monographs in special areas. All proposals submitted in this series will be reviewed by the Editor-in-Chief, in consultation with Editorial Board members and other expert reviewers.

For more information on this series and our other book series, please visit our website at:

www.atlantis-press.com/publications/books

ATLANTIS PRESS

AMSTERDAM – PARIS

Bayesian Theory and Methods with Applications

Vladimir P. Savchuk

National Metallurgical Academy of Ukraine
Gagarina Av. 4, 49600 Dnipropetrovsk, Ukraine

Chris P. Tsokos

University of South Florida
Department of Mathematics and Statistics
1202 Parrilla de Avila, Tampa, FL 33613, USA

ATLANTIS PRESS

AMSTERDAM – PARIS

Atlantis Press

8, square des Bouleaux
75019 Paris, France

For information on all Atlantis Press publications, visit our website at: *www.atlantis-press.com*

Atlantis Studies in Probability and Statistics

ISBNs
Print: 978-94-91216-41-1
E-Book: 978-94-91216-14-5
ISSN: 1879-6893

Softcover reprint of the hardcover 1st edition 2011

Preface

This textbook aimed at the advanced undergraduate and graduate readership is devoted to a systematic account of the fundamentals of the Bayes theory of statistical estimation with applications to the analysis of engineering reliability. Lately, there has been a significant trend toward using the Bayesian approach to develop and analyze problems in different fields of our society. At the same time, the Bayes theory is characterized by an inner logical harmony and simplicity which makes it still more attractive for applied purposes. The application of the bayes theory and methods in the field of reliability gives us the opportunity to save money and time assigned for experiments owing to utilization of relevant prior information instead of the corresponding number of trials.

The subject matter of the book pursues the following double aim:

1. To give an account of the present state of the Bayes theory and methods with emphasis on application.
2. To demonstrate how we can use the Bayes approach for the evaluation of the reliability function in the calculations of reliability which, in practice, covers a great variety of the problems of statistical analysis of engineering reliability.

The distinguishing feature of this monograph is a close unity of fundamental investigation of the main principles of the Bayes theory with clear presentation of its practical applications. The rendering of the fundamentals of the Bayes methodology follows the classical works by Ramsey, Good, Savage, Jefferys, and De Groot, while its present state is represented by the results produced during the last 30 years by a number of scientists from the U.S.A., Canada and countries of Western Europe. The greater part of the monograph is comprised of the presentation of new and original results of the author, the most significant of which are Bayes quasi-parametric estimators, Bayes relative minimax estimators under the conditions of a partial prior information, and the estimators of the working capacity with an additive error. The Bayes procedures suggested in the monograph are distinguished by a simple way of representation of prior information and use of censored samples that undoubtedly testify to their practical usefulness. The subject methodology presented in this monograph is illustrated with a great number of examples.

Chapter 1 of the monograph plays the role of an introduction and is, in fact, a brief excursion into the history of the Bayes approach. The general principles of the Bayes approach and hierarchical Bayes methodology are discussed in this chapter. Also included are the varieties of subjective probability constructions, as well as an application of the Bayes methodology in the reliability field.

Chapter 2 describes the components of the Bayes approach. In particular, forms of loss functions, choice of the prior probability distribution and the general procedure of reliability estimation are considered.

A systematic description of accepted estimation procedures is given in Chapter 3. The authors demonstrate the process of solving the problems of survival probability estimation from accelerated life tests.

Chapter 4 is devoted to non-parametric Bayes estimation which, in our opinion, is the front line of Bayes theory. Nonparametric Bayes estimators in which the Dirichlet processes are not used are discussed. The authors also consider the nonparametric bayes approach of quantile estimation for increasing failure rate.

A detailed presentation of a new method called "quasi-parametric" is given in Chapter 5. Bayes estimators of a reliability function for a restricted increasing failure rate distribution are studied.

Chapter 6 deals with the class of Bayes estimators of a reliability function under the conditions of partial prior information. The setting of the problem and its general solution that yields a new type of estimator are considered.

Chapter 7 is devoted to empirical Bayes estimators first suggested by Robins. The main results are described briefly. The authors present a new method based on the idea of quasi-parametrical estimation.

Chapters 8–10 are united by common contents that are based on a reliability estimation using functional models of working capacity.

The monograph is addressed (first and foremost) to practicing scientists, though it also deals with a number of theoretical problems. The monograph is a blend of thorough, mathematically-strict presentations of the subject matter and it is easily readable. The monograph can be a useful, authoritative and fundamental source of reference for training statisticians, scientists and engineers in different fields.

The authors are grateful to several reviewers for their useful suggestions that we have included in the manuscripts: Dr. M. McWaters, Dr. Dennis Koutras, Dr. S. Sambandham, Dr. G. G. Haritonov, Dr. V. B. Chernjavskii, Dr. G. Aryal and Dr. R. Wooten.

Finally, we would like to thank Taysseer Sharaf for his kind assistance in the preparation of the manuscript. I would also like to thank Ms. Beverly DeVine-Hoffmeyer for her excellent assistance in typing this book.

Contents

Chapter 1

General Questions of Bayes Theory

1.1 A brief excursus into the history of the Bayes approach

The Bayes approach is credited to the well-known paper by Thomas Bayes which was published. Nearly three years after his death. G. Crellin asserts [50] that the Bayes notes concerned with the ideas touching upon the field, named the Bayes approach, were discovered by Richard Price, who sent them to the Royal Society under the title "Note on the Solution of a Problem in a Doctrine about an Event". A current account of this paper can be found in [13]. R.A. Fisher [84] gives an analysis of Bayes' work in terms we use now. Later, some of the opponents of the Bayes approach ascertained that this work was not published in his lifetime because of Bayes' doubt about the validity of the conclusions proposed in it. Such a point-of-view about an event which happened more than 200 years ago may be considered at least strange and, in any case, cannot be used as an argument in a scientific dispute.

We now turn our attention to the importance of the Bayes Theory foundations. In the second part of his work (the first one does not have any new ideas), Bayes considers a speculative trial with a successive rolling of two balls. The rolling of the first ball corresponds to some number from the interval $[0,1]$. The rolling of the second ball forms the sequence of n binomial outcomes with the probabilities of success p and failure $(1-p)$ for each trial. Suppose that X is the number of successes and Y the number of failures. Then we can write

$$P\{p_1 \leqslant p \leqslant p_2,\, X=a,\, Y=b\} = \int_{p_1}^{p_2} \frac{n!}{a!\,b!} p^a (1-p)^b dp. \tag{1.1}$$

Putting $p_1 = 0$, $p_2 = 1$ in (1.1) we obtain

$$P\{X=a,\, y=b\} = \int_0^1 \frac{n!}{a!\,b!} p^a (1-p)^b dp = \frac{1}{n+1}. \tag{1.2}$$

Thus, the parameter p is assumed to be random and the probability of the event of p being in the interval dp is proportional to the length of this segment. In other words, p is distributed uniformly in $[0,1]$. This fact is also emphasized by the corollary of (1.2) which asserts the probability of observing a successes and b failures is a priori independent of the values of a and b but depends on the sum of a and b. The property of uniformness of the prior distribution appears to be somewhat obscure in the Bayes work and is often disregarded. This problem is the subject of the special analysis in the work by A. Edwards [72].

The following Bayes lemma determines the conditional posterior probability of a random parameter p falling into some interval $[p_1, p_2]$:

$$P\{p_1 \leqslant p \leqslant p_2 \mid X = a,\ Y = b\} = \frac{(n+1)!}{a!\,b!} \int_{p_1}^{p_2} p^a (1-p)^b dp. \tag{1.3}$$

1.2 The Philosophy of the Bayes Approach

Philosophic aspects of Bayes theory can be separated into two groups dealing with: 1) the relationship between inductive and deductive ways of thinking; and 2) the interpretation of probability.

The deductive approach of thinking played a major role in scientific practice during the time of formation of the Bayes method. Bayes results have actually shown how one can transform the inductive judgement problem into the problem of probability.

At the present time, the question of the relationship between induction and deduction is being solved more seriously and completely using Bayes theory Jeffrey's book [115] gives a complete analysis of the relationship between induction and deduction, including the leading role of the Bayes approach.

Jeffrey's discusses two basic arguments. First, the deductive method itself cannot build an adequate base for all possible conclusions of any applied science. The second argument of Jeffrey's leans in favor of the arbitrarily-takennon-uniqueness of the tool of deductive logic is that for any drawn observation set there exists a huge number of describing laws.

Broader choice principles are necessary. One of them is the simplicity principle of "Occam's" blade [275]. Therefore, deductive thinking is a very important element of any scientific conclusion of learning experience. Knowledge obtained this way partially contains the results of previous observations that are going to be used for the prediction of a future result. Jeffrey's calls this part of knowledge a generalization or induction. Jeffrey's considers deductive logic as a special case of inductive logic. Two basic terms "true" and "false" are limit cases of the values given by the inductive logic.

Thus, according to Jeffrey's, the main part of induction is a generalization of previous experience and empirical data for the purpose of analysis of observable events and prediction of future events. To order the induction process Jeffrey's states eight rules (five basic and three auxiliary):

1. All the hypotheses must be clearly stated and all conclusions must be derived only from these hypotheses.
2. An inductive theory must not be self-contradictory.
3. Any given law must be practically doable. The definition is useless unless the object defined can be recognized with this definition.
4. An inductive theory must consider the possibility of the fact that conclusions derived with this theory may be wrong.
5. Inductive theory must not reject empirical observation "a-priori".
   The other three auxiliary rules carry the following sense.
6. The number of postulates must be minimized.
7. Although we do not consider the human brain as a perfect thinking instrument, we have to accept it as useful and as the only one available.
8. Taking into account the complexity of induction, we cannot hope to develop it better than deduction. Therefore, we should discard any statement that contradicts one of pure mathematics.

As suggested by Jeffrey's, induction theory looks reasonable and has obvious practical value. However, if we had accepted it as a starting point, we would have come to a contradiction with the most common "frequency" interpretation of probability.
Let us note that from the point of view of mathematics, probability is the function of the set satisfying the axioms of general measure theory. In order to apply the theorems of mathematical probability (including Bayes theory), it is enough to accept the fact that those axioms are fulfilled. At the same time, all the conclusions can have different interpretations depending on the sense of the initial definition of probability.
There are two poles of the probability theory: objective and subjective probability. In the objective sense, a probability of an event A is considered together with the fulfilment of certain conditions [90]. We should select two things here: first, principal regeneration; and second, an infinite number of experiments with conditions remaining constant. Both attributes a rein direct contradiction with the third rule of Jeffrey's. In other words, it becomes unacceptable to describe real or possible events by the objective definition of probability.
In the subjective sense, probability is a qualitative estimate of the possibility of the event given, for example, by the individual experience of the investigator. Subjective probability

is adequate to the theory of inductive conclusions and satisfies the axioms of probability at the same time. It is evident that all the trust levels are very approximate.

Considering the relationship between two interpretations of probability,it is necessary to investigate two important questions. The first approaches concerned with the notion of randomness associated with the Bayes approach, the second with studying the real meaning of the term "objective".

The existing disagreements between "subjectivists" and "objectivists" are of a mostly terminological nature. As a matter of fact, when talking about probability, people always mean frequency.

All the philosophical questions considered in this section justify the use of Bayes' approach as a general system of inductive thinking, and explain the irrelevance of the approach of scientists who firmly stand on objectivist positions.

1.3 The General Principles of Bayes Methodology

We understand the methodology of the Bayes approach as a collection of constructing principles, forms and learning methods. Let us first try to understand the basics of Bayes theory. Often when talking about only Bayes theory people think about only certain aspects of it. At the same time, the modern understanding of Bayes approach is a complete theory naturally containing the following statements.

Statement 1. The parameter of the system studied is random. Moreover, the "randomness" is understood not only in a general sense but also as "uncertainty". A random parameter is assigned prior distribution.

Statement 2. All the observed results and the prior distribution are unified by the Bayes theorem in order to obtain a posterior distribution parameter.

Statement 3. A statistical conclusion or decision rule is accepted with a condition of maximal estimated utility, in particular, the minimization of loss related to this rule.

We shall consider all these statements separately.

1.3.1 *Possible interpretations of probability*

Unlike classical estimate theory dealing with non-random parameters, Bayes'theory assumes random parameters. This randomness is understood in a general sense, when the values of the parameter are generated by the stable real mechanism with known properties or properties that can be obtained by the study of corresponding data.

In most of the cases involving technical problems, all the parameters of the system or model are constants of the special kind that represent in certain idealized form some inner properties of the system or model studied.The meaning of uncertainty can be easily seen in the following example. The correlation between two physical values that are random in a classical sense is studied. The coefficient of the correlation describes the correlation itself and is an adequate characteristic of correlation. However, it is impossible to find, more or less, its precise value without conducting a large number of experiments. From previous experience, we know that this coefficient is non-negative. Hence, we conclude that the coefficient is contained in the interval $[0,1]$ and we don't know which value in this interval it takes. How can we measure its uncertainty? What mathematical instrument can adequately characterize it? One of the possible variants is Jeffrey's' approach based on rational levels of certainty.

An interpretation of judgment in Bayes methodology always has a probabilistic nature. However, randomness is considered not only in a classical sense but also as uncertainty. Probabilistic judgment can be one of three types:

1. By means of objective probability interpretation;
2. By means of rational levels of certainty that mostly are reduced to a mathematical representation of the absence of prior knowledge;
3. By means of subjective levels of confidence that represent the personal relation of the investigator to the event or system being studied.

All these areas of study in practice do not overlap.

1.3.2 *A union of prior information and empirical data*

Bayes theorem gives us the base to transfer from prior to posterior information by adding empirical data. This process can be represented as a consequent gathering of information. At the initial stage of study, one has certain information about the properties of the system being studied based on previous experience. Except for non-formal experience, this contains empirical data obtained before conducting a similar experiment. During the testing the investigator collects new information that changes his judgment about the system properties. By doing this, he reconsiders and re-evaluates his prior information. Moreover, at any moment of time we describe the system properties, and this description is complete in a sense that we used all the information available. This process does not stop; it continues with every new empirical result.

Zelner's probability reconsideration diagram [275] is very illustrative, see Fig. 1.1. Let system properties be represented by, generally speaking, vector parameter θ; I_a stands for the initial information. Formalization of initial information is done by recording prior parameter distribution, which is conditional to I_a that is, $h(\theta \mid I_a)$. All empirical data collected during the test are formalized by the "likelihood" function $\ell(\theta \mid x)$. The former represents the probability (or probability density) of the empirical data observed and written as a function of the parameter. Essentially, to get $\ell(\theta \mid x)$ we need to know the model of the system as a conditional probability distribution of a random variable or some other representation. Bayes' theorem, by means of the transformation

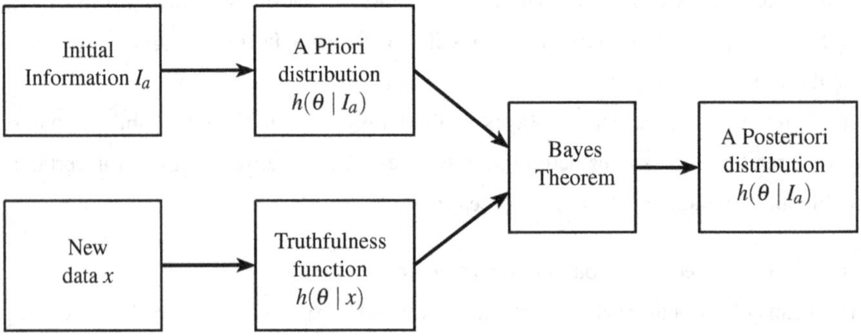

Fig. 1.1 Zelner's probability reconsiderations diagram.

$$h\left(\theta \mid x, I_a = \frac{h(\theta \mid x, I_a)\ell(\theta \mid x)}{\int h(\theta \mid x, I_a\ell(\theta \mid x)d\theta}\right)$$

allows us to obtain posterior probability distribution of the parameter $\theta : h(\theta \mid x, I_a)$, that is conditional with respect to the initial information I_a and empirical data x.

The more information we collect, the more it dominates in the posterior distribution. The distribution density accumulates near the true value of the parameter. If two investigators used different prior information, their a posterior distributions get closer and closer to each other.

This pattern is called an *orthodox Bayes procedure*. Its difference from other modifications is that the prior distribution remains the same during the collection of empirical data. This property was mentioned by De Finetti [61].

Limer [140] gives a more complicated modification of the orthodox scheme that assumes a possibility of correction of prior confidence levels, see Figure 1.2.
This modification is called *rational Bayes procedure.* The main feature of both Bayes procedures, orthodox and rational, is that they always can be used for concrete calculations and for the purposes of applying it to a broad spectrum of problems.

1.3.3 *Optimality of Bayes estimation rules*

The final result of all Bayes procedures described above is the posterior of the distribution parameter characterizing the basic properties of the system or event under study. This distribution gives a clear and complete description of the parameter uncertainty. However, in many situations it is necessary to have a shorter decision rule giving a parameter description of one or several constants estimating an unknown parameter. Examples of such constants are point estimates and Bayes confidence limits.
In a Bayes approach the difference between the parameter and its estimate can be found in its utility function. The former characterizes losses that appear as a consequence of substitution of the true parameter value by its estimate. The estimation rule is chosen so that it minimizes the mathematical expectation of the loss function. This rule is general for all problems of estimation theory, which is a great advantage of the Bayes approach.
The decision function which minimizes the expected losses is called by Vald [257] an *optimal Bayes solution with respect to the chosen prior* distribution.

1.4 Subjective probabilities

The Bayes approach is based essentially on subjective probabilities and, due to this, the conceptions of these probabilities are a part of the Bayes methodology. Below we consider the foundations of the theory of subjective probabilities in connection with the Bayes approach.
It was Jacob Bernulli who proposed, for the first time, to treat probabilities as degrees or levels of confidence. This point-of-view appears in his book "The Skills of Assumptions" which was published in 1713, eight years after his death. In the 19th Century, De Morgan promoted the doctrine that a probability is not an objective characteristic of the external universe, but a subjective quantity which may change from subject to subject. Further development of the theory of subjective probabilities was obtained in the works by Ramsey [203], De Finetti [61], Koopman [126], Savage [216], De Groot [63] and other authors.

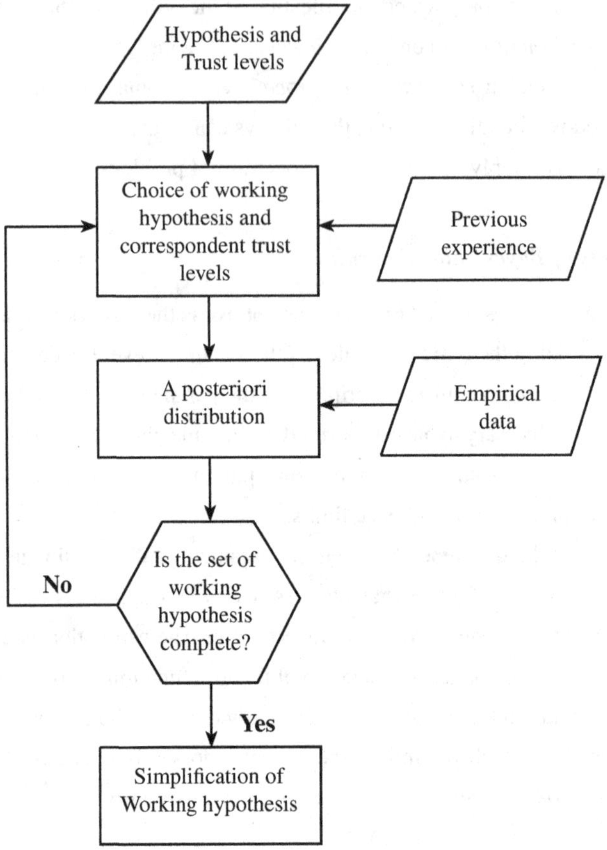

Fig. 1.2 Limer scheme.

Here we set forth the main principles of this theory in accordance with the works by De Finneti and De Groot.

For the ordering of confidence levels we introduce axiomatically the notion of the *relalive likelihood* of an event (or a proposition) compared to another one. Further, $A \prec B$ indicates that the event A is more probable than the event B; the notation $A \sim B$ is used for events with the same likelihoods. Probability, starting from an intuitive point of view, is a numerical measure of the likelihood of an event A. A probability distribution, having been given, not only points out the difference in likelihoods of two events, but also indicates how much one of the events is more probable than another.

It is important that a probability distribution be consistent with the relation $\preccurlyeq$. For any probability distribution, defined on σ-algebra of the events, the property of consistency means that $P\{A\} \leqslant P\{B\}$ iff $A \preccurlyeq B$. Let us suppose that the relation is subjected to the following requirements.

1) For any two events A and B, one and only one of the following relations takes place: $A \prec B$, $B \prec A$, $A \sim B$.
2) If, for A_1, A_2, B_1, B_2, we have $A_1 \cap A_2 = B_1 \cap B_2 = \theta$ and $A_i \preccurlyeq B_i$, then $A_1 \cup A_2 \preccurlyeq B_1 \cup B_2$. If, in addition to this, $A_1 \prec B_1$ or $A_2 \prec B_2$, then $A_1 \cup A_2 \prec B_1 \cup B_2$.
3) Whatever an event A will be, $\theta \preccurlyeq A$. Moreover, $\theta \prec \Omega$, where Ω is a sample space.
4) If $A_1 \supset A_2 \ldots$ is a decreasing sequence of events, besides $A_i \succcurlyeq B_i$, $i = 1, 2, \ldots$, where B is some fixed event, then $\bigcup_{i=1}^{n} A_i \succcurlyeq B$.

These assumptions appear to be axioms of the theory of subjective probabilities. Further, it is proved first that the unique probability distribution associated with the relation $\preccurlyeq$ and, second, the Kolmogorov's probability axioms are valid for the random events, given by the assumptions 1–4.

Subjective probabilities, being a numerical measure of an event likelihood, are found by their comparison with the events having certain probabilities. In view of this circumstance, we have to assume that there exists a class β of events with the following properties: 1) each event from the class β has a certain probability; 2) for each number p ($0 \leqslant p \leqslant 1$) there is an event $B \in \beta$ the probability of which is equal to p. Thus, to determine the probability of some event A, we need to find such an event $B \in \beta$ that $A \sim B$ and to assign to A the same probability as that of B. As events from the class β are chosen, the events of the form $Z \in I$, where X is a random variable having uniform distribution on $[0,1]$, $I = [a,b]$. In particular, if $I_1 \subset I_2$, then $\{X \in I_1\} \succcurlyeq \{X \in I_2\}$. To perform such a passing, we state one last assumption: there exists a random variable with a uniform distribution in the interval $[0,1]$.

The above method of obtaining subjective probabilities was named byDe Groot [63] *an auxiliary experiment.* Clearly, it is not necessary to carry out such an experiment; moreover, even the existence of its establishment is redundant. It is sufficient that a statistician imagine an ideal experiment which determines a random variable with the uniform distribution and be able to compare the relative likelihood of the event he is interested in with that of an arbitrary event of the form $\{X \in I\}$.

The uniqueness of the distribution $P\{A\}$is justified by the following theorem (proved in [63]).

Theorem 1.1. *For any event A there is the unique number a_* ($0 \leqslant a_* \leqslant 1$) such $A \sim G[0, a_*]$. Here $G[a,b] = \{X \in [a,b]\}$. The desired probability distribution, in view of the theorem, is represented by the relation*

$$A \sim G[0, P\{A\}].$$

As follows from this relation, for any two events A and B such that $A \preccurlyeq B$, $G[0, P\{A\}] \preccurlyeq G[0, P\{B\}]$, hence $P\{A\} \leqslant P\{B\}$.

Another way to determine the subjective probability is based on the union of the conceptions of the indeterminacy and usefulness. Ramsey initiated the solution theory which was based on the duality; of interconnected notions of estimating probability and usefulness. In accordance with this theory, the probability appears to be the degree of readiness of the object to perform one or another action in the situation of the decision making with unreliable possible gains. It is required only that all possible outcomes be of equal value.
The work by De Finetti, devoted to the determination of subjective probabilities in the situation of the chance analysis in laying a bet, is a brilliant development of this theory. Let us consider, briefly, the essence of the De Finetti constructions. Suppose that we have to estimate the chances on the set of certain events $A, B, C, \ldots$ and to take any bets from people who want to bet on these events. This means that each event A is associatedwith some probability $P\{A\}$. If now, S_A is the opponent bet (positive or negative), that is, this sum must be paid off in the case when the event A happens, then the cost of the bet participation ticket must be equal to $P\{A\}S_A$. It is natural to raise a question: "What desired properties must be assigned for these probabilities". De Finetti proposed to use the following coherence principle: the *probabilities must be assigned in such a way that there is no loss in general.* This simple principle implies immediately the fulfilment of all probability axioms.

a) $0 \leqslant P\{A\} \leqslant 1$. If the opponent bets on A and A really happens, then his prize will be S, less the ticket price $P\{A\}S_A$, that is $W_1 = S[1 - P\{A\}]$. If the event A doesn't occur, then his prize is $W_2 = -SP\{A\}$. The coherence principle requires that $W_1 W_2 \leqslant 0$ for all S, that is, $[1 - P\{A\}]P\{A\} \geqslant 0$ or $0 \leqslant P\{A\} \leqslant 1$.
b) $P\{\Omega\} = 1$. Whenever an event will occur, it belongs to a sample space Ω. If the opponent bets on Ω, his prize is $W_\Omega = S_\Omega[1 - P\{\Omega\}]$. Due to the coherence condition, there is no such S_Ω, that $W_\Omega > 0$. Hence it follows the relation $P(\Omega) = 1$.
c) If $A \cap B = \theta$, then $P\{A \cup B\} = P\{A\} + P\{B\}$. Let the opponent bet on the event A, B and $C = A \cup B$. The following outcomes with corresponding prizes are possible:

$$\begin{aligned}
&\text{for } A\cap\bar{B}W_1 = S_A(1-P\{A\}) - S_BP\{B\} + S_C(1-P\{C\}),\\
&\text{for } \bar{A}\cap BW_2 = -S_AP\{A\} + S_B(1-P\{B\}) + S_C(1-P\{C\}),\\
&\text{for } \bar{A}\cap\bar{B}W_3 = -S_AP\{A\} - S_BP\{B\} - S_CP\{C\}.
\end{aligned} \tag{1.4}$$

The coherence condition requires the following: there are no such S_A, S_B and S_C that the prizes W_1, W_2 and W_3 are simultaneously positive. If the main matrix of the system of linear equations (1.4) is invertible, then it is possible to make the bet's S_A, S_B and S_C in such a way that the prizes get arbitrary preassigned values.

In order for this not to happen, the determinant of the main matrix of the system (1.4) must be equal to O, that is,

$$\begin{vmatrix} 1-P\{A\} & -P\{B\} & 1-P\{A\cup B\} \\ -P\{A\} & 1-P\{B\} & 1-P\{A\cup B\} \\ -P\{A\} & -P\{B\} & -P\{A\cup B\} \end{vmatrix} = 0,$$

or $-P\{A\cup B\} + P\{A\} + P\{B\} = 0$.

Hence

$$P\{A\cup B\} + P\{A\} + P\{B\}.$$

From the De Finetti construction we may conclude: as far as the confidence degrees (for the estimation of the bet chances in the subject case) are subjected to the Kolmogorov axioms and have a probability interpretation, they can be represented in a probability form. Limer [140] ascertains that there is only one answer to a question about the requirements imposed on the confidence levels: "They must be only probabilities and there are no other needed requirements. If a relative frequency is given and all events are equiprobable, then, in view of such a confluence of circumstances, the individual probability is found to be equal to the frequency."

The theorem on interchangeability of events is an important result of the De Finetti theory. First of all, De Finetti ascertains that the notion of independence, broadly used in classical statistics, appears to be only a mathematical abstraction and cannot be related to the chain of events which are recognized intuitively or empirically. Instead of the notion "independence" he introduces the notion "interchangeability": a sequence of random events is called *interchangeable* if the corresponding (to events) probabilities are independent of the successive order of the events. For example, $A\bar{A}\bar{A}$ and $\bar{A}A\bar{A}$ have the same probabilities.

The following important theorem is proved byDe Finetti [62].

Theorem 1.2. *Any coherent assignment of probabilities for the finite interchangeable sequence of binomial events is equivalent to the limit assignment of these events with the help of the simultaneous distribution for which:*

a) *if it is considered as conditional with respect to p, then the events appear to be mathematically independent and*

$$P\{AA\ldots\bar{A}A\ldots\bar{A}\} = p^r(1-p)^{n-r};$$

b) *there is a unique prior distribution $h(p)$. A marginal distribution has, in this case, the following form:*

$$P\{AA\ldots\bar{A}A\ldots\bar{A}\} = \int_0^1 p^r(1-p)^{n-r}h(p)dp.$$

This theorem gives the important methodological result of the prediction of the happening of possible events. For example, given some true assignment of probabilities of an infinite sequence of interchangeable events and if the number of successes in the first n trials is r, then the success probability in the next trial equals

$$\begin{aligned} P\{A_{n+1}\,|\,A_1A_2\bar{A}_3\cdots A_n\} &= \frac{P\{A_1A_2\bar{A}_3\cdots A_nA_{n+1}\}}{P\{A_1A_2\bar{A}_3\cdots A_n\}} \\ &= \frac{\displaystyle\int_0^1 p^{r+1}(1-p)^{n-r}h(p)dp}{\displaystyle\int_0^1 p^r(1-p)^{n-r}h(p)dp} = \int_0^1 p\hbar(p)dp, \end{aligned}$$

where

$$\hbar(p) = \frac{p^r(1-p)^{n-r}h(p)}{\displaystyle\int_0^1 p^r(1-p)^{n-r}h(p)dp}.$$

Thus, the probability of foreseeing the outcome of the next trial is such that as it would be some true part of successes p and some prior distribution $\hbar(p)$ which transforms, in view of Bayes theorem, into the posterior distribution $\hbar$, starting from the results of independent sampling.

There is a theory of subjective probabilities which concentrates on the guarantee of the possibility to transmitting the subjective information. It was developed in the works by Cox [49], Tribus [250] and was philosophically substantiated by Crellin [50]. The possibility of the subjective information to be transmitted and the use of likelihood for the acceptance of decisions are the source of this theory. The system, consisting of likelihoods, must be subjected to the following requirements:

1) The system must not be ambiguous, that is, the assertion, for which the likelihood is used, must be precise.
2) The system must guarantee comparability in general. Likelihoods of different statements must have the possibility of comparison in order to transfer subjective information about which of the events is more probable. The system must be admissible for any assertion.
3) The system must be noncontradictory, that is, if we have different ways of likelihood estimating, it is necessary that their results be the same.
4) The system must possess the property of continuity of the method of likelihood estimating.

The first requirement is satisfied due to the use of symbol logic and logical propositions, the second one because of the real number range for the quantity likelihood measure. The third and the fourth conditions require that numerical representation of likelihood for composite statements be subjected to the functional relations which use the likelihoods of components. Reasoning intuitively one comes to the conclusion that the likelihood measure $\Theta(\cdot)$ must satisfy the relations

$$\Theta\{A\cap B \mid C\} = \Theta\{A \mid C\}\Theta\{B \mid A\cap C\} = \Theta\{B \mid C\}\Theta\{A \mid B\cap C\}, \tag{1.5}$$

and

$$\Theta\{A \mid C\} + \Theta\{\bar{A} \mid C\} = 1. \tag{1.6}$$

In the works [49, 250] the necessity of using these relations precisely for the likelihood measure is substantiated. They are also fundamental in probability theory. There is, however, the principal difference in sense between the classical interpretation of probability and the one given by the relations (1.5) and (1.6). Crelin [50] brings up a justified proposal that such a notion of “probability” is needed only in order to obtain the possibility of manipulation by the usual rules of probability theory and has a deductive form.
We conclude here that the theories of subjective probabilities are based on Kolmogorov’s axioms.

1.5 The Hierarchical Bayes Methodology

This methodology (developed from the orthodox Bayes methodology) is the subject of investigation in the works by Good [93, 94]. The considered phenomenon is associated with different probability levels subjected to each other. The relation among these levels is ensured by means of successive conditional distributions. In this case the Bayes rule is applied as many times as the number of levels, in addition to the initial one, are given. We illustrate the hierarchical Bayes approach in the following example.

Let X follow a normal distribution with unknown mean μ and known standard deviation σ, that is, $f(x) = f(x;\mu) = N(\mu;\sigma)$. This probability level we will consider as the lowest or initial. According to Bayes setting we let $\mu \in M$ be a random parameter, having a prior distribution $h(\mu)$. If we use a prior distribution, and conjugate to the kernel of the "likelihood" function, then for $h(\mu)$ we should take the normal density with parameters a and s, i.e., $h(\mu) = h(\mu;a,s,) = N(a,s)$. With respect to the value of X, a and s are hyper parameters (Good [94], Deely, Lindley [59] and others). So, how do we choose hyper parameters a and s? To do this we have to go one step up in the Bayes hierarchy, that is, let a and s be random parameters and define their a priori distribution $h_1(a,s)$. Then the prior probability density for the parameter μ can be written with the help of a mixed density, if we accept that $h(\mu)$ is conditional density with respect to a and s:

$$h(\mu) = \iint_{\Omega_{as}} h(\mu;a,s)h_1(a,s)da\,ds \tag{1.7}$$

where Ω_{as} is the range for a and s. Then the representation for the marginal density of X has the form

$$\begin{aligned} f(x) &= \int_M f(x;\mu)h(\mu)d\mu \\ &= \int_M f(x;\mu)d\mu \iint_{\Omega_{a,s}} h(\mu;a,s)h_1(a,s)da\,ds \end{aligned} \tag{1.8}$$

It seems obvious that (1.7) can be written for the posterior probability density $\hbar(\mu \mid \cdot)$ as well, if according to the Bayes theorem we add an observation vector of empirical data to the conditional prior density $h(\mu;a,s)$.

1.6 Use of the Bayes methodology in reliability theory

Can we apply the Bayes approach in the reliability theory? This question doesn't have a unique answer among the specialists in this area. If a reliability conclusion has to be considered as an element of the solution process, then empirical data must be added by subjective knowledge related to the subject. This is a direct consequence of an engineering practice. Construction of the new technical device involves on one hand an individual experience, mathematical modeling and analog devices, and on the other experimental work. The set of factors of the first group delivers an a priori judgement about reliability, while experimental work gives empirical data. Both are relevant to the process of making a decision about reliability. Indeed, if we can use our experience while working on a device, why can't we rely on that experience when estimating the quality of the device?

Many scientists and specialists indicate the usefulness of Bayes methodology in reliability theory (see [14], [30], [43]). It will be discussed extensively throughout the development of this book.

Chapter 2

The Accepted Bayes Method of Estimation

2.1 The components of the Bayes approach

We give a brief description of the structure of Bayes estimates with the help of formal mathematical constructions of the Bayes theory. The Bayes scheme of the decision theory includes the following four components.

1) The statistical model, represented by the probability space $(\Omega, \mathscr{L}, P)$. Here Ω is the set of all possible data in some design of experiments Π, $\Omega = \{x\}$. The data x appear to be the data of a random experiment, thus on Ω it is determined some σ-algebra $\mathscr{L}$ of random events; $P \in \mathscr{B}$, where $\mathscr{B}$ is the family of probability measures on Ω, $\mathscr{L}$. In the traditional Bayes approach, the probability measure P is defined by the representation of some parameter θ (vector or scalar), that is, $\mathscr{B} = \{P_\theta\, ;\, \theta \in \Theta\}$ is a parameterized family of probability measures.

2) The probability space $(\Theta, \mathscr{E}, H)$ for the parameter θ which is assumed to be random. Here $\mathscr{E}$ is σ-algebra on Θ, H is a probability measure on $(\Theta, \mathscr{E})$. The measure H is called a prior probability measure of the parameter θ. The prior measure H belongs to some given family of probability measures $\mathscr{H}$.

3) The set of such possible decisions D that each element d from D is a measurable function on Ω. In estimation theory the set of decisions D may contain all estimates of the parameter θ or some function $R(\theta)$ measurable on Ω.

4) The loss functions $L(\theta, d)$ (or $L(R(\theta), d)$) determined on $\Theta \times D$. This loss function determines the losses caused by an erroneous estimation, that is, by the replacement of the parameter θ by the decision element d. It is assumed later that the families $\mathscr{B}$ and $\mathscr{H}$ are dominated by some σ-finite measures μ and ζ respectively. If we denote the densities

$$f(x \mid \theta) = P_\theta\{dx\}/\mu\{dx\}, \quad h(\theta) = H\{d\theta\}/\zeta\{d\},$$

which exist in a view of the Radon-Nikodym theorem, the joint density of the probability distribution for the random variables X and θ takes on the form

$$g(x,\theta) = f(x \mid \theta)h(\theta).$$

In accordance with the Bayes theorem, the conditional density for θ given $X = x$ is called the *posterior probability density function* (p.d.f.) of the parameter θ and is written as

$$\hbar(\theta \mid X = x) = \frac{f(x \mid \theta)h(\theta)}{\int_\Theta f(x \mid \theta)H\{d\theta\}}, \qquad \theta \in \Theta, \tag{2.1}$$

for each $x \in \Omega$ such that

$$f(x) = \int f(x \mid \theta)h(\theta)\zeta\{d\theta\} > 0.$$

If Y is a statistic on $(\Omega, \mathscr{L}, P_\theta)$, then the probability measure P_θ can be obtained by transformation into P_θ^Y. If $f^Y(y \mid \theta) = P_\theta^Y\{dy\}/\mu\{dy\}$ is the density of the probability measure P_θ^Y, then the posterior p.d.f. of the parameter θ given $Y(X) = x$ has the form

$$\hbar^Y(\theta \mid Y = y) = \frac{f^Y(y \mid \theta)h(\theta)}{\int_\Theta f^Y(y \mid \theta)h(\theta)\zeta\{d\theta\}}. \tag{2.2}$$

Further, for the sake of simplicity, we will use for the prior and posterior p.d.f. appearing in the Bayes formulas (2.1) and (2.2) the notations $h(\theta)$ and $h(\theta \mid x)$, respectively. Since the denominator in (2.1) and (2.2) is independent of θ and is determined only by the observation x (or by the statistic y), we will determine only the kernel of the prior density using the symbol of proportionality "$\backsim$". So, instead of the expression (2.1), we will write

$$\hbar(\theta \mid x) \backsim f(x \mid \theta)h(\theta) \tag{2.3}$$

taking into account the fact that the normalizing factor of the p.d.f., $\hbar(\theta \mid x)$ has been found from the integral

$$\beta = \left[\int_\Theta f(x \mid \theta)h(\theta)\zeta\{d\theta\}\right]^{-1}. \tag{2.4}$$

In the case when the parameter θ takes on the discrete values $\theta_1, \theta_2, \ldots, \theta_k$, the prior distribution is given in the form of prior probabilities $p_j = P\{\theta = \theta_j\}$, $j = 1, \ldots, k$. The expressions (2.3) and (2.4) are also valid for this case, if one represents $h(\theta)$ and $\hbar(\theta)$ by means of a delta-function. In particular,

$$h(\theta) = \sum_{j=1}^k p_j \delta(\theta - \theta_j).$$

The Bayes formula (2.3) lets us find the posterior density of the parameter θ in the form

$$\hbar(\theta \mid x) = \sum_{j=1}^{k} \bar{p}_j \delta(\theta - \theta_j).$$

where $\bar{p}_j = P\{\theta = \theta_j \mid x\}$, $j = 1, \ldots, k$, are the posterior probabilities.
For the discrete values of the parameter θ, the Bayes formula is often written in the form

$$p_j = \frac{p_j f(x \mid \theta_j)}{\sum_{i=1}^{k} p_i f(x \mid \theta_i)}, \quad j = 1, 2, \ldots, k. \tag{2.5}$$

The choice of a *loss function* plays an important role in the theory of Bayes estimating. In most cases the loss function is represented in the following form:

$$L(\theta, d) = C(\theta) W(|d - \theta|), \tag{2.6}$$

where $W(0) = 0$, and $W(t)$ is a monotonically increasing function for $t > 0$; $C(\theta)$ is assumed to be positive and finite. The prior Bayes estimate $\hat{\theta}_H$ is defined as an element from D which minimizes the prior risk [272]

$$G(H, d) = \int_{\Omega} f(x) \mu\{dx\} \int_{\Omega} C(\theta) W(|d(x) - \theta|) H\{d\theta \mid x\} C(\theta) W(|d - \theta|), \tag{2.7}$$

After the X has been observed, the most handy function (from the Bayes point-of-view) for further consideration is not the prior risk (2.7) but the posterior one, having the form

$$\bar{G}(H, d) = \int_{\Theta} C(\theta) W(|d(x) - \theta|) H\{d\theta \mid X\}. \tag{2.8}$$

The Bayes estimate of the parameter θ with respect to the prior distribution H should be the element $\theta_H(X)$ of the set D, minimizing the posterior risk with given X:

$$\int_{\Theta} C(\theta) W(|\hat{\theta}_H(x) - \theta|) H\{d\theta \mid X\} = \inf_{d \in D} \int_{\Theta} C(\theta) W(|d(x) - \theta|) H\{d\theta \mid X\}. \tag{2.9}$$

The analysis of the problem in the above-given setting shows that investigation of the specific solution with the given testing scheme is based on the following three questions:

1) a choice of the family of probability measures $\mathscr{B}$;
2) a choice of the prior distribution H;
3) a choice of the loss function $L(d, \theta)$.

The first question, having a practical significance, is associated with completeness of the statistical model, used by the researcher. The other two are less specific. Some recommendations on a choice of H and $L(d, \theta)$ will be given below.
In applied statistical analysis, the interval estimates are frequently used. The Bayes theory operates with an analogous notion having, however, interpretation which differs from the

classical one. In the simplest case of a scalar parameter θ, a Bayes confidence interval $\underset{\sim}{\theta}$ is introduced by the expression

$$\int_{\underset{\sim}{\theta}} \hbar(\theta \mid x) d\theta = \gamma,$$

where γ is the confidence probability. Since the choice of $\underset{\sim}{\theta}$ can be established in many ways, one adds an additional requirement: the interval $\underset{\sim}{\theta}$ must have the minimal length. In the case of a vector parameter θ, the confidence interval is chosen from the condition

$$\int_{\underline{R} \leqslant R(\theta) \leqslant \overline{R}} \hbar(\theta \mid x) d\theta = \gamma;$$

moreover, the difference $\overline{R} - \underline{R}$ must be the smallest. As seen from the definition above, the classical and the Bayes confidence intervals have different interpretations. In the classical form, the confidence interval, "covering" with a given probability an unknown parameter, is random. In the Bayes approach the parameter is random, while the confidence interval has fixed limits, defined by the prior density and confidence probability γ.

2.2 Classical properties in reference to Bayes estimates

According to classical statistics the quality of statistical estimates may be characterized by: how much these estimates satisfy the requirements of consistency, unbiasedness, effectiveness and sufficiency. As a rule, a classical estimate, approved in each particular case, appears to be a compromise, that is, we give preference to some property to the detriment of the others. As was mentioned, the leading property of the Bayes estimate is its optimality. The classical properties, indicated above, are not adequate to the Bayes methodology. Many authors use them only to keep up the tradition. Here we present some results which modify the classical estimates in the Bayes approach.

2.2.1 *Sufficiency*

The property of sufficiency works smoothly. The Bayes formula (2.1) (or (2.2)) is connected with the Bayes definition of the sufficient statistics. A posterior p.d.f. of the parameter θ, generated by the sufficient statistics $S(X)$, is equivalent (from the Bayes point-of-view) to the posterior p.d.f. of the parameter θ, constructed on the initial observation, that is:

$$\hbar^s(\theta \mid S(X)) = \hbar(\theta \mid X).$$

At the same time, this proves the equivalence of the Bayes and traditional definitions of sufficiency (see, e.g., [272]). Thus, the property of sufficiency in the Bayes estimating theory keeps its classical form.

2.2.2 *Consistency*

With respect to the property of consistency we cannot draw the previous conclusion. Reasoning rigorously, we can ascertain that a traditional analysis of an estimate behavior with the sample size tending to infinity contradicts the essence of the Bayes approach. Indeed, if it is assumed that θ is a random parameter with nondegenerating prior p.d.f., $h(\theta)$, then it is senseless to investigate the asymptotical properties of convergence of the estimate $\hat{\theta}_H$ with respect to $\theta = \theta_0$. By the same reason, it is incorrect when computing the mean value, to compare it with the random variable θ. There are, however, representations that make possible the investigation of the estimate $\hat{\theta}_H$ for large samples. If we assume that a chosen prior distribution is not exact, then one can get the estimate with the help of the Bayes scheme, and, later on, investigate it, digressing from the method used in obtaining the estimate (bearing in mind classical theory). In many cases the Bayes estimates are consistent and converge frequently to the maximum likelihood estimate, MLE.

Zacks [272] provides an example when the estimate of the Poisson cumulative distribution function $p(i \mid \lambda) = \mathrm{e}^{-\lambda}\lambda^i/i!$ with the prior $\lambda \backsim \Gamma(1,1)$ (gamma p.d.f.) is consistent. Lindley [146] proves that, if $\hat{\theta}_n$ is the best normal asymptotical estimate, then one can ascertain that Bayesian estimates and MLE are equivalent. The exact form of the prior distribution in this case is not significant, since for the samples with a large size MLE can be replaced with the unknown parameter θ. Bickel and Yahow present [24] the strict proof for the assertion, analogous to the case of the one-parametric exponential family and a loss function having a quadratic form. Asymptotical properties of the Bayes estimators for the discrete cumulative distribution functions were investigated by Freedman [87].

We give the part of Jeffrey's' reasoning's [115] with respect to the properties of the posterior p.d.f. for large-size samples. For a scalar parameter θ, and in accordance with (2.3), let p.d.f.

$$\hbar(\theta \mid x) \backsim h(\theta)\ell(\theta \mid x) = h(\theta)\mathrm{e}^{\ln \ell(\theta|x)}, \tag{2.10}$$

where $\ell(\theta \mid x)$ is the likelihood function, being, by essence, a p.d.f. of the observed values $x = (x_1, x_2, \ldots, x_n)$ of a trial and coinciding with $f(x \mid \theta)$.

(The parameter θ is assumed to be an argument of a likelihood function.) It is supposed that $h(\theta)$ and $\ell(x \mid \theta)$ $(\theta \in \Theta)$ are nondegenerating and have continuous derivatives; moreover,

$\ell(x \mid \theta)$ has a unique maximum at the point $\hat{\theta}_{\text{m.l.}}$, which is the MLE, generally speaking, $\ln[\ell(\theta \mid x)]$ has the order n, and $h(\theta)$ is independent on the sample size. Thus, it is intuitively clear that for the large-size samples, the likelihood cofactor is dominating in the posterior p.d.f.

Bernstein [169] and Mizes [166] prove the more general statement. The main thrust of this theorem is that, if the prior p.d.f. of the parameter θ is continuous, then, while the number of observations is increasing, the posterior p.d.f. is tending to a limit (which can be found analytically) independent of the prior distribution. Furthermore, since under the more common conditions, the p.d.f. form approaches, with a growth of n, the normal distribution curve centered on the MLE and the posterior p.d.f. for the case of the large-size samples appears to be normal also with the mean value $\hat{\theta}_{\text{m.l.}}$.

The proof of the asymptotical normality of the posterior p.d.f., $\hbar(\theta \mid x)$, can be carried out as follows. Let us expand into a Taylor series the functions $h(\theta)$ and $\ell(\theta \mid x)$ and at the MLE $\hat{\theta}_{\text{m.l.}}$:

$$h(\theta) = h(\hat{\theta}_{\text{m.l.}}) + (\theta - \hat{\theta}_{\text{m.l.}})h'(\hat{\theta}_{\text{m.l.}}) + \frac{1}{2}(\theta - \hat{\theta}_{\text{m.l.}})^2 h''(\hat{\theta}_{\text{m.l.}}) + \cdots$$

$$= h(\hat{\theta}_{\text{m.l.}}) \left[1 + \frac{(\theta - \hat{\theta}_{\text{m.l.}})h'(\hat{\theta}_{\text{m.l.}})}{h(\hat{\theta}_{\text{m.l.}})} + \frac{1}{2}\frac{(\theta - \hat{\theta}_{\text{m.l.}})^2 h''((\hat{\theta}_{\text{m.l.}})}{h(\hat{\theta}_{\text{m.l.}})} + \cdots\right]$$

Denoting by $g(\theta) = \ln \ell(\theta \mid x)$ and taking into account the relation $g'(\hat{\theta}_{\text{m.l.}}) = 0$, we obtain

$$\exp[g(\theta)] \backsim \exp\left[\frac{1}{2}(\theta - \hat{\theta}_{\text{m.l.}})^2 g''(\hat{\theta}_{\text{m.l.}})\right] \times \left[1 + \frac{1}{6}(\theta - \hat{\theta}_{\text{m.l.}})^3 g'''(\hat{\theta}_{\text{m.l.}}) + \cdots\right],$$

where the last equation is obtained by the expansion $e^x = 1 + x + \cdots$.

Multiplication of these expansions gives us

$$\hbar(\theta \mid x) \backsim \exp\left[\frac{1}{2}(\theta - \hat{\theta}_{\text{m.l.}})^2 g''(\hat{\theta}_{\text{m.l.}})\right]$$

$$\left[1 + \frac{(\theta - \hat{\theta}_{\text{m.l.}})h'(\hat{\theta}_{\text{m.l.}})}{h(\hat{\theta}_{\text{m.l.}})} + \frac{1}{2}\frac{(\theta - \hat{\theta}_{\text{m.l.}})^2 g''(\hat{\theta}_{\text{m.l.}})}{h(\hat{\theta}_{\text{m.l.}})} + \frac{1}{6}(\theta - \hat{\theta}_{\text{m.l.}})^3 g'''(\hat{\theta}_{\text{m.l.}}) + \cdots\right] \tag{2.11}$$

The dominating factor has the form of a normal p.d.f. with the mean value equal to MLE $\hat{\theta}_{\text{m.l.}}$ and the variance

$$[-g''(\hat{\theta}_{\text{m.l.}})]^{-1} = \left[-\frac{d^2 \ln \ell(\theta \mid x)}{d\theta^2}\right]^{-1}_{\theta = \hat{\theta}_{\text{m.l.}}}$$

Thus, if we use only the dominating cofactor, the approximation of the posterior p.d.f. of θ for large sizes of the sample n takes the form

$$\hbar(\theta \mid x) = \frac{1}{\sqrt{2\pi}} |g''(\hat{\theta}_{\text{m.l.}})|^{\frac{1}{2}} \exp\left[-\frac{1}{2}(\theta - \hat{\theta}_{\text{m.l.}})^2 |g''(\hat{\theta}_{\text{m.l.}})|\right] \tag{2.12}$$

Since $|g''(\hat{\theta}_{\text{m.l.}})|$ usually is a function of n, then with the growth of n, the posterior p.d.f. takes on the more pointed form. Jeffrey's [115] points out the fact that this approximation gives errors of order $n^{-1/2}$. Koks and Hinkly [125] generalize these results to the case of a vector parameter θ.

To justify (2.12), one may only use the fact that the likelihood must concentrate with increasing order about its maximum. Hence, these conclusions can be used more broadly than the case of independent random variables with the same distributions. Dawid [54] and Walker [262] carry out a scrupulous investigation of a set of regularity conditions under which the posterior distribution with the probability equal to unity is asymptotically normal. These conditions are almost alike as regularity conditions which are necessary for the asymptotic normality of the MLE. The research on the application of the expansion (2.11) for statistical outcomes may be found in works by Lindley [143] and Johnson [117].

The relation between the consistency of Bayes estimates and MLE is studied in the work by Strasser [242]. The point is that there is an example by Schwartz [231] in which the MLE is nonconsistent, but the Bayes estimate, under the same conditions, possesses the property of consistency. Strasser [242] complemented the regularity conditions up to the strict consistency of the MLE [272] by the conditions for the prior measure H so that the consistency of the maximal likelihood estimator implies the consistency of a Bayes estimator. The investigation of the relations between the consistency of a Bayes estimator and MLE is carried on by Le Cam [136].

If it is assumed that the parameter θ is fixed but unknown, then the consistency of a Bayes estimator can be investigated more naturally and nearer to the classical interpretation. These questions are considered by De Groot [63], Berk [19], Mizes [166] and by other authors. They may be interpreted as follows: if $x_1, x_2, \ldots, x_n$ is a sample from the distribution with the unknown parameter θ and if the value of θ is actually equal to θ_0, then, as $n \to \infty$, $\hbar(\theta \mid x)$ will concentrate more strongly about the value θ_0. The estimate of the parameter constructed on such a posterior distribution may be named, to all appearances, as consistent.

We give a brief explanation for this phenomenon. Let the parameter θ take only the finite set of values $\theta_1, \theta_2, \ldots, \theta_k$. Suppose that $P\{\theta = \theta_i\} = p_i$ for $i = 1, 2, \ldots, k$, and for each given value $\theta = \theta_i$, the random variables $x_1, x_2, \ldots, x_n$ generate a sample from the distribution with the p.d.f., f_i. It is assumed also that all f_i are different in such a sense that, if Ω is a sample space corresponding to the single observation, then

$$\int_\Omega |f_i(x) - f_j(x)| d\mu(x) > 0, \quad \forall\, i \neq j.$$

Let, for the observed values $x_1, x_2, \ldots, x_n$, $\bar{p}_i$ denote the posterior probability of the event $\theta = \theta_i$ for which, due to the Bayes theorem, we have

$$\bar{p}_i = \frac{p_i \prod\limits_{j=1}^{n} f_i(x_j)}{\sum\limits_{r=1}^{k} \Pr \prod\limits_{j=1}^{n} f_r(x_j)}, \qquad i = 1, 2, \ldots, k.$$

Suppose now that $x_1, x_2, \ldots, x_n$ is the sample from the distribution with the p.d.f., f_t, where t is some of the values $1, 2, \ldots, k$. As was shown in [63], the following limit relations are valid with the probability equal to one:

$$\lim_{n\to\infty} \bar{p}_t(x) = 1, \quad \lim_{n\to\infty} \bar{p}_i(x) = 0, \quad \forall\, i \neq t.$$

We give another example with a continuous distribution of the parameter θ which will be a mean value of the Gaussian random variable with a given measure of exactness r (the variance is equal to r^{-2}). Suppose that a prior distribution θ is Gaussian with a mean value μ and exactness measure τ ($-\infty < \mu < \infty$, $\tau > 0$). It is easy to check that the posterior distribution θ is Gaussian with the mean value

$$\mu' = \frac{\tau\mu + nr\hat{\mu}}{\tau + nr}, \quad \text{where } \hat{\mu} = \frac{1}{n}\sum_{i=1}^{n} x_i,$$

with the exactness measure $\tau + nr$. Let us rewrite the expression for μ' in the form

$$\mu' = \frac{\tau\mu}{\tau + nr} + \hat{\mu}\,\frac{nr}{\tau + nr}.$$

Assume now that the sample $x_1, x_2, \ldots, x_n$ is factually taken from the Gaussian distribution with the mean value θ_0. In accordance with the law of large numbers (see, for example, Kolmogorov's second theorem [208]), $\hat{\mu} = \theta_0$ with the probability 1. At the same time, it follows from the formula for μ', $\mu' \to \hat{\mu}$ as $n \to \infty$. In this sense, μ' is consistent. Furthermore, since the posterior variance of the parameter θ tends to zero, the posterior distribution of θ converges to the degenerated distribution, concentrated at the point θ_0.

2.2.3 *Unbiasedness*

Here, evidently, we meet a situation analogous to those in the above investigation of consistency. Since the parameter θ appears to be random, it is absurd to attempt to find the estimate $\hat{\theta}$ in the form $E[\hat{\theta}]$. Due to this circumstance, many authors, including Ferguson [80], proceed in the following way: at first they obtain the Bayes estimate in some definite form, thereafter they "forget" about the parameter randomness and investigate unbiasedness in the usual interpretation of this term.

Sage and Melsa attempt to give the Bayes definition of unbiasedness. In particular, they give two definitions:

1) a Bayes estimate $\hat{\theta}(x)$ is called *unbiased*, if

$$E[\hat{\theta}] = E[\theta(x)]; \text{ and}$$

2) a Bayes estimate $\hat{\theta}(x)$ is called *conditionally unbiased*, if

$$E[\hat{\theta}(x) \mid \theta] = E[\theta].$$

The second definition is more essential, since, in the first place, it is closer (by sense) to the classical one, and in the second place, is clearer than the first definition. Since $E[\hat{\theta}]$ is a mean value with respect to the prior measure, the equality $E[\hat{\theta}(x)] = E[\theta]$ corresponds to that ideal scheme when the posterior distribution coincides with the prior one (it is, however, not necessary). According to this, the Bayes estimate cannot be unbiased. Bland [25] gives the example of the statistical model which proves the incorrectness of the first definition.

The second definition of unbiasedness, mentioned above, is used by Hartigan in his work [102]. The estimate $\hat{\theta}(x)$, obeying the condition $E[\hat{\theta}(x) \mid \theta] = E[\theta]$.

The possibility of using the first definition is not even discussed. Moreover, he introduces the definition of the exact Bayes estimate which must satisfy the condition $P\{\hat{\theta}(x) \neq \theta\} = 0$. Hartigan proves that an unbiased Bayes estimator is exact.

2.2.4 *Effectiveness*

We say that one Bayes estimate is more effective than the other bearing in mind the following reason. If the posterior probability is chosen as a measure of effectiveness, its value, for identical observations, will be defined by the prior distribution (on the whole by the prior variance of the parameter). Consequently, the comparison criterion is not objective, since the prior distribution may be chosen, in some sense, arbitrarily. If we use the same prior distribution, then in view of the uniqueness of the Bayes solution, there are no two Bayes estimates for the same observation.

2.3 Forms of loss functions

As was mentioned in § 2.1, the loss function $L(d,\theta)$, where usually $d = \hat{\theta}$, is frequently represented in the form

$$L(d,\theta) = C(\theta)W(|d-\theta|). \tag{2.13}$$

Here $W(0) = 0$ and $W(t)$ is a monotonically increasing function; $C(\theta)$ is assumed to be positive and finite. As mentioned by Le Cam [136], the loss function of the form (2.13) was proposed by Laplace who understood that the exact expression for the function W cannot be found analytically.

The choice of the loss function is an important question in the theory of Bayes statistical estimating. Accuracy of such a choice stipulates the estimate quality. Frequently authors use a squared-error loss function, for which $W(|d-\theta|) = (\theta - d)^2$. This function gives a good approximation for any loss function of the form $C(\theta)W(|d-\theta|)$ having a smooth character in the neighborhood of the origin. Another function which is the convex loss function satisfying the condition $W(|d-\theta|) = (d-\theta)^k$, $k \geqslant 1$.

It is well known that the Bayes estimator of the function $R(\theta)$ for the squared-error loss function has a form of the posterior mean value

$$\hat{R}^* = \int_{\Theta} R(\theta)\hbar(\theta \mid x)d\theta.$$

For $k = 1$, the median of the posterior distribution appears to be the Bayes estimator. The theory of Bayes estimating for convex loss functions was developed by De Groot and Rao [64]. Rukhin [214] proves a theorem for which the estimate of the parameter θ is the same for any convex loss function, if only the posterior density is unimodal and symmetric with respect to θ. The loss functions represented above are unbounded. This circumstance may be a reason for misunderstanding. In particular, Girshik and Savidge [88] give an example in which the Bayes estimate, minimizing the posterior risk, has an infinite prior risk.

In a number of works there are also other loss functions whose properties are connected with the properties of the statistical models and peculiarities of the phenomena investigated by researchers. The direct generalization of the squared-error loss function will be the relative squared-error loss function given by:

$$L_{S_1}(\hat{\theta},\theta) = \left(\frac{\theta - \hat{\theta}}{\theta}\right)^2 \tag{2.14}$$

and its modification

$$L_{S_2}(\hat{\theta},\theta) = \left(\frac{\theta^\beta - \hat{\theta}^\beta}{\theta^\beta}\right)^2, \quad \beta > 0, \tag{2.15}$$

Which are broadly used when the investigations are directed precisely toward the relative errors. As shown by Higgins and Tsokos [108], the Bayes estimator of $R(\theta)$ under some loss function, minimizing the posterior risk with the loss function (2.15), is computed in the following manner:

$$\hat{R}^*_\beta = \left[\frac{\displaystyle\int_\theta \frac{\hbar(\theta \mid x)}{[R(\theta)]^\beta} d\theta}{\displaystyle\int_\theta \frac{\hbar(\theta \mid x)}{[R(\theta)]^{2\beta}} d\theta} \right]^{1/\beta}.$$

Harris [99] proposes to use for the investigation of probability of a nonrenewal system being operated without breakdowns with a loss function given by:

$$L_H(\hat{\theta}, \theta) = \left| \frac{1}{1-\hat{\theta}} - \frac{1}{1-\theta} \right|^k. \tag{2.16}$$

Thereafter he states: "If the reliability of a system is 0.99, then it fails, in the average, only once in 100 trials; if, at that time the system reliability is 0.999, then it fails only once in 1,000 trials, that is, this is ten times better. Therefore, the loss function must depend on how well we can estimate the quantity $(1-\theta)^{-1}$."

Higgins and Tsokos [108] propose to use the loss function of the form

$$L_e(\hat{\theta}, \theta) = \frac{f_1 \mathrm{e}^{-f_2(\hat{\theta}-\theta)} + f_2 \mathrm{e}^{-f_1(\hat{\theta}-\theta)} f_1 + f_2}{-1}, \quad f_1 > 0,\ f_2 > 0, \tag{2.17}$$

which enforces the losses, if the estimate is substantially different from the parameter. It is interesting that for small $\theta - \hat{\theta}$,

$$L_e(\hat{\theta}, \theta) = \frac{f_1 f_2}{2} (\theta - \hat{\theta})^2 + \mathrm{O}((\theta - \hat{\theta})^3).$$

The authors compare Bayes estimator of probability of failures, the mean time prior to failures with the reliability function for squared-error loss function with those having the form (2.15), (2.16), (2.17), and a linear loss function of the following form:

$$L_p(\hat{\theta}, \theta) = \begin{cases} p|\theta - \hat{\theta}|, & \hat{\theta} \leqslant \theta, \\ (1-p)|\theta - \hat{\theta}|, & \hat{\theta} > \theta, \end{cases} \tag{2.18}$$

Which generalizes the function $L(\hat{\theta}, \theta) = |\theta - \hat{\theta}|$ mentioned above on the case for unequal significance for exceeding and underestimating of the estimate $\hat{\theta}$ with respect to the parameter θ. The conclusions given by Tsokos and Higgins may be interpreted as follows:

1) The quadratic loss function is less stable in comparison with the others we have considered. If the quadratic loss function is used for approximating, then the obtained approximation of the Bayes estimate is unsatisfactory.
2) The Bayes estimator is very sensitive with respect to the choice of loss function.
3) The choice of loss function should be based, not on the mathematical conveniences, but on the practical significance.

The loss function which uses the fact that exceeding the parameter is worse than decreasing (this is intrinsic, for example, for the reliability measure) is written by Cornfield [47] in the form

$$L(\hat{\theta},\theta) = \begin{cases} K_1\left(\dfrac{\hat{\theta}}{\theta}-1\right)^2, & \hat{\theta}\leqslant\theta, \\ K_1\left(\dfrac{\hat{\theta}}{\theta}-1\right)^2+K_2\left(\dfrac{\hat{\theta}}{\theta}-1\right)^2, & \hat{\theta}>\theta. \end{cases} \tag{2.19}$$

In order to ensure for the loss function the different significance for the positive and negative errors, Zelner [274] introduces the so called linearly-exponential loss function

$$L_{\text{EX}}(\hat{\theta}-\theta) = b\left[e^{a(\hat{\theta}-\theta)}-a(\hat{\theta}-\theta)-1\right] \tag{2.20}$$

This function is asymmetric and is nearly symmetric for small a and can be well approximated by the quadratic functions. We give an example of the estimator which is obtained from the loss function (2.20). If X is a Gaussian random variable with the given mean value θ and given variance σ^2, and the prior distribution density θ satisfies the condition $h(\theta) \backsim$ const., then

$$\hat{\theta}^* = \bar{x} = \frac{a\sigma^2}{2n},$$

where $\bar{x}$ is a sample mean value. It is not difficult to verify that for small a and/or for large sample sizes n, the estimator $\hat{\theta}^*$ is near the MLE. The loss function (2.20) solves actually almost the same problem as that in (2.19). But the last loss function is not so handy in calculations because we cannot find with it the desired estimates in close analytical form; instead we have to use special numerical methods to obtain the desired approximation.

El-Sayyad [73] uses, in addition to the loss functions given above, the following loss function:

$$L_{\alpha\beta}(\hat{\theta},\theta) = \theta^{\alpha}(\hat{\theta}^{\beta}-\theta^{\beta})^2, \tag{2.21}$$

and

$$L_{\ln}(\hat{\theta},\theta) = (\ln\hat{\theta}-\ln\theta)^2, \tag{2.22}$$

Smith [235] determines the class of bounded loss functions A given by the conditions: the loss unction is symmetric with respect to $|\hat{\theta}-\theta|$, decreases with respect to $|\hat{\theta}-\theta|$ and satisfies the conditions

$$\sup_{\hat{\theta},\theta} L(\hat{\theta},\theta) = 1, \quad \inf_{\hat{\theta},\theta} L(\hat{\theta},\theta) = 0.$$

Smith scrupulously investigates the Bayes estimates of the so-called step loss function

$$L_b(\hat{\theta},\theta) = L_b(\hat{\theta}-\theta) = \begin{cases} 0 & \text{if } |\hat{\theta}-\theta| < b, \\ 1 & \text{if } |\hat{\theta}-\theta| \geqslant b, \end{cases} \tag{2.23}$$

Estimators were found for many parametric families. These estimators differ substantially from the Bayes estimators with the squared-error loss function.

2.4 The choice of a prior distribution

The choice of prior distribution in applied problems of Bayes estimating is one of the most important questions. At the same time, the solution of this problem doesn't touch the essence of the Bayes approach. The existence of a prior distribution is postulated. All further arguments are based on this postulation. Some authors, however, investigate the question of choice of a prior distribution being in the framework of the Bayes approach. We propose the following three recommendations for the choice of a prior distribution. They are, correspondingly, based on: 1) the conjugacy principle; 2) the absence of information; and 3) the information criterion. We shall discuss individually each of these recommendations.

2.4.1 *Conjugated prior distributions*

Each prior distribution, due to the Bayes theorem, can be used together with any likelihood function. It is convenient, however, to choose a prior distribution of a special form giving the simple estimators. For a given distribution $f(x \mid \theta)$ we may find such families of prior p.d.f. that a posterior p.d.f. will be the elements of the same family. Such a family is called *closed with respect to the choice or conjugated with respect to* $f(x \mid \theta)$. It is said sometimes: "naturally-conjugated family of prior distributions". Most of the authors state that this approach is dictated by the convenience of theoretical arguments and practical conclusions. Haifa and Shleifer [202] attempt to give a more convincing justification of a conjugated prior distribution. We discuss this question in detail.

Assume that sample distributions are independent and allowing the sufficient statistics $\mathbf{y}$ of fixed dimension with the domain $\Omega_{\mathbf{y}}$. A family $\mathscr{H}$ of all prior distributions is constructed in the following way: each element $\mathscr{H}$ is associated with the element $\Omega_{\mathbf{y}}$. If, prior to a trial, for θ is chosen the element from $\mathscr{H}$ corresponding to $\mathbf{y}' \in \Omega_e$ and a sample gives the sufficient statistics $\mathbf{y}$, then the posterior distribution also belongs to $\mathscr{H}$ and assigns to some element $\mathbf{y}'' \in \Omega_e$. For the definition of $\mathbf{y}''$ with the help of $\mathbf{y}$ and $\mathbf{y}'$ a binary operation $\mathbf{y}'' = \mathbf{y}' * \mathbf{y}$ is introduced. We consider below the formalization of a conjugated prior distribution given in [202].

It is supposed that for arbitrary samples $x = (x_1, x_2, \ldots, x_n)$ with each fixed n there is a sufficient statistic

$$\mathbf{y}_n = (x_1, x_2, \ldots, x_n) = \mathbf{y} = (y_1, y_2, \ldots, y_s),$$

where y_j is a real number and the dimension of the vector $\mathbf{y}$ is independent of n.

For any given n and arbitrary sample $(x_1, x_2, \ldots, x_n)$, there exists a function k and s-dimensional vector $\mathbf{y} = (y_1, y_2, \ldots, y_s)$ consisting of real numbers, that the likelihood function satisfies the relation

$$\ell_n(\theta \mid x_1, x_2, \ldots, x_n) \backsim k(\theta \mid \mathbf{y}).$$

The function $k(\theta \mid \mathbf{y})$ is called a *likelihood kernel*. We will touch upon an important property of the kernel $k(\theta \mid \mathbf{y})$.

Theorem 2.1. *Let* $\mathbf{y}^{(1)} = y_p(x_1, x_2, \ldots, x_p)$ *and* $\mathbf{y}^{(2)} = y_{n-p}(x_{p+1}, \ldots, x_n)$. *Then we can find such a binary operation* $*$ *that satisfies the relation*

$$\mathbf{y}^{(1)} * \mathbf{y}^{(2)} = \mathbf{y}^* = (y_1^*, y_2^*, \ldots, y_s^*)$$

and possesses the following properties:

$$\ell_n(\theta \mid x_1, x_2, \ldots, x_n) \backsim k(\theta \mid \mathbf{y}^*),$$

and

$$k(\theta \mid \mathbf{y}^*) \backsim k(\theta \mid \mathbf{y}^{(1)})\, k(\theta \mid \mathbf{y}^{(2)}).$$

As it follows from the theorem, $\mathbf{y}^*$ can be found only by using $\mathbf{y}^{(1)}$ and $\mathbf{y}^{(2)}$, without $(x_1, x_2, \ldots, x_n)$.

The posterior p.d.f., is constructed with the help of the kernel function $k(\theta \mid \mathbf{y})$ in the following way:

$$h(\theta \mid \mathbf{y}) = N(\mathbf{y})\, k(\theta \mid \mathbf{y}), \tag{2.24}$$

where $\mathbf{y}$ is some statistic, $N(\mathbf{y})$ is a function which needs to be defined.

In order for the function $h(\theta \mid \mathbf{y})$, defined on Θ by the relation (2.24), to be a p.d.f., it is necessary and sufficient that this function be nonnegative everywhere, and the integral from this function over Θ will be equal to unity. Since $k(\theta \mid \mathbf{y})$ is a kernel function of a joint p.d.f. of observations, defined on Θ for all $\mathbf{y} \in \Omega_{\mathbf{y}}$, is necessarily nonnegative for all

$(\mathbf{y},\theta)$ from $\Omega_{\mathbf{y}} \times \Theta$. Consequently, if there exists the integral of $k(\theta \mid \mathbf{y})$ over Θ, then $N(\mathbf{y})$ is determined by the relation

$$[N(\mathbf{y})]^{-1} = \int_{\Theta} k(\theta \mid \mathbf{y}) d\theta$$

and $h(\theta \mid \mathbf{y})$, represented by the expression (2.24), will be a p.d.f.

Suppose now that $\mathbf{y}$ is a sufficient statistic, determined with the help of the observed sample $(x_1, x_2, \ldots, x_n)$, and $h(\theta)$ is a prior p.d.f. In accordance with the Bayes theorem for the posterior distribution density we have

$$\hbar(\theta \mathbf{y}) \backsim h(\theta) k(\theta \mid \mathbf{y})$$

If now $h(\theta)$ is a p.d.f., conjugated to the kernel k with the parameter $\mathbf{y}' \in \Omega_{\mathbf{y}}$, that is, $h(\theta) \backsim k(\theta \mid \mathbf{y}')$, then, in accordance with the Bayes theorem,

$$h(\theta \mid \mathbf{y}) \backsim k(\theta \mid \mathbf{y}') k(\theta \mid \mathbf{y}) \backsim k(\theta \mid \mathbf{y}' * \mathbf{y}).$$

Thus: 1) the kernel of a prior p.d.f. is combined with the kernel of a sample in a manner similar to the combination of two sample kernels; 2) both a prior and posterior p.d.f. are induced by the same likelihood kernel, but their generating statistics are different. These conclusions may be interpreted as a follows: the prior distribution is a result of processing some nonexistent data (or data which exist but are lost) for the same statistical model as a likelihood function.

Let us consider the following example. A Bernoulli process with the parameter $\theta = p$ induces independent random variables $(x_1, x_2, \ldots, x_n)$ with the same probabilities $p^x(1-p)^{1-x}$, where $x = 0, 1$. If n is the number of observed values and $r = \sum x_i$, then the likelihood of a sample is written as

$$\ell_n(p \mid x_1, x_2, \ldots, x_n) \backsim p^r (1-p)^{n-r}.$$

In addition to this, $\mathbf{y} = (\mathbf{y}_1, \mathbf{y}_2) = (r, n)$ is a sufficient statistic whose dimension is equal to 2, independently of n. A prior p.d.f. conjugated with the likelihood kernel and induced by the statistics $y' = (r', n')$ is a density of the beta distribution

$$h(p) = \frac{p^{r'}(1-p)^{n'-r'}}{B(r'+1, n'-r'+1)}, \quad 0 \leqslant p \leqslant 1,$$

where

$$B(\alpha, \beta) = \int_0^1 x^{\alpha-1}(1-x)^{\beta-1} dx = \frac{\Gamma(\alpha+\beta)}{\Gamma(\alpha)\Gamma(\beta)}.$$

In view of the Bayes theorem

$$\hbar(p \mid \mathbf{y}) \backsim h(p) p^r (1-p)^{n-r} \backsim p^{r'+r}(1-p)^{n+n'-(r+r')},$$

that is, the kernels of the prior and posterior p.d.f. coincide, and the beta distribution with the parameters $r'' = r + r'$ and $n'' = n + n'$ appears to also be posterior.

A family of conjugated posterior d.d. may be enlarged by the extension of the domain $\Omega_{\mathbf{y}}$ up to and including all values for which $k(\theta \mid \mathbf{y})$ is nonnegative for all θ, and the integral of $k(\theta \mid \mathbf{y})$ over the domain Θ is convergent.

In the example we have considered, the parameters r and n take the values of positive integers. At the same time, an integral of $k(\theta \mid \mathbf{y})$ over $\Theta[0,1]$ converges for all real $r > -1$ and $n > -1$ to the complete beta function. Therefore, we can obtain, assuming that the parameter $\mathbf{y} = (r, n)$ may take an arbitrary value from the domain determined in such a way, the family of densities which is substantially broader.

A complicated report on naturally conjugated p.d.f. is given in the monographs [91] and [202]. Dawid and Guttman [55] investigate the question of obtaining conjugated distribution in foreshortening of singularities of models. In particular, it is shown that simple forms of conjugated distributions are an implication of a group structure of models.

2.4.2 *Jeffrey's introduces prior distributions representing a "scantiness of knowledge"*

These distributions are the subject of consideration in the work by Zelner [272] and also are investigated by other authors. This assumption is an implication of the desire not to leave the Bayes approach in the cases when an investigator doesn't have enough knowledge about the properties of the model parameters or knows nothing at all. Jeffrey's [115] proposes two rules for the choice of a prior distribution, which, in his opinion, "embrace the most widespread situations", when we don't have the information on the parameter:

1) if the parameter exists in the finite segment $[a, b]$ or in the interval $(-\infty, +\infty)$ then its prior probability should be supposed to be uniformly distributed;
2) if the parameter takes the value in the interval $[0, \infty)$, then the probability of its logarithm should be supposed to be uniformly distributed.

Consider the first rule. If the parameter interval is finite, then for obtaining the posterior distribution we may use the standard Bayes procedure.

In so doing, a prior distribution is not conjugated with the kernel of a likelihood function. If the interval for the parameter θ is infinite, we deal with improper prior p.d.f. The rule of Jeffrey's for the representation of the fact of ignorance of the parameter value should be interpreted in this case as

$$h(\theta)\,d\theta \backsim d\theta, \quad -\infty < \theta < \infty, \tag{2.25}$$

that is, $h(\theta) \backsim$ const. Thus, we have

$$\int_{-\infty}^{\infty} h(\theta)\,d\theta = \infty.$$

Jeffrey's proposes to use for the representation of a probability of a certain event instead of 1. Exactly this fact, in his opinion, allows us to obtain a formal representation of ignorance. For any two intervals (a,b) and (c,d) the relation

$$\frac{P\{a<\theta<b\}}{P\{c<\theta<d\}} = \frac{0}{0},$$

that is, represents indeterminacy, and thus we cannot make a statement about the chances of θ being in some finite pair of finite intervals.

The second rule of Jeffrey's touches upon the parameters whose nature lets us make an assumption on their having a value lying in the interval $[0,\infty)$ for example, a standard deviation. He proposes for such a parameter its logarithm having a uniform distribution, that is, if one puts $\vartheta = \log\theta$, then the prior d.d. for ϑ will be chosen in the form

$$h(\vartheta)\,d\vartheta \backsim d\vartheta, \quad -\infty < \vartheta < \infty. \tag{2.26}$$

Since $d\vartheta = d\theta/\theta$ (2.26) yields

$$h(\theta) \backsim \theta^{-1}, \quad 0 \leqslant \theta < \infty. \tag{2.27}$$

corresponding to the absence of information about the parameter θ.

An important property of (2.27) is its invariance with respect to the transformations $K = \theta^n$. Actually,

$$dK = n\theta^{n-1}d\theta \implies \frac{dK}{K} \backsim \frac{d\theta}{\theta}.$$

This property is very important because some research parameterizes the models in terms of the standard deviation σ, others in terms of a variance σ^2 or in terms of the parameter of exactness $\tau = \sigma^2$. It is easy to show that, if we choose the quantity $d\sigma/\sigma$ as the prior d.d. for σ, the relation will be

$$\frac{d\sigma}{\sigma} \backsim \frac{d\sigma^2}{\sigma^2} \backsim \frac{d\tau}{\tau},$$

a logical implication. This prior distribution is also improper, whence we may conclude that the relation $P\{0<\theta<a\}/P\{a<\theta<\infty\}$ is indeterminacy, that is, we can say nothing about the chances of the parameter being in the intervals $(0,a)$ and (a,∞). Indeterminacy similar to this one is considered again a formal representation of ignorance.

A question of representation of an improper prior p.d.f. is considered by Akaike [2–4]. He proposes the following interpretation: an improper prior p.d.f. can be represented in the form of a limit of a proper prior p.d.f. in such a way that the corresponding posterior p.d.f. converges point wisely to the posterior p.d.f., responding to an improper prior distribution. A mutual entropy is considered their nearness measure. It is shown also that the most appropriate choice is a choice of approximating eigenvalues, depending on a sample.
In spite of the fact that prior p.d.f.s, in accordance with the assumption of Jeffrey's are improper, corresponding to them the posterior distributions are proper and allow us to obtain the desired estimates. Let $(x_1, x_2, \ldots, x_n)$ be a sample from $N(\mu, \sigma)$ where μ and σ are unknown. If we have no prior information about μ and σ we may apply the principles of Jeffrey's and use as a prior d.d. a function of the form

$$h(\mu,\sigma)\,d\mu\,d\sigma \backsim \frac{1}{\sigma}\,d\mu\,d\sigma, \quad -\infty<\mu<\infty,\ 0<\sigma<\infty.$$

Using the Bayes theorem, we can easily obtain the posterior d.d. That is,

$$\begin{aligned}\hbar(\mu,\sigma \mid x) &\backsim h(\mu,\sigma)\ell(\mu,\sigma \mid x)\\ &\backsim \frac{1}{\sigma^{n+1}}\exp\left\{-\frac{1}{2\sigma^2}\left[vs^2+n(\mu-\hat{\mu})^2\right]\right\},\end{aligned} \tag{2.28}$$

where $\ell(\mu,\sigma \mid x) = \sigma^{-n}\exp\left[-\sum(x_i-\mu)^2/(2\sigma^2)\right]$ is a likelihood function, $v = n-1$, $\hat{\mu} = \frac{1}{n}\sum x_i$, $vs^2 = \sum(x_i-\hat{\mu})^2$. The posterior density we have written is proper. In the same manner, a marginal posterior d.d. of the parameter μ

$$\begin{aligned}\hbar(\mu \mid x) &= \int_0^\infty \hbar(\mu,\sigma \mid x)\,d\sigma\\ &\backsim \int_0^\infty \frac{1}{\sigma^{n+1}}\exp\left\{-\frac{1}{2\sigma^2}\left[vs^2+n(\mu-\hat{\mu})^2\right]\right\}d\sigma\\ &\backsim \left[vs^2+n(\mu-\hat{\mu})^2\right]^{-\frac{v+1}{2}}\end{aligned} \tag{2.29}$$

is proper. As seen from (2.29), $\hbar(\mu \mid x)$ has a form of Student d.d. with a mean value $\hat{\mu}$. Analogously to $\hbar(\sigma \mid x)$,

$$\hbar(\sigma \mid x) \backsim \frac{1}{\sigma^{v+1}}\exp\left(-\frac{vs^2}{2\sigma^2}\right).$$

This posterior d.d. for σ has a form of the inverse gamma-distribution.
Some authors decide not to use improper d.d., preferring instead to introduce "locally-uniform" and "sloping" distribution densities. Box and Tico [28] propose the functions which are "sufficiently-sloping" in that domain where a likelihood function takes greater values. Outside of this domain, the form of the curve of a prior p.d.f. doesn't matter,

since, if one finds a kernel of the posterior p.d.f., he multiplies it by the small values of a likelihood function.

The most interesting and important peculiarity of the proposed improper prior p.d.f. is the property of invariance. Jeffrey's gives it an interesting interpretation. He proves the following statement. Suppose that a prior p.d.f. for the vector θ is chosen in the form

$$h(\theta) \backsim \left|\mathrm{Inf}_\theta\right|^{1/2}. \tag{2.30}$$

Here Inf_θ is a Fisher information matrix for the vector of parameters $\theta = (\theta_1, \theta_2, \ldots, \theta_K)$, that is,

$$\mathrm{Inf}_\theta = -E_X\left[\frac{\partial^2 \log f(X \mid \theta)}{\partial\theta_i \partial\theta_j}\right],$$

where the mean value is taken over the random variable X. Then a prior p.d.f. of the form (2.30) will be invariant in the following sense. If a researcher parameterizes his model with the help of the component of the vector η, where $\eta = F(\theta)$, and F is single-valued differentiable transformation of the components of the vector θ, and chooses a prior p.d.f. for θ so that

$$h(\eta) \backsim |\mathrm{Inf}_\eta|^{1/2}.$$

then the posterior probability statements, obtained in this way, don't contradict the posterior statements obtained with the help of parameterization of the components of the vector θ and a prior p.d.f. of the form (2.30). The proof of this statement can be found in the book by Zelner [275]. Hartigan [101] develops the idea of representing a prior p.d.f. in the form (2.30) and formulates six properties of invariance. The property (2.30) is a particular case among them. Hardigan's interpretation of invariance is more common and includes the invariance relative to transformations of a sample space, repeated performance of samples, and contraction of a space for the parameter θ.

2.4.3 *Choice of a prior distribution with the help of information criteria*

This is the subject of investigation in many works devoted to the Bayes estimation. In this connection, [46, 60, 65, 108, 275] should be distinguished.

The approach proposed by Zelner [275] may be interpreted as follows. As information measure, contained in the p.d.f. of the observation $f(x \mid \theta)$ for a given θ, is used in the integral

$$I_x(\theta) = \int_\Omega f(x \mid \theta) \ln f(x \mid \theta)\, dx. \tag{2.31}$$

A priori mean information contents is defined as

$$\bar{I}_x = \int_{\Theta} I_x(\theta)h(\theta)\,d\theta.$$

If now, from a prior information contents $\bar{I}_x$ associated with the observation x, we subtract information contents of the prior information, then it is possible to represent a measure of information gained by

$$G = \bar{I}_x - \int_{\Theta} h(\theta)\,\ln h(\theta)\,d\theta.$$

Then it is assumed (in the situation of there being no exact information about a prior p.d.f.) to choose $h(\theta)$ from the maximization condition for G. Zelner calls such a function a prior p.d.f. with "minimal information". Now consider the following example. Suppose

$$f(x \mid \theta) = \frac{1}{\sqrt{2\pi}}\exp\left[-\frac{(x-\theta)^2}{2}\right], \quad x \in (-\infty,\infty).$$

Then it is easy to obtain

$$I_x(\theta) = -\int_{-\infty}^{\infty} f(x \mid \theta)\,\ln f(x \mid \theta)\,d\theta = -\frac{1}{2}(\ln 2\pi + 1),$$

that is, $I_x(\theta)$ is independent of θ, hence for the proper $h(\theta)$

$$I_x = -\frac{1}{2}(\ln 2\pi + 1)$$

and

$$G = -\frac{1}{2}(\ln 2\pi + 1) - \int_{\Theta} h(\theta)\,\ln h(\theta)\,d\theta.$$

The value of G will be maximal if one minimizes a portion of the information contained in a prior distribution

$$I_\theta = \int_{\Theta} h(\theta)\,\ln h(\theta)\,d\theta$$

The solution of this problem is a uniform p.d.f. on Θ, that is, $h(\theta) \backsim$ const. It should be noted that this result is in full accord with the form of a prior p.d.f. obtained using the rule of Jeffrey's [114].

If one considers (see Lindley [143]) a functional G in the asymptotical form

$$G_A = \int_{\Theta} h(\theta)\,\ln\sqrt{n|\mathrm{Inf}_\theta|}\,d\theta - \int_{\Theta} h(\theta)\,\ln h(\theta)\,d\theta,$$

where n is the number of independent samples from a general population, distributed by the probability law $f(x \mid \theta)$, and finding a prior p.d.f., $h(\theta)$ maximizing G_A under the condition $\int \theta\, h(\theta)d\theta = 1$, then we can obtain

$$h(\theta) \backsim |\mathrm{Inf}_\theta|^{1/2},$$

that is, a prior p.d.f. corresponding to the generalized rule of Jeffrey's, considered above, giving the invariant p.d.f. At the same time, as was shown by Zelner [275], if G is represented in the nonasymptotical form, then an invariant prior p.d.f. of Jeffrey's does not always appear to be a p.d.f. with "minimal information". In the case when a prior p.d.f. of Jeffrey's doesn't maximize G, its use makes us bring additional information into the analysis in contrast to the case when it uses prior information to maximize G. As can be seen from the above conclusions, the desire of Jeffrey's to ensure the property of invariance of the statistical deductions with respect to the parameter transformation deviates from the principle of "scantiness of knowledge". Convert [46], Deely, Tierney and Zimmer [60], Jaynes [113] investigate the question about the choice of a prior distribution with the minimization of the direct portion of information I_θ (Shennon), contained in a prior p.d.f. A rule of choice of $h(\theta)$ from the condition $I_\theta \longrightarrow \min$ is called an *entropy maximum principle* because the entropy $S_\theta = -I_\theta$ is used instead of I_θ. They introduce the term "*a least favorable distribution*". If $\mathscr{H}$ is a family of prior distributions, then $H \in \mathscr{H}$ is the least favorable distribution under the condition, that is, its corresponding minimum of the expected losses is greater than that one for the other elements of a family.

It should be noted that the estimate obtained in such a way coincides with a minimax one [257].

Deely, Tierney and Zimmer consider the use of a maximum entropy principle for the choice of a prior distribution in the binomial and exponential models. They show, in particular, that a least favorable distribution may be the best one in accordance with a maximum entropy principle.

Jaynes [113] modified this principle to a more general form. He introduces the measure

$$S_K = -\int_\Theta h(\theta) \ln \left[\frac{h(\theta)}{K(\theta)} \right] d\theta,$$

where K, as noted by El-Sayyad [73], is a suitable monotonic function. El-Sayyad proposes the use of a group theory approach for a choice of $K(\theta)$. Such an approach results in a change of the parameters of $h(\theta)$, which is very essential and doesn't change the entropy measure. For example, if θ_1 is a position parameter, θ_2 is a scale parameter ($\theta_2 > 0$), then the prior density is found so that $h(\theta_1, \theta_2) = ag(\theta_1 + b, a\theta_2)$, and the solution takes the form $h(\theta_1, \theta_2) \backsim \theta_2^{-1}$. Thus, we again have obtained the invariant prior p.d.f. of Jeffrey's.

For the binomial model, as shown by Jaynes [113], the use of the generalized maximum entropy principle gives the equation $\theta(1-\theta)h'(\theta) = (2\theta - 1)h(\theta)$, whence $h(\theta) \backsim [\theta(1-\theta)]^{-1}$.

Devjatirenkov [65] uses the information criterion

$$I(\hat{\theta}) = \int_{\Theta}\int_{\Omega} \hbar(\theta \mid x)p(x)\ln q(\theta \mid \hat{\theta})dx d\theta,$$

where $q(\theta \mid \hat{\theta})$ is the p.d.f. of the parameter with the given estimate, for the determination of the best (in the sense of minimum of I estimate $\hat{\theta}$. The estimate obtained in such a way appears to be less sensitive (in comparison with the usual one) with respect to the deviation of a prior distribution. It is interesting that a variance of the estimate for the Gaussian distribution attains the lower limit of the Cramer-Rao inequality.

In the work [46] information quality was used not as a criterion of a choice of a prior distribution, but as a method of indeterminacy elimination for the determination of the parameters of a prior distribution density. Arguments given in [46] are of an intuitive nature, but seem to be reasonable and may be used in practice. We give the main results of [46]. Suppose $f(x \mid \theta)$ is p.d.f. of observation x and $h(\theta;\gamma)$ is a prior p.d.f. with the parameter γ.

Analogous to a Fisher information $I_x(\theta)$ one introduces the so called *Bayes information*, contained in $h(\theta;\gamma)$:

$$BI_{\gamma}(\theta) = E_{\theta}\left[\left|\frac{\partial \ln h(\theta;\gamma)}{\partial \theta}\right|^2\right]. \tag{2.32}$$

Next one determines a weight significance w of a prior information with respect to an empirical one: $w = BI_{\gamma}(\theta)/I_x(\theta)$. Suppose now that θ_p is a prior estimate of the parameter θ. If the vector γ consists of two parameters γ_1 and γ_2, then we need to solve a system of two equations:

$$E_{\gamma}[\theta] = \theta_p,$$
$$BI_{\gamma}(\theta) = wI_x(\theta).$$

In the case when the number of parameters γ exceeds two, it is necessary to use additional arguments (see [46]). For example, for the binomial model

$$f(x \mid \theta) = \binom{n}{x}\theta^x(1-\theta)^{n-x}$$

and a prior p.d.f. beta $h(\theta) \backsim \theta^{a-1}(1-\theta)^{b-1}$, we have

$$I_x(\theta) = \frac{n}{\theta(1-\theta)}.$$

It also follows from (2.32),

$$BI_{\gamma}(\theta) = \frac{(a+b-4)(a+b-2)(a+b-1)}{(a-2)(b-2)}.$$

The system of equations for the determination of a and b has the form

$$\frac{a}{a+b} = \theta_p,$$

$$BI_\gamma(\theta) = wI_x(\hat{\theta}),$$

where θ_p and $\hat{\theta}$ is prior and empirical estimates of the parameter θ.

The methods for a choice of a prior distribution which are based on an information criterion fall outside the limits of the traditional Bayes approach and are drawn either to minimax or to empirical Bayes methods. In the works of some authors there are many efforts to construct fundamental theories directed to justification of a choice of prior distributions. We single out the works by Japanese statistician Akaike [2–4] who proposes the methods of effective use of Bayes models. The goal of constructions proposed by him is a change of the role of a prior distribution in the Bayes models. Akaike [2] proposes to use prior distributions adaptive to empirical data. They are called *modificators*.

In the problem of prediction of a density for the distribution $g(z)$ of future observations based on a sample of obtained data, which is being solved with the help of Bayes theory, a prior distribution (modificator) is chosen from the correspondence between the $g(z)$ and estimate $\hat{g}(z)$, expressed with the help of *Kulbak information measure*

$$B(g,\hat{g}) = -\int \ln[g(z)/\hat{g}(z)]g(z)\,dz.$$

In this capacity a mean value of entropy is used, that is $E_x[B(g(z), g(z \mid x))]$, where,

$$g(z \mid x) = \int_\Theta f(z \mid \theta)\hbar(\theta \mid x)d\theta \ \text{ and } \ \hbar(\theta \mid x) \backsim f(x \mid \theta)h(\theta).$$

Thus, a prior p.d.f. is chosen by minimization of the mean value of entropy. It is interesting to note that Akaike's method gives the improper prior p.d.f. of Jeffrey's in some cases (in particular, in the problem of prediction of a distribution of the Gauss random vector).

Another interesting attempt to exclude the arbitrariness in the choice of a prior p.d.f. is proposed by Bernardo [20]. He recommends choosing standard prior and posterior distributions that describe a situation of "insignificant prior information", and deficient information is found from empirical data. His criterion of a choice of a prior p.d.f., $h(\theta)$ is constructed with the help of expected information about θ proposed by Lindley:

$$I^\theta\{\in, h(\theta)\} = \int_\Omega f(x)dx \int_\Theta \hbar(\theta \mid x)\ln\frac{\hbar(\theta \mid x)}{h(\theta)}\,d\theta,$$

where $\in$ denotes an experiment during which a random variable X with p.d.f., $f(x \mid \theta)$, $\theta \in \Theta$, is observed. It is also assumed that $h(\theta)$ belongs to the class of admissible prior distributions $\mathscr{H}$. The main idea is interpreted in the following way. Consider a random variable $I^\theta\{\in (k), h(\theta)\}$ determining a portion of information about θ, expected in k recurrences of an experiment. We may achieve, by infinite recurrence, the exact value of θ. Thus, $I^\theta\{\in (\infty), h(\theta)\}$ measures a portion of deficient information about θ with a prior p.d.f., $h(\theta)$. The standard prior distribution $\pi(\theta)$, which corresponds to "indefinite prior knowledge", is defined as minimizing deficient information in the class $\mathscr{H}$. The standard posterior distribution after the observation x is defined with the help of Bayes theorem:

$$\pi(\theta \mid x) \backsim \pi(\theta) f(x \mid \theta).$$

Since the exact knowledge of a real number requires the knowledge of an infinite quantity of information, in the continuous case we obtain $I^\theta\{\in (\infty), h(\theta)\} = \infty$, for all $h(\theta) \in \mathscr{H}$. Standard posterior distributions for this case are defined with the help of a limit passing:

$$\pi(\theta \mid x) = \lim_{k\to\infty} \pi_k(\theta \mid x);$$

moreover, $\pi_k(\theta \mid x) \backsim \pi_k(\theta) f(x \mid \theta)$, and $\pi_k(\theta) = \arg\max I^\theta\{\in (k), h(\theta)\}$.
For the case of binomial trials a standard prior p.d.f., $\pi(\theta) \backsim \theta^{-1}(1-\theta)^{-1}$.
That is, we have the same result as the one in the work by Jaynes [113] obtained with the help of maximum of entropy.
The attractive feature of Bernardo theory is that this theory is free of some difficulties which are peculiar to a standard Bayes approach, in particular, the use of standard prior distributions doesn't give any marginal paradoxes (see the works by Stone and Dawid [243], and by Dawid, Stone and Zidek [56]) peculiar to non-informative prior distributions.
An interesting approach for a choice of prior distributions, based on geometrical probabilities, is proposed by Fellenberg and Pilz [79]. They consider a problem of the choice of a prior distribution in the estimation of a mean value of the time-to-failure for the exponential distribution with the cumulative distribution function $F(t;\lambda) = 1-\exp(-\lambda t)$. For prior information a segment of uncertainty $[\lambda_1, \lambda_2]$ is used for the parameter A corresponding to the space of c.d.f. $\mathscr{B} = \{F(t;\lambda_1) \leqslant F(t;\lambda) \leqslant F(t;\lambda_2)\}$, consisting of the unknown cumulative distribution function $F(t;\lambda)$. It is assumed that a probability of λ being in $[\lambda_1, \lambda_2]$ is equal to unity. A prior p.d.f., $h(\lambda)$, is determined from the condition that a probability of a parameter λ getting into the interval $[\lambda_1, x]$ equals the probability of $F(t;\lambda)$ getting into the space $\mathscr{B}_x = \{F(t;\lambda_1) \leqslant F(t;\lambda) \leqslant F(t;\lambda_2)\}$. The equality of probabilities

$$P\{\lambda_1 \leqslant \lambda \leqslant x\} = P\{F(t;\lambda) \in \mathscr{B}_x\}$$

is valid because of monotonicity of $F(t;\lambda)$ on the parameter λ. The probability $P\{F(t;\lambda) \in \mathscr{B}_x\}$ is determined from geometrical reasoning (having used a principle of equal chances) as a ration of the area contained between $F(t;\lambda_1)$ and $F(t;x)$. The resulting expression for the prior density of the parameter A has the form

$$h(\lambda) = \frac{\lambda_1\lambda_2}{\lambda_2-\lambda_1}\cdot\frac{1}{\lambda_2} \quad \lambda_1 \leqslant \lambda \leqslant \lambda_2.$$

2.5 The general procedure of reliability estimation and the varieties of relevant problems

This section is connected conceptually with the preceding four paragraphs. However, there are no references for the ideas discussed in them. The reader who doesn't want to learn the Bayes approach from the formal mathematical positions may skip them and start with the consideration of the general problems of the Bayes theory of estimation discussed below.

2.5.1 *Reliability estimation*

The setting of a problem of reliability estimation consists of the following four elements:

a) *distribution of probabilities of the basic random variable* characterizing the reliability of a technical device or system (for example, a cumulative distribution function of time-to-failure $F(t;\theta)$, where θ is a vector of parameters;
b) *a prior probability distribution*, represented, for example, in the form of p.d.f., $h(\theta)$, of the vector of parameters θ, characterizing the uncertainty of the given prior information I_a about reliability;
c) *loss function*, $L(\hat{R},R)$ characterizing the losses involved when one replaces the reliability R by its estimate $\hat{R}$;
d) *testing plan*, II, prescribing the method of obtaining experimental data I_e.

The problem may be interpreted as follows: we need to find the estimates of reliability R by using a priori information I_a and experimental data I_e. We consider below two forms of representation of the estimate for the reliability

a) the set of the point estimate R and standard deviation (s.d.) which is a characteristic of exactness of the estimate $\hat{R}$;
b) confidence interval $[\underline{R},\overline{R}]_\gamma$ with a given confidence probability .

The principal scheme for obtaining Bayes estimates is represented in Fig. 2.1. It consists of three steps.

Step 1 *Composition of likelihood function* $\ell(\theta, I_e)$. To do this we use some statistical model describing the distribution of the basic random variable $F(t;\theta)$ and experimental data I_e obtained after a realization of a testing plan II

Step 2 *Construction of a posterior distribution* $h(\theta \mid I_a, I_e)$. Here we use the Bayes formula

$$h(\theta \mid I_a, I_e) = \frac{h(\theta \mid I_a)\ell(\theta \mid I_e)}{\int_{\Theta} h(\theta \mid I_a)\ell(\theta \mid I_e)d\theta}, \tag{2.33}$$

where Θ is a range of the parameter θ.

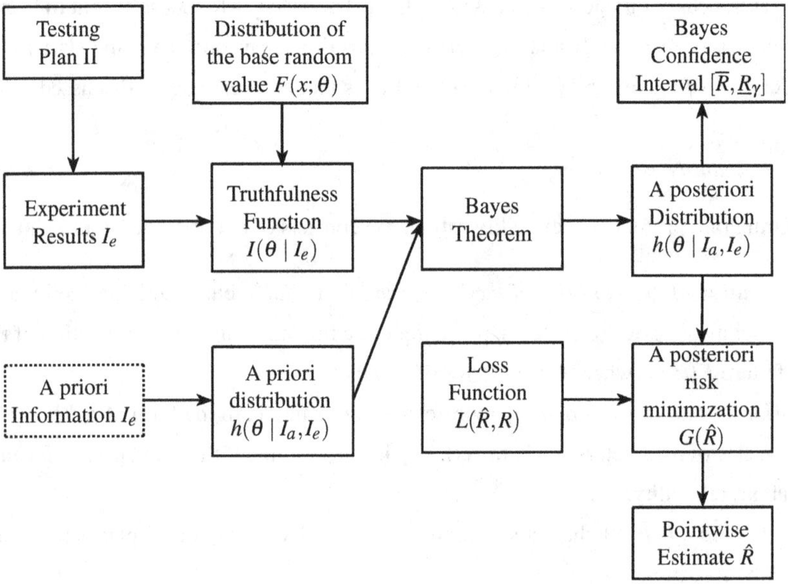

Fig. 2.1 The general scheme of obtaining the Bayes estimates

Step 3 *Obtaining Bayes estimates.* The Bayes confidence interval is defined by the condition $P\{\underline{R} \leqslant R \leqslant \overline{R}\} = \gamma$, or

$$\int_{\underline{R} \leqslant R(\theta) \leqslant \overline{R}} \hbar(\theta \mid I_a, I_e)d\theta = \gamma. \tag{2.34}$$

To obtain the Bayes point estimate $\hat{R}^*$, we should write the function of the posterior risk

$$G(\hat{R}) = \int_{\Theta} (\hat{R}, R(\theta))\hbar(\theta \mid I_a, I_e)d\theta \tag{2.35}$$

and choose among all estimates $\hat{R}$ such that one minimizes the function (2.35), that is,

$$\hat{R}^* = \arg \min_{\hat{R}\in[0,1]} G(\hat{R}). \tag{2.36}$$

If a squared-error loss function is chosen of the form $L(\hat{R},R) = (R-\hat{R})^2$, then the Bayes estimate is determined in the form of the posterior mean value

$$\hat{R}^* = \int_{\Theta} R(\theta)\bar{h}(\theta \mid I_a, I_e)d\theta. \tag{2.37}$$

The error of estimation of the value of $\hat{R}^*$ is assessed by the posterior s.d., $\sigma_{\hat{R}^*}$, which satisfies the relation

$$\sigma_{\hat{R}^*}^2 = \int_{\Theta} R^2(\theta)\bar{h}(\theta \mid I_a, I_e)d\theta - \hat{R}^{*2}. \tag{2.38}$$

Example 2.1. The device time-to-failure is subjected to the exponential distribution with the probability density

$$f(t;\lambda) = \lambda\, \mathrm{e}^{-\lambda t}, \quad t \geqslant 0,\ \lambda \geqslant 0. \tag{2.39}$$

As a prior distribution, a gamma-distribution with the likelihood kernel [202] has been chosen. The distribution density of the parameter λ has the form

$$h(\lambda \mid I_a) = \frac{\rho^{\delta}\lambda^{\delta-1}\mathrm{e}^{-\rho\lambda}}{\Gamma(\delta)}, \quad \lambda \geqslant 0,\ \delta \geqslant 0,\ \rho \geqslant 0, \tag{2.40}$$

and the parameters δ and ρ are assumed to be known. A mean square-error loss function, $L(\hat{R},R) = (R-\hat{R})^2$. As a testing plan $[n,U,T]$ (see [91]) has been chosen. We shall discuss the solution of the problem in detail including finding the estimates of the failure rate λ. The solution will be given in the form of the three steps:

1) Composing a likelihood function we bear in mind the fact that as a result of testing by the plan $[n,U,T]$ we have observed a censored sample.

   Suppose, for definiteness, that d of the tests have ended by failures at the instants $t_1^*, t_2^*, \ldots, t_d^*$ and that $n-d$ of those remaining were interrupted before failure after T units of time from the beginning. The likelihood function describing this situation is chosen (see [91]) in the form

$$\ell(\lambda \mid I_e) = \prod_{i=1}^{d} f(t_i^*;\lambda) \prod_{j=1}^{n-d} \int_T^{\infty} f(x;\lambda)\, dx. \tag{2.41}$$

   Substitution of p.d.f. (2.39) into (2.41) and simplifying, we have

$$\ell(\lambda \mid I_e) = \prod_{i=1}^{d} \lambda\, \mathrm{e}^{-\lambda t_i^*} \left(\mathrm{e}^{-\lambda T}\right)^{n-d} = \lambda^d \mathrm{e}^{\lambda K}, \tag{2.42}$$

   where $K = t_1^* + t_2^* + \cdots + t_d^* + (n-d)T$. Thus, the sufficient Bayes testing statistics appears to be as a pair of numbers (d,K).

2) Substituting the likelihood function (2.42) and a prior p.d.f. (2.40) in the Bayes formula (2.33), we have the posterior distribution density

$$\hbar(\lambda \mid I_a, I_e) = \frac{(\rho+K)^{\delta+d}}{\Gamma(\delta+d)} \lambda^{d+\delta+1} e^{-(\rho+K)}. \tag{2.43}$$

The obtained expression is a gamma-function. Consequently, the chosen prior distribution is conjugated.

3) Determine the point estimate $\hat{\lambda}^*$. For the squared-error loss function, the minimum of the posterior risk $G(\hat{\lambda})$ is attained at the point of the posterior mean value of the estimated parameter, that is,

$$\hat{\lambda}_* = \int_0^\infty \lambda \hbar(\lambda \mid I_a, I_e) d\lambda = \frac{d+\delta}{\rho+K}.$$

The posterior s.d., which may be interpreted as exactness characteristic of the estimate λ^*, is defined by the variance of the gamma-distributed random variable, that is,

$$\sigma_{\hat{\lambda}^*} = \frac{\sqrt{d+\delta}}{\rho+K}.$$

An interval estimate of the failure-rate is often used as the upper λ confidence limit. Define the Bayes analog of this estimate $\bar{\lambda}_\gamma$ and putting $\underline{\lambda}_\gamma = 0$. By definition, $P\{\lambda \leqslant \bar{\lambda}_\gamma\}$ and since the posterior distribution is a gamma-distribution, the transformation $z = 2\lambda(\rho+K)$ gives us the chi-square distribution with $2(\delta+d)$ degrees of freedom, we have

$$P\{2\lambda(\rho+K) \leqslant X_{\gamma;2(\delta+d)}\} = \gamma, \tag{2.44}$$

where $X_{\gamma;2(\delta+d)}$ is a quantile of the chi-square distribution of the probability . From this relation (2.44) we finally obtain

$$\bar{\lambda}_\gamma = \frac{X_{\gamma;2(\delta+d)}}{2(\rho+K)}.$$

2.5.2 *Varieties of problems of Bayes estimation*

When one solves practical problems, it is very difficult to establish all the above-mentioned elements for Bayesian reliability analysis and modeling. Therefore, we need to improve the classification of all possible varieties. From the methodological point-of-view, the most essential elements can be classified as follows:

1) the forming of a reliability model;
2) completeness of information on a prior distribution (or completeness of a prior uncertainty);

3) completeness of information on the main random variable.

We consider, in brief, each of these classifications. From the point-of-view of the first characteristic, we will distinguish two types of reliability models, giving the base for a corresponding approach for reliability determination. The first one (which is used more often) we will name "formal" and write it in the form

$$\xi > t_{\text{req}} \tag{2.45}$$

where ξ is a random time to-failure, t_{req} is the time which is necessary, in accordance with technological assignment of the device or system functioning. The model (2.45) doesn't touch upon real technical peculiarities of the device or system and enables us to analyze different (by nature) devices in a standard way, based only on the observable properties of the device (results of trials).

In addition to this model, we will use a model which is based on the mathematical description of real processes of the device collapse. This model, represented in the form

$$Z_j(t) = \phi(X(t)) > 0, \quad t \geqslant t_{\text{req}}, \ j = 1, 2, \ldots, m, \tag{2.46}$$

will be named "functional". $Z_j(t)$ denotes a random process of the initial device variables (loading factors, physically-mechanical characteristics, geometrical parameters, etc.); the function $\phi(\cdot)$ is called the *survival function.*

The set of conditions (2.46) symbolizes the time of the device being operable. There are many works devoted to the investigation of reliability of technical devices in the framework of this modeling which don't use the Bayes approach [26, 32, 89, 135, 173, and 260].

The questions connected with using the formal models of the device reliability will be discussed in the following five chapters, from the third to the seventh one, inclusive. Chapters 8–10 are devoted to the methods in reliability analysis based on the functional models.

From the point-of-view of a prior uncertainty (the second classification property) we will discuss the following cases:

(A1) The case of a complete prior determinacy, when the prior distribution density is determined uniquely;

(A2) The case of an incomplete priori determinacy, when a prior density is not given, and is determined only by finite number of restrictions, imposed on some functions defined on a prior distribution (for example, only a mean prior value of the parameter θ may be given);

(A3) The case of a complete a priori indeterminacy, when only the finite number of estimates of the parameter θ are known.

The first case is the most frequently encountered and will be discussed in Chapters 3, 4, 5, 8, 9. The case (A2) is the least studied in Bayes literature.

In Chapter 6 we give the description of the general formal representation of a partial a priori information and solve many concrete problems. The case (A3) is known as empirical Bayes estimation and is discussed in Chapter 7.

With respect to the third property, we will discuss the following two cases:

(C1) Parametric, when a parametric family is given for the cumulative distribution function of the main random variable, that is, $F(t) = F(t;\theta)$, where $\theta \in \Theta$;

(C2) Nonparametric, when this cumulative distribution function is determined on some nonparametric class (for example, a class of all continuous cumulative distribution functions).

Furthermore, we will use, as a rule, parametric estimates, since they are simpler and broadly applied. Nonparametric Bayes estimates will be studied in Chapter 4 and partially in Chapter 7. In Chapter 5 we will use the so called quasiparametric estimates. They use different methods for an approximate solution of a problem of estimation which is set as a parametric one, but are solved by means of nonparametric methods.

Chapter 3

The Methods of Parametric Bayes Estimation Based on Censored Samples

3.1 General description of the accepted estimation procedure

Under the analysis of reliability of technical devices, the essential role is played by the characteristics of the device capacity for work, in particular, by the time-to-failure, TTF, of the device during some time interval t:

$$R = R(t) = P\{\xi > t\} \tag{3.1}$$

where ξ is a random time to-failure function. Throughout what follows, the characteristic (3.1) will be used for the investigation of the peculiarities of the Bayesian approach, taking into account the fact that other Bayes characteristics (for example, those of a quantile type) can be obtained analogously.

The principal feature of all parametric Bayes methods is such that it is determined up to the parameters $\theta = (\theta_1, \theta_2, \ldots, \theta_t)$ whether a cumulative distribution function $F(t;\theta)$ or a distribution density $f(t;\theta)$ of a random variable ξ, is given, so that

$$R = R(t;\theta) = 1 - F(t;\theta) = \int_t^\infty f(x;\theta)dx \tag{3.2}$$

In the case when we are interested only in the dependence of the survival probability, SP, on the parameter θ, for arbitrary t, we will write $R(\theta)$. The vector of parameters θ is determined on the set Θ. The problem is that one has to estimate the SP having prior information and empirical data.

Frequently, prior information is determined as a prior distribution density, $h(\theta)$, of the model parameters of the reliability. In many important cases (from the point-of-view of practice), described below, one uses another parameterization: as model parameters will be used t as the valuesof the TTF at some given time instants $t_1, t_2, \ldots, t_\ell$, $R(t_j;\theta)$. Such a method of representation of a parameter vector is preferred for the following practical reason: an engineer can form a prior representation (subjective or frequency) without using the parameter θ which doesn't have, as a rule, a technical interpretation. He obtains it directly from the TTF. There is also a form of dual representation of a priori information in the form of a joint p.d.f. of the TTF at some instant t and $(\ell-1)$ component of the vector θ. When one chooses a parameterization method, he should use the following evident principle: the parameters of reliability models must have a clear physical interpretation. Only in this case, the researcher, using his informal experience, can assign a prior distribution adequate to real processes of functioning of a technical device.

In this chapter and the later ones, we will investigate the Bayes procedures of the TTF estimation for the plan of testing with censoring the failure data. This plan is applied in many practical engineering situations. For example, a tested technical device is a part of a composite system. The halting of testing may be caused either by the failure of the testing object or by the failure of some other object. The last case will be called a *standstill.* In autonomous tests, the standstill may be caused by a failure of the testing equipment. The typical situation we meet is estimation of the equipment with the help of results of the exploitation. Some of the equipment elements are put into operation at different moments of time. One should estimate the TTF at the given moment of time.

Let us enumerate the testing devices. For each i, the test may be ended by a failure at time t_i^* or by a standstill at the moment t_i, $i=1,2,\ldots,n$. If a failure occurs at the moment $t_i^* \leqslant t_i$, then the value t_i^* will be known after the trial. Provided that $t_i^* > t_i$, the exact value of t_i^* is unknown. It is known only that a failure may occur after the moment t_i. The random moments of failures or standstills are assumed to be mutually independent and have a density $f(t;\theta)$. After we have enumerated the moments of failures and standstills, the result of testing may be represented as a vector $\tau = \{t^*, t\}$, where $t^* = \{t_1^*, t_2^*, \ldots, t_d^*\}$, $t = \{t_1, t_2, \ldots, t_k\}$.

The technique of the Bayes TTF estimation is defined completely by the standard methods of Bayes estimation, discussed in Chapter 2. Starting from the sample τ and using p.d.f., $f(t;\theta)$ we write the expression of the likelihood function $\ell(\theta \mid \tau)$. The questions touching upon the determination of $\ell(\theta \mid \tau)$ for the censored samples are discussed in the next section. Further, using the Bayes theorem, one writes the kernel of the posterior density

$$\hbar(\theta \mid \tau) \sim \ell(\theta \mid \tau) h(\theta) \tag{3.3}$$

and determines the normalizing constant β:

$$\beta = \int_{\Theta} \ell(\theta \mid \tau) h(\theta)\, d\theta. \tag{3.4}$$

Then, a posterior p.d.f. takes on the form

$$\hbar(\theta \mid \tau) = \frac{1}{\beta} h(\theta) \ell(\theta \mid \tau). \tag{3.5}$$

Choosing the loss function $L(\hat{R},R)$in the form proposed in the previous chapter, where $\hat{R}$ is the estimate, and $R = R(\theta)$ is the true reliability measure and solving the minimization problem

$$\hat{R}^* = \arg \min_{\hat{R}\in(0,1)} \int_{\Theta} L\left(\hat{R},R(\theta)\right) \hbar(\theta \mid \tau)\, d\theta \tag{3.6}$$

one finds the point Bayes estimate of the reliability, $\hat{R}^*$. It should be mentioned that, if there are no empirical data τ, one can't use (3.6) instead ofthe posterior p.d.f., $\hbar(\theta \mid \tau)$, of a prior p.d.f., $h(\theta)$ is used. In this case $\hat{R}^*$ is a prior Bayes estimator.

If a squared-error loss function has been chosen, then the solution of the problem (3.6) is written explicitly:

$$\hat{R}^* = \int_{\Theta} R(\theta)\hbar(\theta \mid \tau)\, d\theta, \tag{3.7}$$

that is, the estimate $\hat{R}^*$ is the posterior mean value of the function $R(\theta)$. The exactness of the estimate we have obtained can be characterized by the posterior variance (or by s.d.) which coincides with the minimal value of a risk function

$$\sigma^2_{\hat{R}^*} = \int_{\Theta} \left[R(\theta) - \hat{R}^*\right]^2 \hbar(\theta \mid \tau)\, d\theta. \tag{3.8}$$

Since a SP is a positive characteristic of reliability, it is interesting to construct the lower confidence limit $\underline{R}^*_\gamma$, represented by the equation

$$P\left\{R(\theta) > \underline{R}^*_\gamma \mid \tau\right\} = \gamma,$$

where γ is the given confidence level. Finally, the determination of $\underline{R}^*_\gamma$ is reduced to the solution of the transcendent equation

$$\int_{R(\theta)\geqslant \underline{R}^*_\gamma} \hbar(\theta \mid \tau) d\theta - \gamma = 0, \tag{3.9}$$

in which the unknown estimate $\underline{R}^*_\gamma$ belongs to the integration domain. Thus, the standard parametric approach of estimating reliability is carried out as the successive application of the expressions (3.3)–(3.9). We can encounter, using different parametric families $f(t;\theta)$ and different prior p.d.f., $h(\theta)$ for the problem solution, some definite peculiarities and difficulties which don't have, however, a principal value. If one estimates reliability of some system, the solution of a problem may be more complicated In this case, the parameter θ contains many components (depending on the number of elements) and the function $R(\theta)$ is cumbersome.

Systematization of known parametric Bayes estimates. The recent works of many authors pay thorough attention to the obtaining of Bayesian estimates of reliability. Even a brief excursion in this field would be very cumbersome. Besides, the necessity of such an excursion appears to be dubious, because most of the results obtained in this field don't have a principled character. Below we give a systematization of the main results with the corresponding references. The reader who wants to learn some concrete results more deeply can find them in the works we cite. There are two complicated reviews on the application of Bayes methods to reliability. The first one [232] gives the analysis of works that were published until 1976; the second [249] is from 1977 to 1981. We present, in addition to these books, the systematization of the later most interesting works. We include works that have appeared since 1981 and a series of publications which were not mentioned in [232, 249].

The following principle is taken as a basis of classification: all the works divided into groups characterized by:

a) a form of the parametric family;
b) a form of a loss function;
c) a choice of a prior distribution;
d) plans testing for obtaining estimates;
e) structure type of the technical system, the reliability of which is being tested.

In accordance with the first characteristic, all works are divided into the following subgroups: binomial models [68, 71, 88, 197, 201, 234, 263, 268], models with a constant failure rate [11, 22, 147, 149, 164, 185, 255], Poisson models [37, 103, 107, 189, 230, 267, 268, 271], the case of normal distribution [96, 264], the case of gamma-distribution [66, 104, 116, 157, 255, 264], models based on a Weibull distribution [7, 33, 40, 44, 78, 119,186, 237, 251], and models with a log-normal distribution [175, 182]. In all these works, the authors use a natural parameterization of the corresponding distribution families. This means that if, for example, the Weibull cumulative distribution function is written in the form $F(t;\alpha,\sigma)-\exp\left[-(t/\sigma)^{\alpha}\right]$, then as a priori information is used the prior p.d.f. $h(\alpha,\sigma)$ of the variableswhich are model parameters. The use of corresponding results is impeded in practice, because the engineer-researcher usually meets some difficulties, when he forms a priori representation with respect to parameters having an often abstract nature. What actually happens is that a researcher has direct information on the degree of reliability. For example, for the above-mentioned above Weibull model, the interval of TTF values at the moment to: $R_{t_0}-1-F(t_0;\alpha,\sigma)$, is given and, having this information, one should obtain the Bayes estimate. Similar situations will be considered at the end of this chapter.

In accordance with the second characteristic (a form of a loss function), the publications are considered more distinct. The most of works use a quadratic loss function [17, 22, 37, 40, 44, 48, 96, 100, 105, 107, 150, 167, 184, 189, 230, 238, 258, 268] which gives the Bayes estimate in the form of the posterior m.v. In the work [157] a loss function $|\hat{R}-R(\theta)|$ is used. Some authors (see [60, 230, 258] accentuate the quadratic loss functions $[\hat{R}-R(\theta)]^2/R(\theta)$ and $[\hat{R}-R(\theta)]^2/R(\theta)^2$, giving the estimates $\{E[R^{-1} \mid \tau]\}$ and $E[R^{-1} \mid \tau]/E[R^{-2} \mid \tau]$ respectively. In the works [73, 258] the authors introduce and substantiate the usefulness of a loss function having the forms

$$C(R(\theta))\left[\hat{R}^{\beta}-R^{\beta}(\theta)\right]^2, \quad C(R(\theta))\left[\ln\hat{R}-\ln R(\theta)\right]^2.$$

In accordance with the third characteristic, we divide the works into four subgroups. To the first group belongs the works [1, 2, 29, 31, 36, 37, 38, 44, 66, 68, 96, 97, 100, 105, 109, 139, 147, 157, 163, 167, 183, 189, 190, 228, 234,237-241, 267, 272] which deal with conjugated systems of prior distributions. In the second group we include publications [17, 40, 44, 48, 95, 105, 141, 150, 186, 263] in which the authors attempt to use objective prior distributions. They either construct prior distributions based on the given statistical data of previous information, assuming that statistical mechanisms possess the property of stability, or apply the empirical Bayes approach. In the works [29, 100, 105, 157, 175, 189, 215, 230], the authors use the subjective discrete or uniform prior distributions. And, at last, in the fourth group we include a few publications [6, 60, 75] which use a principle of entropy maximum, considered in Chapter 2. Thus, we may come to the conclusion that in these works the authors attempt to avoid the assignment of the subjective prior distribution, doing this only in the case of the discrete representation.

In accordance with the fourth characteristic, the following four plans are used most often:

1) n articles are tested with fixing of a failure moment, the testing's are interrupted, when $r \leqslant n$ of failures have occurred [8, 22, 44, 69, 157, 163, 167, 236–240, 258];
2) n articles are being tested during the given time interval T and fixed the number of the articles which failed [103, 107, 268];
3) n articles are tested with fixing of the time they have failed, the testing are interrupted, when all articles have failed [184, 186];
4) during the testing of n articles failure moments are fixed, the testing is interrupted after the given time T has been ended [22, 31, 69, 155].

The last, and, fifth, characteristic enables us to subdivide the publications in the following way. In the works [29, 234, 241, 248, 271], the authors estimate the reliability of parallel systems, in the works [97, 148, 158, 159, 190, 197, 238–240, 261, 271] the reliability of sequential systems. Composed (parallel-sequential) schemes are considered in the works [31, 138, 139].

Finally, in the works [119, 268], the authors consider systems which differ from the above-mentioned.

Taking into account our arguments, mentioned above, we can make the following conclusion. In spite of the great variance of the solved problems, the questions of TTF estimation by the censored samples under the assumption that a priori information is given in the form of a prior distribution of the investigated reliability degree remain open. We complete it in the following section.

3.2 Likelihood function for Bayes procedures

One of the compound parts of any Bayes procedure of estimation is the composition of a likelihood function. In the simplest case for the testing plans without censoring, the likelihood function is written in the form

$$\ell(\theta \mid \tau) = \prod_{i=1}^{n} f(\tau_i; \theta) \tag{3.10}$$

Questions concerning construction of a likelihood function for the censored samples are discussed by many authors (see, for example, [31, 123]. The most complete formalization of the procedure of random censoring is done in [14, 15]. We represent below the main principles of this formalization.

Suppose that n are tested. Each i-th testing is associated with twonumbers t_i and t_i^* $(i = 1, 2, \ldots, n)$, t_i^* is a failure moment, t_i is a censoringmoment. Failure moments t_i^*, with the gap of censoring, are assumed to be mutually independent, equidistributed random variables with a c.d.f. $F(t;\theta)$. A sample $\tau = (\tau_1, \tau_2, \ldots, \tau_n)$, corresponding to the general plan of testing, has form

$$\tau = \left(\tau_{i_1}^*, \tau_{i_2}^*, \ldots, \tau_{i_d}^*, \tau_{j_1}^*, \tau_{i_2}^*, \ldots, \tau_{j_k}^*\right), \quad d + k = n, \tag{3.11}$$

where the set $I = (i_1, i_2, \ldots, i_d)$ is compounded by numbers of articles for which failures are observed, and the set $J = (j_1, j_2, \ldots, j_d)$ numbers of articles for which the failures are being censored. The set $\tau_1^*, \tau_2^*, \ldots, \tau_n^*, \tau_1, \ldots, \tau_n$ is considered a random vector.

Further it is supposed that a cumulative distribution function of the whole set of random variables possesses the following property: the conditional distribution $t_1, t_2, \ldots, t_n$ (under the condition that nonobserving values of failure moments $\tau_{j_1}^* > \tau_{i_2}^*, \ldots, \tau_{j_k}^* > t_{j_k}$, and observing ones $\tau_{i_1}^* \leqslant \tau_{j_1}, \ldots, \tau_{i_d}^* \leqslant t_{i_d}$ is independent of θ and may depend only on the values

$\tau^*_{i_1}, \ldots, \tau^*_{i_d}$. Under the assumption of the existence of joint p.d.f. values t_i,this means that for the conditional p.d.f., the relation

$$p\left(t_1, t_2, \ldots, t_n \mid t^*_1, \ldots, t^*_n\right) = p\left(t_1, t_2, \ldots, t_n \mid t^*_{i_1}, \ldots, t^*_{i_d}\right), \tag{3.12}$$

holds, where

$$t^*_i \leqslant t_i, \quad \forall i \in I, \quad t^*_j > t_j, \quad \forall j \in J.$$

The plan of testing with censoring, satisfying the relation (3.12), is called in [14] a *plan of testing with noninformative censoring* (NC-plan).

Note that the condition (3.12) is fulfilled, if the sets of all failure moments $\left(\tau^*_1, \tau^*_2, \ldots, \tau^*_n\right)$ and the sets of all censoring moments $t_1, t_2, \ldots, t_n$ are mutually independent. This exact situation occurs when t^*_i are independent with respect to i and don't depend on all t_j $(i,\ j = 1, 2, \ldots, n)$. Such an assumption looks natural when one carries out a testing of articles with two types of failures, when each test is continuing up to the moment until a failure occurs. We indicate the type of occurred failure. The sample, obtained in this way, has a form $\tau = (\tau_1, \tau_2, \ldots, \tau_n)$, where $\tau_i = \min\{t^*_i, t_i\}$. The event $\tau_i = t^*_i\ (\tau_i = t_i)$ responds to the case when the first (second) type failure has been occurred before the occurring of the second (first) one.

For the establishment of the likelihood function, we write a joint density of the observed data:

$$p(\tau) = p\left(t^*_{i_1}, \ldots, t^*_{i_d}, t_{j_1}, \ldots, t_{j_k}\right) = \int_{t^*_{i_1}}^{\infty} dt_{i_1}$$
$$\cdots \int_{t^*_{i_d}}^{\infty} dt_{i_d} \int_{t_{j_1}}^{\infty} dt^*_{j_1} \cdots \int_{t_{j_k}}^{\infty} dt^*_{j_k} \prod_{\ell=1}^{n} f\left(t^*_\ell; \theta\right) p\left(t_1, \ldots, t_n \mid t^*_1, \ldots, t^*_n\right).$$

Integrating $t^*_{j_1}, \ldots, t^*_{j_k}$ over, in accordance with (3.12), yields

$$p(\tau \mid \theta) = \prod_{m=1}^{d} f\left(t^*_{i_m}; \theta\right) \prod_{\ell=1}^{k} \left[1 - F\left(t_{j_\ell}; \theta\right)\right] c(\tau), \tag{3.13}$$

where

$$c(\tau) = \int_{t^*_{i_1}}^{\infty} dt_i \cdots \int_{t^*_{i_d}}^{\infty} dt_{i_d} p\left(t_1, \ldots, t_n \mid t^*_{i_1}, \ldots, t^*_{i_d}\right)$$

is independent of the parameter θ and defined only by the obtained data. We rewrite the expression (3.13) in a more suitable form in order to determine reliability degrees. To this end we use the function of a failure rate

$$\lambda(t; \theta) = \frac{f(t; \theta)}{1 - F(t; \theta)} \tag{3.14}$$

and the resource function (or the integral function of intensity)

$$\Lambda(t;\theta) = \int_0^t \lambda(x;\theta)dx = \int_0^\infty \chi(t-x)\lambda(x;\theta)dx \tag{3.15}$$

where $\chi(z) = 0$ for $z < 0$, and $\chi(z) = 1$ for $z \geqslant 0$.

Note that, since

$$R(t;\theta) = 1 - F(t;\theta) = \exp\left[-\int_0^t \lambda(x;\theta)dx\right]$$

for the resource function we obtain

$$\Lambda(t;\theta) = -\ln[1 - F(t;\theta)]. \tag{3.16}$$

Let us transform the expression (3.13), using the relations (3.14) and (3.16):

$$p(\tau \mid \theta) = c(\tau)\prod_{i\in I}\lambda(t_i^*;\theta)\exp\left\{-\left[\sum_{i\in I}\Lambda(t_i^*;\theta) + \sum_{j\in J}\Lambda(t_j;\theta)\right]\right\}. \tag{3.17}$$

The expression (3.17) can be simplified with the help of (3.15) in the following way:

$$\begin{aligned}\sum_{i\in I}\Lambda(t_i^*;\theta) + \sum_{j\in J}\Lambda(t_j;\theta) &= \int_0^\infty \left[\sum_{i\in I}\chi(t-t_i^*) + \sum_{j\in J}\chi(t-t_j)\right]\lambda(t;\theta)dt \\ &= \int_0^\infty N(t)\lambda(t;\theta)dt \end{aligned} \tag{3.18}$$

where $N(t)$ is the number of articles being tested at the moment t. By using the relation (3.18), we can rewrite (3.17) as

$$p(\tau \mid \theta) = \prod_{i\in I}\lambda(t_i^*;\theta)\exp\left\{-\int_0^\infty N(t)\lambda(t;\theta)dt\right\}c(\tau). \tag{3.19}$$

The distribution density $p(\tau \mid \theta)$, represented as a function of the parameter θ, by definition is a likelihood function for the (NC)-plan, corresponding to the censoring data τ of the form (3.11). Throughout what follows we will use the notations $t^* = (t_1^*, \ldots, t_d^*)$, $t = (t_1, \ldots, t_k)$ for the moment of failure and moment of censoring, respectively, observed in $n = d + k$ independent testing's.

Following these notations, we can rewrite the likelihood function $\ell(\theta \mid \tau)$ as one of the following equivalent expressions:

$$\ell(\theta \mid \tau) = c(\tau)\prod_{i=1}^{d} f(t_i^*;\theta)\prod_{j=1}^{k}[1 - F(t_2;\theta)], \tag{3.20}$$

$$\ell(\theta \mid \tau) = c(\tau)\prod_{i=1}^{d}\lambda(t_i^*;\theta)\exp\left[-\sum_{j=1}^{n}\Lambda(t_j;\theta)\right], \tag{3.21}$$

$$\ell(\theta \mid \tau) = c(\tau)\prod_{i=1}^{d}\lambda(t_i^*;\theta)\exp\left[-\int_0^\infty N(t)\lambda(t;\theta)dt\right]. \tag{3.22}$$

We use one or another of these expressions, depending on convenience, giving the posterior p.d.f. $\hbar(\theta \mid \tau)$ and on the manner of representation of the parametric family of distributions the random variable of a trouble-free time of functioning. In concluding this section we note that the assumption about the randomness of the censoring moments doesn't play an essential role in the above reasoning. In the case more general than those considered earlier, for each testing is planned the duration t_i' $(i = 1, 2, \ldots, n)$ that cannot be exceeded. Thus, in each testing it is observed the minimal of three quantities $\tau_i = \min\{t_i^*, t_i, t_i'\}$, and the sample has a form $\tau = \left(t_1^*, \ldots, t_d^*, t_1, \ldots, t_{k'}, t_k', \ldots, t_{k''}'\right)$, where $k' + k'' = k$, $n = d + k$. To formalize the given testing plan mentioned above, one should consider the set of random variables $\left\{t_1^*, \ldots, t_n^*, t_1, \ldots, t_n, t_1', \ldots t_n'\right\}$, having a joint density

$$p = \prod_{\ell=1}^{n} f\left(t_\ell^*; \theta\right) p\left(t_1, \ldots, t_n \mid t_1^*, \ldots, t_n^*\right) \prod_{j=1}^{n} \delta_j\left(t_j'\right),$$

where $\delta_j(t_j')$is the delta-function. Applying the transformations, analogous to those that have been used for $p(\tau \mid \theta)$, we obtain

$$p(\tau \mid \theta) = \prod_{m=1}^{d} f\left(t_{i_m}^*; \theta\right) \prod_{\ell=1}^{k'} \left[1 - F\left(t_{j_s}; \theta\right)\right] \prod_{s=1}^{k''} \left[1 - F\left(t_{j_\ell}; \theta\right)\right].$$

This expression coincides with (3.13), if one puts $k' + k'' = k$ and supposes that the moments of random and determinate censorings don't differ. Therefore, the relation for the likelihood function (3.20)–(3.22) remains valid, not only for the random censoring, but also for the determinate one.

3.3 Survival probability estimates for the constant failure rate

The case of the constant failure rate $\lambda(t) = \lambda = \text{const.}$) is associated with the exponential distribution of the TTF with p.d.f.

$$f(t; \lambda) = \lambda \, \mathrm{e}^{-\lambda t}$$

and with the cumulative distribution function

$$F(t; \lambda) = 1 - \mathrm{e}^{-\lambda t}.$$

This distribution is one-parametric. The probability of the trouble-free time at some moment t_0 is written in the form

$$R = R(t_0; \lambda) = \mathrm{e}^{-\lambda t_0}.$$

In view of the arguments mentioned above, we consider a situation when the prior distribution is defined directly for the estimated TTF, i.e., $h(r)$ is given. Represent p.d.f. $f(t;\lambda)$ and c.d.f. $F(t;\lambda)$ in accordance with the parameter $r = \exp(-\lambda t_0)$. This yields

$$\lambda = \lambda(r) = -\frac{\ln r}{t_0},$$

whence

$$f(t;\lambda(r)) = -\frac{\ln r}{t_0} r^{t/t_0} \tag{3.23}$$

and

$$F(t;\lambda(r)) = r^{t/t_0}. \tag{3.24}$$

Substituting the expressions (3.23) and (3.24) into (3.20), we obtain the likelihood function which corresponds to the sample τ for the NC-plan oftesting:

$$\ell(r \mid \tau) = c(\tau)\left(-\frac{1}{t_0}\right)^n r^{\omega} \ln^d r, \tag{3.25}$$

where

$$\omega = \omega(\tau) = \frac{1}{t_0}\left(\sum_{i=1}^{d} t_i^* + \sum_{j=1}^{k} t_j\right)$$

is a total respective operating time of testing that generates, together with the number of failures d, the sufficient statistic with respect to the sample τ under the NC-plan.

In accordance with the Bayes theorem (3.3), for the posterior p.d.f. of the parameter τ we have

$$\hbar(r \mid \tau) \sim h(r) r^{\omega} \ln^d r. \tag{3.26}$$

For further investigation we choose a quadratic loss function. It enables us to write the following expressions for the Bayes estimate $\hat{R}^*$ and posterior variance, respectively:

$$\hat{R}^* = \frac{1}{\beta}\int_0^1 h(r) r^{\omega+1} \ln^d r dr, \tag{3.27}$$

$$\sigma_{\hat{R}^*}^2 = \frac{1}{\beta}\int_0^1 h(r) r^{\omega+2} \ln^d r dr - \hat{R}^{*2}, \tag{3.28}$$

where $\beta = \int_0^1 h(r) r^{\omega} \ln^d r dr$ is the normalizing constant. The lower confidence TTF limit, in accordance with the expression (3.9), can be found from the equation

$$\int_{\underline{R}_\gamma^*}^1 h(r) r^{\omega} \ln^d r dr = \gamma \int_0^1 h(r) r^{\omega} \ell \ln^d r dr \tag{3.29}$$

where γ is a confidence level.

In the general case for the practical application of the relations (3.27)–(3.29), we need to use numerical methods of integration and numerical methods for the solution of transcendent equations. Often we can meet such situations when $h(r)$ is chosen by the frequency relations and appears to bean approximation of some empirical equation. (We'll represent below, from the point-of-view of practical interests, some of the most important cases.)

3.3.1 *The case of uniform prior distribution*

Suppose that R is subjected to a prior distribution with p.d.f.

$$h(r) = \begin{cases} \dfrac{1}{R_u - R_\ell}, & R_\ell \leqslant r \leqslant R_u, \\ 0, & r < r_\ell, \quad r > R_u. \end{cases} \tag{3.30}$$

This case is typical for the practical situation when a researcher, using the previous experiment, can guarantee that a value of TTF of the created device will not fall outside the interval $[R_\ell, F_u]$. In accordance with (3.27) we obtain

$$\hat{R}^* = \frac{\displaystyle\int_{R_\ell}^{R_u} r^{\omega+1} \ln^d r dr}{\displaystyle\int_{R_\ell}^{R_u} r^{\omega} \ln^d r dr}. \tag{3.31}$$

For the application of formula (3.31) we use the following integral, which can be easily found:

$$\int x^\theta \ln^n x dx = x^{\theta+1} \sum_{k=0}^{n} (-1)^k n^{(k)} \frac{\ln^{n-k} x}{(\theta+1)^{k+1}} + C, \tag{3.32}$$

where $n^{(k)} = \frac{n!}{(n-k)!}$is the number of arrangements of k elements from n elements. The expression (3.31) is written as

$$\hat{R}^* = \frac{I_E(R_u, \omega+1, d) - I_E(R_\ell, \omega+1, d)}{I_E(R_u, \omega, d) - I_E(R_\ell, \omega, d)}, \tag{3.33}$$

where the function $I_E(x,a,n)$ is given follows:

$$I_E(x,a,n) = s^{a+1} \sum_{k=0}^{n} \frac{1}{(n-k)!} \cdot \frac{|\ln^{n-k} x|}{(a+1)^k}. \tag{3.34}$$

The expression for the posterior variance can be found analogously:

$$\sigma_{\hat{R}^*}^2 = \frac{I_E(R_u, \omega+2, d) - I_E(R_\ell, \omega+2, d)}{I_E(R_u, \omega, d) - I_E(R_\ell, \omega, d)} - \hat{R}^{*2}. \tag{3.35}$$

In this case the equation (3.29) has a form

$$I_E(R_\gamma^*, \omega, d) = (1-\gamma) I_E(R_u, \omega, d) + \gamma I_E(R_\ell, \omega, d). \tag{3.36}$$

The case $R_\ell = 0$, $R_u = 1$, i.e., a TTF is distributed uniformly on the segment $[0,1]$, will be of interest to us. We name it as the case of trivial a priori information. The formulas (3.33)–(3.35) are simplified substantially:

$$\hat{R}^* = \left(1 - \frac{1}{\omega+2}\right)^{d+1}, \quad \sigma_{\hat{R}^*}^2 = \left(\frac{\omega+1}{\omega+3}\right)^{d+1} - \hat{R}^{*2}, \tag{3.37}$$

$$\underline{R}_\gamma^{*\omega+1} \sum_{k=0}^{d} \frac{\omega+1}{(d-k)!} |\ln \underline{R}_\gamma^*|^{d-k} = \beta(1-\gamma). \tag{3.38}$$

Let us compare the estimates (3.37) with the maximum likelihood estimates. To this end we use the likelihood function (3.25). After solving the likelihood equation $\partial \ln \ell(r \mid \tau)/\partial r$, we obtain

$$R_{\mathrm{ml}} = \mathrm{e}^{-d/\omega}. \tag{3.39}$$

Next we find the minimal estimate of the variance. Then, in accordance with the Kramer–Rao inequality,

$$D\left[R_{\mathrm{ml}}\right] \geqslant \mathrm{e}^{-d/\omega},$$

where

$$I(r) = \int_0^\infty \frac{\left[\frac{\partial}{\partial r} f(t;\lambda(r))\right]^2}{f(t;\lambda(r))} dt.$$

For the given case

$$I(r) = \frac{1}{r^2 \ln^2 r},$$

whence,

$$D\left[R_{\mathrm{ml}}\right] \geqslant \mathrm{e}^{-2n/\omega}(n/\omega)^2 = D_{\min}. \tag{3.40}$$

Let us compare (3.37) with (3.39) and (3.40) respectively. It is easily seen from the expression (3.39) that $R_{\mathrm{ml}} = 1$ for $d = 0$, i.e., we cannot apply the maximum likelihood estimate for the case of completely successful tests. At the same time, the substitution $d = 0$ into the expression (3.37) gives us $\hat{R}^* = (\omega+1)/(\omega+2)$ and the case $\hat{R}^* = 1$ is realized only in the asymptotic $n \to \infty$. Analogously, for $d = 0$ in the expression (3.40) we obtain $D_{\min} = 0$ and $\sigma^2_{\hat{R}^*}$, as it follows from (3.37) is always positive and tends to zero onlyas $n \to \infty$.
In Table 3.1 we represent the results of numerical comparison of $\hat{R}^*$ with R_{ml} and $\sigma^2_{\hat{R}^*}$ with $D_{\min}$ for a broad range of values of sufficient statistics. As can be seen from the given numerical values, $\sigma^2_{\hat{R}^*} < D_{\min}$ for $d > 1$.
Compare now the lower Bayes confidence limit for the case of trivial a priori information with a usual confidence limit (for $d = 0$)

$$\underline{R}'_\gamma = (1-\gamma)^{1/n}, \tag{3.41}$$

which holds for the plan $[N,U,T]$ under completely trouble free tests. For $d = 0$, equation (3.39) gives us

$$\underline{R}^*_\gamma = (1-\gamma)^{1/(\omega+1)}. \tag{3.42}$$

If one reduces the formula (3.42) for the plan $[N,U,T]$, it yields

$$\underline{R}^*_\gamma = (1-\gamma)^{1/(n+1)}.$$

Table 3.1

ω	$\hat{R}_{ml}$	$\hat{R}^*$	D_{min}	$\sigma^2_{\hat{R}^*}$	d
2	0.367879	0.421875	0.135335	0.038022	
3	0.513417	0.512000	0.117154	0.034153	
4	0.606531	0.578704	0.091970	0.029534	
5	0.670320	0.629748	0.071893	0.025306	
10	0.818731	0.770255	0.026813	0.012534	
20	0.904836	0.869741	0.008187	0.004708	
30	0.935507	0.909149	0.003890	0.002426	2
40	0.951229	0.930259	0.002262	0.001474	
50	0.960789	0.943410	0.001477	0.000988	
100	0.980199	0.970876	0.000384	0.000272	
200	0.990050	0.985222	0.000098	0.000071	
300	0.993356	0.990099	0.000044	0.000032	
400	0.995012	0.992556	0.000025	0.000019	
500	0.996008	0.994036	0.000016	0.000012	
3	0.367879	0.409600	0.135335	0.029759	
4	0.472367	0.482253	0.125511	0.027740	
5	0.548812	0.539775	0.108430	0.025049	
10	0.740818	0.706067	0.049393	0.014092	
20	0.860700	0.830207	0.016668	0.005726	
30	0.904837	0.880738	0.000081	0.003037	
40	0.927743	0.908109	0.004841	0.001873	3
50	0.941763	0.925268	0.003193	0.001268	
100	0.970446	0.961357	0.000948	0.000355	
200	0.985112	0.980344	0.000218	0.000094	
300	0.990650	0.986821	0.000098	0.000043	
400	0.992528	0.990087	0.000055	0.000024	
500	0.996008	0.992056	0.000036	0.000016	

In the work [120] the estimate for the plan $[N, U, (r, T)]$ was obtained which, for a constant failure rate, results in the sufficient statistic (d, ω).This estimate has form

$$\underline{R}^*_\gamma = \exp\left(-\frac{\chi^2_{1-\gamma;2(d+1)}}{2\omega}\right) \tag{3.43}$$

where $\chi^2_{1-\gamma;2(d+1)}$is a quantile of the chi-square distribution.

In Table 3.2 we represent the values of the estimate (3.43) and the lower Bayes confidence limit in accordance with the equation (3.38) for a broad range of sufficient statistic values. Having compared the results of the table, we may conclude that $\underline{R}^*_\gamma > \underline{R}'_\gamma$, that is, the Bayes confidence interval is always smaller than the usual one. At the same time, the estimates $\underline{R}^*_\gamma$ and $\underline{R}'_\gamma$ have equal limits as $n \to \infty$ and their values almost don't differ beginning with $\omega = 40$.

The analysis we have performed lets us as certain that the Bayes estimates are more effec-

Table 3.1 (continued)

ω	$\hat{R}_{ml}$	$\hat{R}^*$	$D_{\min}$	$\sigma^2_{\hat{R}^*}$	d
2	0.367879	0.421875	0.135335	0.038022	
3	0.513417	0.512000	0.117154	0.034153	
4	0.606531	0.578704	0.091970	0.029534	
5	0.670320	0.629748	0.071893	0.025306	
10	0.818731	0.770255	0.026813	0.012534	
20	0.904836	0.869741	0.008187	0.004708	
30	0.935507	0.909149	0.003890	0.002426	2
40	0.951229	0.930259	0.002262	0.001474	
20	0.960789	0.943410	0.001477	0.000988	
100	0.980199	0.970876	0.000384	0.000272	
200	0.990050	0.985222	0.000098	0.000071	
300	0.993356	0.990099	0.000044	0.000032	
400	0.995012	0.992556	0.000025	0.000019	
500	0.996008	0.994036	0.000016	0.000012	
3	0.367879	0.409600	0.135335	0.029759	
2	0.472367	0.482253	0.125511	0.27740	
5	0.548812	0.539775	0.108430	0.025049	
10	0.740818	0.706067	0.049393	0.014092	
20	0.860700	0.830207	0.016668	0.005726	
30	0.904837	0.880738	0.0081	0.003037	
40	0.927743	0.908109	0.004841	0.001873	3
50	0.941763	0.925268	0.003193	0.001268	
100	0.970446	0.961357	0.000948	0.000355	
200	0.985112	0.980344	0.000218	0.000094	
300	0.990650	0.986821	0.000098	0.000043	
400	0.992528	0.990087	0.000055	0.000024	
500	0.996008	0.992056	0.000036	0.000016	

tive. Therefore, by using them in practice we can substantially reduce the number of tests necessary for the confirmation of the given reliability requirements. In order to clarify the quantity relations between the necessary volume of tests ω^*_{req} which we need to carry out by using the Bayes methodology and the volume ω_{req} of tests which we have to perform by using non-Bayes methods, one performs a numerical modeling of the process of experimental functioning of the object on the given reliability level R_{req}. The values ω^*_{req} and ω_{req} were defined from the conditions $\underline{R}^*_\gamma = R_{\text{req}}$ and $\underline{R}'_\gamma = R_{\text{req}}$.

Figure 3.1 shows the behavior of the relative gain in the number of tests $\omega_{\text{req}}/\omega^*_{\text{req}}$ depending on a prior confidence level R_ℓ (when $R_u = 1$) for different R_{req}. As can be seen from Figure 3.1, the gain may substantially increase.

Table 3.2

	$d=0$		$d=1$		$d=1$	
ω	$\underline{R}^*_{0.9}$	$\underline{R}'_{0.9}$	$\underline{R}^*_{0.9}$	$\underline{R}'_{0.9}$	$\underline{R}^*_{0.9}$	$\underline{R}'_{0.9}$
1	0.316229	0.100009	0.0	0.0	0.0	0.0
2	0.464160	0.316241	0.273468	0.143023	0.0	0.0
3	0.562342	0.464172	0.378163	0.273488	0.264325	0.169625
4	0.630958	0.562353	0.459350	0.378184	0.344914	0.264312
5	0.681292	0.630968	0.5229742	0.459370	0.411686	0.344900
10	0.811131	0.794335	0.702148	0.677768	0.616408	0.587282
15	0.865964	0.857701	0.784187	0.771592	0.717025	0.701290
20	0.896151	0.891255	0.830918	0.823267	0.776124	0.766343
30	0.928415	0.926121	0.882078	0.878403	0.842242	0.837431
35	0.938042	0.936332	0.897584	0.894824	0.862567	0.858927
45	0.951177	0.950120	0.918917	0.917197	0.890740	0.888449
55	0.959716	0.959001	0.932898	0.931724	0.909335	0.907762
65	0.965714	0.965197	0.942768	0.941917	0.922525	0.921378
75	0.970157	0.969766	0.950107	0.949462	0.932366	0.931493
85	0.973581	0.97327	0.955778	0.955272	0.939989	0.939303
95	0.976300	0.976054	0.960292	0.959885	0.946068	0.945514
100	0.977460	0.977238	0.962290	0.961852	0.948668	0.948167
150	0.984867	0.984767	0.974569	0.974403	0.965367	0.965139
200	0.988610	0.988554	0.980834	0.980740	0.973868	0.973738
300	0.992380	0.992354	0.987160	0.987119	0.982473	0.982415
400	0.994275	0.884260	0.990347	0.990323	0.986816	0.986782
500	0.995415	0.995406	0.992266	0.992251	0.989433	0.989411

3.3.2 *The case of a prior beta-distribution*

There are practical situations when an engineer has information about a pointwise prior estimate R_0 of the TTF and information about the error of itsdetermination in the form of a prior variance σ_0^2. In this case, as ascertainedin [43], a prior distribution can be approximated by a beta distribution with the p.d.f.

$$h(r) = \frac{r^{\alpha-1}(1-r)^{\beta-1}}{B(\alpha,\beta)}, \quad 0 \leqslant r \leqslant 1, \tag{3.44}$$

where $B(\alpha,\beta) = \int_0^1 x^{\alpha-1}(1-x)^{\beta-1}$ is a beta function and parameters α, β are defined as

$$\alpha = R_0\left[\frac{R_0(1-R_0)}{\sigma_0^2} - 1\right], \quad \beta = (1-R_0)\left[\frac{R_0(1-R_0)}{\sigma_0^2} - 1\right].$$

Due to the Bayes theorem on a prior distribution density, we have

$$h(r \mid \tau) \sim r^{\alpha+\omega}(1-r)^{\beta-1}\ln^d r, \tag{3.45}$$

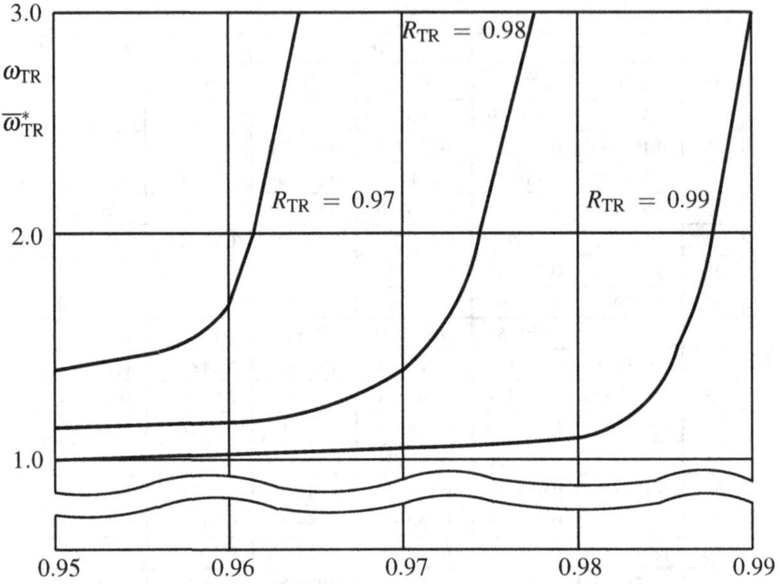

Fig. 3.1 Illustration of the gain in the testing volume under using of Bayes procedures.

whence one obtains the following Bayes estimates:

$$\hat{R}^* = \frac{I_B(\omega+1)}{I_B(\omega)}, \quad \sigma_{\hat{R}^*} = \frac{I_B(\omega+2)}{I_B(\omega)} - \hat{R}^{*2}, \tag{3.46}$$

where the function $I_B(v)$ is defined by the integral

$$I_B(v) = \int_0^1 x^{\alpha+y-1}(1-x)^{\beta-1}|\ln x|^d dx. \tag{3.47}$$

For the highly-reliable articles $\alpha+\omega \geqslant 100$, in the integral (3.47) we can use the approximation $\ln r \cong (1-4)$. The point is that for $\alpha+\omega \geqslant 100$, the posterior density concentrates in the domain, adjacent to the unity, so that its values outside of the interval $[0.9;1]$ are negligibly small and the approximation, indicated above, gives satisfactory results for practical use.

Finally we have

$$\begin{aligned} \hat{R}^* &\approx \frac{B(\alpha+\omega+1,\beta+d)}{B(\alpha+\omega,\beta+d)} = \frac{\alpha+\omega}{\alpha+\omega+\beta+d}, \\ \sigma^2_{\hat{R}^*} &\approx \frac{(\alpha+\omega)(\beta+d)}{(\alpha+\beta+d+\omega)^2(\alpha+\beta+d+\omega+1)}. \end{aligned} \tag{3.48}$$

It should be noted that the expressions we have obtained give us the exact values of the required estimates for $d = 0$.

3.4 Reliability estimates for the linear failure rate

The case of a linearly increasing intensity function $\lambda(t)$, corresponding tothe deterioration of exploitation conditions or wear of the article, is a development of the previous model. Suppose, as before, that we have to estimate the TTF, $R = P\{\xi > t_0\}$. Because the failure rate during the time interval $[0,t_0]$ is changing linearly, it becomes z-times worse:

$$z = \frac{\lambda(t_0)}{\lambda(0 \geqslant 1)}. \tag{3.49}$$

We name the quantity z as a degradation degree of the intensity function.Clearly, provided that $z = 1$, we have the previous case $\lambda(t) = \text{const}$.
Represent the function $\lambda(t)$in the form of the following linear function:

$$\lambda(t) = 2\alpha t + \lambda_0,$$

where α and λ_0 are the parameters of linear function. The function $\lambda(t)$ associates with the density of the time to failure, TTF,

$$f(t) = f(t;\alpha,\lambda_0) = (2\alpha t + \lambda_0)\exp\left[-(\alpha t^2 + \lambda_0 t)\right] \tag{3.50}$$

and with the distribution function

$$F(t) = F(t;\alpha,\lambda_0) = 1 - \exp\left[-(\alpha t^2 + \lambda_0)\right]. \tag{3.51}$$

The estimating reliability index is written in the form

$$R = R(\alpha,\lambda_0) = \exp(-\alpha t_0^2 + \lambda_0 t_0). \tag{3.52}$$

This parameterization is a natural generalization of the previous model. However, the parameters of the functions (3.50)–(3.52) don't have a sufficiently technical interpretation. It is more suitable, for these reasons, to use the parameters r and z, where r coincides with the estimating TTF and z has been defined earlier in (3.49). As was mentioned above, it is substantially easier to form a priori representation immediately about reliability index; the parameter z has a clear interpretation and indicates how many times the failure rate has increased in the interval $[0,t_0]$. It is also suitable that r and z are dimensionless parameters. Throughout what follows it is assumed that we are given a prior distribution $h(r,z)$, $(r,z) \in \Omega$, where Ω is the given domain of parameters. Solving (3.49) and (3.52), we obtain

$$\alpha = \frac{\ln r}{t_0^2} \cdot \frac{z-1}{z+1}, \qquad \lambda_0 = -\frac{2\ln r}{t_0(z+1)}. \tag{3.53}$$

After that we can express p.d.f. $f(t)$ and c.d.f. $F(t)$ in terms of dimensionless parameters z and r:

$$f(t)f(t;r,z) = -\frac{2\ln r}{(z+1)t_0}\left[(z-1)\frac{t}{t_0} + 1\right] r^{\frac{z-1}{z+1}\cdot\frac{t^2}{t_0^2} + \frac{2}{z+1}\cdot\frac{t}{t_0}},$$

$$F(t) = F(t;r,z) = 1 - r^{\frac{z-1}{z+1}\cdot\frac{t^2}{t_0^2} + \frac{2}{z+1}\cdot\frac{t}{t_0}}.$$

After substitution of these expressions into (3.20) and some arithmetical transformation, we obtain the likelihood function for the reliability model with a linear intensity function and NC-plan, giving the sample τ:

$$\ell(,z \mid \tau) = c(\tau)\left(-\frac{2}{t_0}\right)^d a(z) r^{b(z)} \ln^d r, \tag{3.54}$$

where

$$a(z) = \frac{1}{(z+1)^d}\prod_{i=1}^{d}[(z-1)v_i^* + 1]$$

$$b = \frac{1}{z+1}\left[(z-1)k + 2_\omega\right],$$

$$\omega = \sum_{i=1}^{d} v_i^* \sum_{j=1}^{k} v_j, \quad k = \sum_{i=1}^{d} v_i^{2*} + \sum_{j=1}^{k} v_j^2,$$

$$v_i^* = \frac{t_i^*}{t_0}, \quad v_j = \frac{t_j}{t_0}.$$

The quantities v_i^* and v_j' have, respectively, the sense of reduced dimensionless moments of failure and censoring. As seen from the expression (3.54), one can use instead of the vector τ the union of vectors v^* and v, composed of the outcomes of the tests. The quantities $\{v_1^*, v_2^*, \ldots, v_d^*, d, \omega, k\}$ form the sufficient statistic.

In accordance with the Bayes theorem for the posterior density of the parameters s and z, we have

$$\hbar(r,z \mid r) \sim h(r)a(r)r^{b(z)} \ln^d r. \tag{3.55}$$

If the value of the degradation index $z = 1$ is taken exactly, we need only a prior distribution of the parameter r. In this case for the posterior p.d.f. of the parameter r, we obtain

$$\hbar(r \mid \tau) \sim h(r) r^b \ln^d r. \tag{3.56}$$

Besides, provided that $z = 1$, we have $b = \omega$, and relation (3.56) coincides with (3.26), obtained for the case $\lambda = \text{const}$. The sufficient statistic for the case, represented by (3.56), has a simpler form than the one for the general case, where it is settled by the three quantities $\{d, \omega, k\}$.

Consider the wide spread case when an engineer can guarantee some interval $[R_\ell, R_u]$ for the estimating reliability R before the beginning of testing.

In accordance with this, we'll assume a priori that $R \in [R_\ell, R_u]$, and the degradation coefficient of the failure rate z belongs to the interval $[z_1, z_2]$.

Let us take for z and r uniform prior distributions in the intervals $[R_\ell, R_u]$ and $[z_1, z_2]$ respectively; moreover, we'll assume that r and z are a priori independent. The expressions for the Bayes estimate $\hat{R}^*$ and posterior variance $\sigma^2_{\hat{R}^*}$ are written as

$$\hat{R}^* = \frac{1}{\beta}\int_{z_1}^{z_2} dz \int_{R_\ell}^{R_u} ra(z)r^{b(z)} \ln^d r dr,$$
$$\sigma^2_{\hat{R}^*} = \frac{1}{\beta}\int_{z_1}^{z_2} dz \int_{R_\ell}^{R_u} r^2 a(z)r^{b(z)} \ln^d r dr - \hat{R}^{*2},$$

where

$$\beta = \int_{z_1}^{z_2} dz \int_{R_\ell}^{R_u} a(z) r^b(z) \ln^d r dr.$$

Using the integral (3.32), we can reduce these expressions to one dimensional integrals which can be numerically integrated. Introduce the function

$$I_\ell(z, R_\ell, R_u, m, d) = \int_{R_\ell}^{R_u} x^{b(z)+m} \ln^d x dx$$
$$= I_E(R_u, b(z)+m, d) - I_E(R_\ell, b(z)+m, d), \tag{3.57}$$

and the desired estimates can be expressed by

$$\begin{aligned} \hat{R}^* &= \frac{1}{\beta}\int_{z_1}^{z_2} a(z) I_\ell(z, R_\ell, R_u, 1, d) dz, \\ \sigma^2_{\hat{R}^*} &= \frac{1}{\beta}\int_{z_1}^{z_2} a(z) I_\ell(z, R_u, R_\ell, 2, d) dz - \hat{R}^{*2}, \end{aligned} \tag{3.58}$$

where

$$\beta = \int_{z_1}^{z_2} a(z) I_\ell(z, R_u, R_\ell, 0, d) dz.$$

For the determination of the lower Bayes confidence limit we have to solve the equation

$$\int_{z_1}^{z_2} a(z) I_\ell\left(z, \underline{R}^*_\gamma, R_u, 0, d\right) dz = \gamma\beta. \tag{3.59}$$

The calculations based on (3.57)–(3.59) require special numerical methods. We have solved this problem with the help of an algorithm written in FORTRAN-IV.

Example 3.1. The following relative operating times $\nu^* = (1,3)$, $\nu = (2,4;\ 3,1;\ 2,8;\ 1,6;\ 2,4;\ 3,4;\ 4,2;\ 1,8;\ 2,5;\ 3,0)$ were fixed during the statistical testing, that is, one test was ended by failure and ten by standstills. We know (taking into consideration a priori information) that a reliability index is not less than 0.9, and a degradation coefficient takes on a value from the interval $[1.0;\ 2.0]$. Calculation base on (3.57)–(3.59) gives the following values of the posterior estimates: $\hat{R}^* = 0.9576$, $\sigma_{\hat{R}^*} = 0.0242$, a lower confidence limit (as $\gamma = 0.9$) $\underline{R}^*_{0.9} = 0.9216$.

The more simple case (bearing in mind the numerical analysis) is one that corresponds to the fixed value of the parameter z, having the posterior density of the type (3.56).
The final formulas for the desired estimates are written with the help of the function (3.57) as:

$$\hat{R}^* = \frac{I_\ell(z,R_\ell,R_u,1,d)}{I_\ell(z,R_\ell,R_u 0,d)}, \quad \sigma^2_{\hat{R}^*} = \frac{I_\ell(z,R_\ell,R_u,2,d)}{I_\ell(z,R_\ell,R_u 0,d)} - \hat{R}^{*2}. \tag{3.60}$$

The value of $\underline{R}^*_\gamma$ is found from the equation

$$I_\ell\left(z,\underline{R}^*_\gamma,R_u,0,d\right) - \gamma I_\ell(z,R_\ell,R_u,0,d) = 0. \tag{3.61}$$

Example 3.2. The initial data for this example differ from those in the previous case only by the condition that gives the exact value of the degradation coefficient $z = 2$. The calculations by formulas (3.60) and (3.61) yield: $\hat{R}^* = 0.9729$, $\sigma_{\hat{R}^*} = 0.0181$, $\underline{R}^*_{0.9} = 0.9476$.

We have performed a lot of computations using the formulae (3.60), (3.61) in order to learn peculiarities of the Bays estimates. In Figures 3.2–3.4 you can see, respectively, the behavior of $\hat{R}^*$, $\sigma_{\hat{R}^*}$ and $\underline{R}^*_\gamma$ as functions of the lower bound R_ℓ of the indeterminacy interval (as $R_u = 1$) and degradation coefficient z. The calculations were performed with the help of the special algorithm for three samples:
Sample 1: $\nu^* = (0.80; 0.85)$;

$$\nu = (1.10; 0.95; 0.90; 1.15; 0.75; 0.90; 0.85; 1.20; 1.15; 1.20);$$

Sample 2: $\nu^* = (1.10; 1.80)$;

$$\nu = (1.30; 1.20; 1.10; 0.30; 1.15; 1.40; 1.20; 1.70; 1.50; 2.00);$$

Sample 3: $\nu = (1.30)$;

$$\nu = (2.40; 3.10; 2.80; 1.60; 2.40; 3.40; 4.20; 1.80; 2.50; 3.00).$$

The order of the decreasing of a number of the samples corresponds to improvement of the experiment results.
In Figures 3.2–3.4, solid lines correspond to the estimate of TTF for the first sample, dotted lines are for the second one, dot-and-dash lines are for the third sample. Analysis of the graphs enables us to draw the following conclusions:

1) While the number of samples is increasing, estimates of the reliability index is improving;
2) For each sample there exists its own dead zone for the change of R_ℓ,moreover, this zone moves to the right as results of experiments improve;

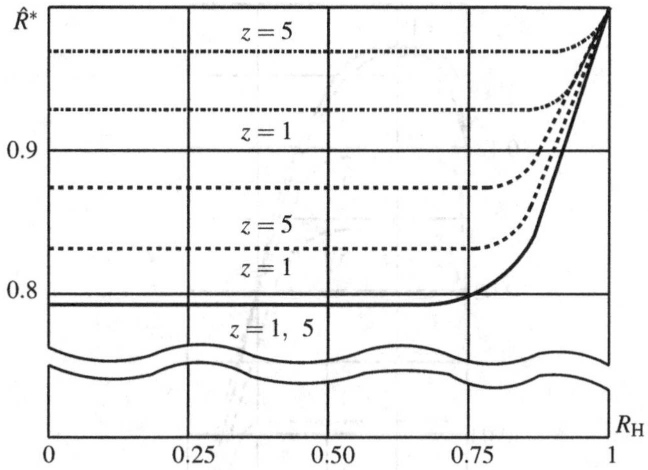

Fig. 3.2 The pointwise Bayes Estimate.

3) If one increases the degradation coefficient, the posterior estimates improve for the same samples.

The last conclusion is logically interpreted in the following way. Suppose two tested articles with the degradation coefficients z_1 and z_2 ($z_1 > z_2$) give the same results. Clearly, that the most reliable will be article whose degradation coefficient is larger.

3.5 Estimation of reliability for the Weibull distribution of a trouble-free time

Consider the case when the trouble-free time ξ is subjected to the Weibull distribution with the density

$$f(t;\lambda,\alpha) = \lambda\alpha t^{\alpha-1}\exp(-\lambda t^{\alpha}), \tag{3.62}$$

and c.d.f.

$$f(t;\lambda,\alpha) = 1 - \exp\left(-\lambda t^{\alpha}\right). \tag{3.63}$$

Then the estimating parameter of reliability during the period of time t_0 iscomputed by the formula

$$R = R(\lambda,\alpha) = \exp\left(-\lambda_0^{\alpha}\right). \tag{3.64}$$

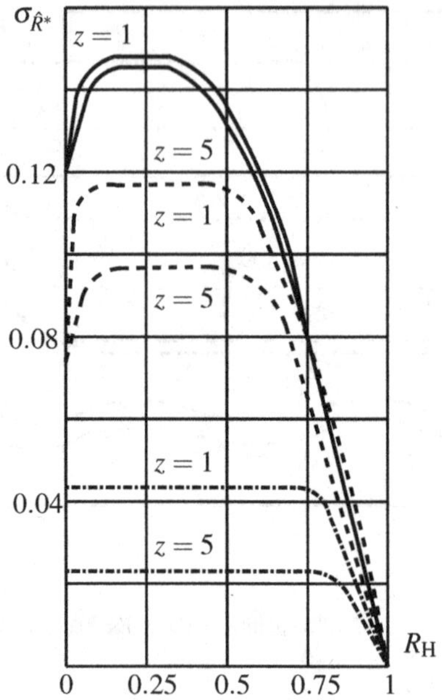

Fig. 3.3 The posterior mean squared value of the TTF.

The expression for the reliability function, when one realizes an NC-plan,may be obtained after we have substituted the relations (3.62) and (3.63) into (3.20):

$$\ell(\lambda,\alpha \mid \tau) = c(\tau)\lambda^d\alpha^d\left(\prod_{i=1}^{d} t_i^*\right)^{\alpha-1} \exp\left(-\lambda\varpi t_0^\alpha\right). \tag{3.65}$$

where

$$\omega = \omega(\alpha) = \sum_{i=1}^{d}(v_i^*)^\alpha + \sum_{j=1}^{k} v_j^\alpha, \quad v_i^* = \frac{t_i^*}{t_0}, \ v_j = \frac{t_j}{t_0}.$$

Reasoning analogously as in the previous paragraph, we may conclude that the given parameterization is not suitable in practice. Therefore, instead of λ, we will use the parameter r introduced earlier. Let us express the likelihood function in terms of r and α. To do this we use the dependence (3.65). It yields

$$\lambda = -\frac{1}{t_0^\alpha}\ln r. \tag{3.66}$$

Next we substitute (3.66) into (3.65) and obtain

$$\ell(r,\alpha \mid \tau) = c(\tau)\left(-\frac{1}{t_0}\right)^d \alpha^d\mu^{\alpha-1}r^\omega\ln^d r. \tag{3.67}$$

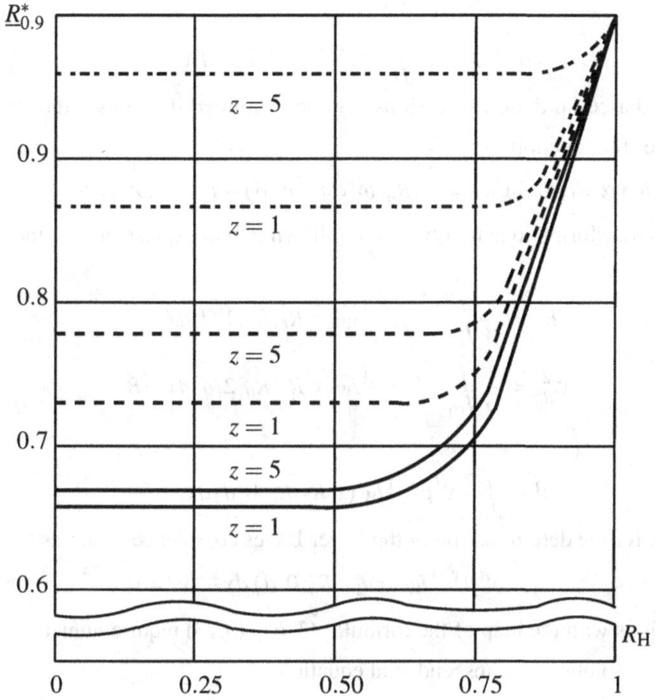

Fig. 3.4 The lower Bayes confidence limit of the TTF.

where

$$\mu = \prod_{i=1}^{d} v_i^*.$$

It should be noted that for $\alpha = 1$, the Weibull distribution model changes into an exponential one, and the likelihood function (3.67) coincides with (3.25).
Assuming that p.d.f. $h(r, \alpha)$ is a priori given and using the Bayes theorem, we obtain

$$\hbar(r, \alpha \mid \tau) \sim h(r, \alpha)\alpha^d \mu^{\alpha-1} r^{\omega} \ln^d r. \tag{3.68}$$

The dependence (3.68) appears to be initial for obtaining any estimates of reliability R. In particular, if the parameters r and α are distributed uniformly in the intervals $[R_\ell, R_u]$ and $[\alpha_1, \alpha_2]$, we obtain

$$\hbar\,(r, \alpha \mid \tau) \sim \alpha^d \mu^{\alpha-1} r^{\omega} \ln^d r, \quad r \in [R_\ell, R_u]\,, \alpha \in [\alpha_1, \alpha_2]\,,$$

whence

$$\hat{R}^* = \frac{1}{\beta} \int_{R_\ell}^{R_u} dr \int_{\alpha_1}^{\alpha_2} \alpha^d \mu^{\alpha-1} r^{\omega+1} \ln^d r d\alpha,$$

where

$$\beta = \int_{R_\ell}^{R_u} dr \int_{\alpha_1}^{\alpha_2} \alpha^d \mu^{\alpha-1} r^{\omega} \ln^d r d\alpha.$$

Calculations, based on these expressions, can be simplified if one uses the integral (3.32) and introduces the function

$$I_W(\alpha, R_\ell, R_u, m, d) = I_E(R_u, \omega(\alpha)+m, d) - I_E(R_\ell, \omega(\alpha)+m, d). \tag{3.69}$$

After tedious transformations we obtain the following final expressions for the estimates of R:

$$\hat{R}^* = \frac{1}{\beta} \int_{\alpha_1}^{\alpha_2} x^d \mu^{x-1} I_W(x, R_\ell, R_u, 1, d) dx, \tag{3.70}$$

$$\sigma^2_{\hat{R}^*} = \frac{1}{\beta} \int_{\alpha_1}^{\alpha_2} x^d \mu^{x-1} I_W(x, R_\ell, R_u, 2, d) dx - \hat{R}^{*2}, \tag{3.71}$$

where

$$\beta = \int_{\alpha_1}^{\alpha_2} x^d \mu^{x-1} I_W(x, R_\ell, R_u, 0, d)\, dx. \tag{3.72}$$

The equation for the determination of the lower Bayes confidence limit has the form

$$\int_{\alpha_1}^{\alpha_2} x^d \mu^{x-1} I_W\left(x, \underline{R}^*_\gamma, R_u, 0, d\right) dx - \beta\gamma = 0. \tag{3.73}$$

The calculations with the help of the formulas (3.70)–(3.73) require numerical methods of integration and solution of transcendental equations.

Example 3.3. The results of testing are represented by the following relative operating time: $v^* = (2.7)$, $v = (1.9; 3.5; 2.4; 3.1; 2.8; 1.6; 2.4; 3.4; 4.2; 1.8; 2.5; 3.0)$. It is known a priori, that the TTF is distributed uniformly in the interval $[0.9; 1]$, and parameter α is in the interval $[1; 1.8]$. Calculations by formula (3.70)–(3.73) with $\gamma = 0.9$ enable us to obtain $\hat{R}^* = 0.9666$, $\sigma_{\hat{R}^*} = 0.0202$, $\underline{R}^*_{0.9} = 0.9291$.

In the case when the value of the parameter α is given exactly (not in the Bayes sense), the formulas for the TTF estimates are simplified substantially. For example, for the posterior p.d.f. of the parameter r, the followingrelation holds:

$$\hbar(r \mid \tau) \sim h(r) r^{\omega} \ln^d r.$$

One can easily obtain the expressions for the TTF Bayes estimates from the relations (3.70)–(3.73) if one multiplies their integrands by the delta-function, taking on the values in all points but the given value α. Using the filter property of the delta-function, we obtain

$$\hat{R}^* = \frac{I_W(\alpha, R_\ell, R_u, 1, d)}{I_W(\alpha, R_\ell, R_u, 0, d)}, \tag{3.74}$$

$$\sigma^2_{\hat{R}^*} = \frac{I_W(\alpha, R_\ell, R_u, 2, d)}{I_W(\alpha, R_\ell, R_u, 0, d)} - \hat{R}^*. \tag{3.75}$$

The equation for $\underline{R}^*_\gamma$ has the following form:

$$I_W\left(\alpha,\underline{R}^*_\gamma,R_u 0,d\right)-\gamma I_W(\alpha,R_\ell,R_u 0,d)=0. \tag{3.76}$$

Example 3.4. The article has been tested 13 times under the same conditions; relative operating times, fixed in the testing, coincide with those in Example 3.3. A priori TTF R is distributed uniformly in the interval $[0.9;1]$. The value of the parameter α is given exactly: $\alpha=1.8$. The calculations by formulas (3.74)–(3.76) give $\hat{R}^*=0.9766$, $\sigma_{\hat{R}^*}=0.0163$, $\underline{R}^*_{0.9}=0.9546$.

We have carried out numerous calculations by formulas (3.70)–(3.76), in particular, for the samples 1, 2, and 3, mentioned in the previous paragraph. They have shown that we meet the same conformities for the TTF estimates as in the case of the linearly increasing intensity function.

In conclusion, we consider the model of the Weibull distribution in connection with the frequently encountered binomial scheme of testing. This scheme may be reduced to the NC-plan, if one assumes that all empirical data coincide with the required time of functioning t_0 : $t_i^*=t_0$ $(i=1,\ldots,d)$, $t_j=t_0$ $(j=1,\ldots,k)$. For the posterior p.d.f., the following relation holds:

$$\hbar(r,\alpha\mid\tau)\sim h(r,\alpha)\alpha^d r^n\ln^d r.$$

Following the usual scheme of the Bayes procedure for the case of a priori independent parameters α and r we obtain

$$\hat{R}^*=\frac{\int_{\alpha_1}^{\alpha_2}\alpha^d h(\alpha)d\alpha\int_{R_\ell}^{R_u}rh(r)r^n\ln^d r\,dr}{\int_{\alpha_1}^{\alpha_2}\alpha^d h(\alpha)d\alpha\int_{R_\ell}^{R_u}h(r)r^n\ln^d r\,dr}=\frac{\int_{R_\ell}^{R_u}r^{n+1}h(r)\ln^d r\,dr}{\int_{R_\ell}^{R_u}r^n h(r)\ln^d r\,dr}, \tag{3.77}$$

i.e., the Bayes posterior TTF estimate is independent of the interval of values of the parameter α. The final expressions for the Bayes estimates with a uniform $h(r)$ in the interval $[R_\ell,R_u]$ coincide with the expressions (3.74)–(3.76), if one substitutes into them $\omega=n$. The same conclusion may be drawn for the model with a linearly increasing intensity function, considered in the previous paragraph. Namely,for $v_i^*=v_j=1$ and a priori independent parameters z and r, from (3.54) and (3.55) it follows

$$\hbar(r,z\mid\tau)\sim h(z)\left(\frac{z}{z+1}\right)^d h(r)r^n\ln^d r,$$

i.e., a prior density may be represented as a product of two functions each of which depends on z and r respectively. Consequently, for the Bayes pointwise TTF estimate the relation (3.77) holds.

The generalization of the considered peculiarities enables us to draw the following conclusion: the Bayes estimates for the binomial testing scheme are non-parametrical for the class of all models with linear and power intensity functions (of the form t^{α}), if the model parameters are a priori independent.

3.6 The Bayes estimate of time to failure probability from accelerated life tests

At present for the experimental testing of many technical devices authors use methods of accelerated life tests. The detailed analysis and modern approach to the theory of accelerated life tests is given in [122]. The essence of these methods may be interpreted as follows: we reduce the testing time due to the increasing severity of operating conditions. In practice we often meet a situation when it's impossible to find the relationships between the operating conditions and reliability characteristics, since the operating conditions may have a random nature.

In such a situation it will be useful to apply the Bayes approach which gives us the possibility to make decisions under uncertain conditions which are considered the best with respect to minimizing a certain specific loss function (see the work [199]). Unfortunately, representation of a priori information is chosen in an arbitrary form in an awkward form.

We represent the procedure of probability for TTF estimating, proposed in [221]. The tests are carried out by the scheme of step-loading [122]. It is assumed that testing conditions have a random nature and a priori information has a comparatively simple representation.

Suppose that during the process of accelerated life tests we have to find the TTF estimate for some time interval $t : R = R(t) = P\{\xi > t\}$. The article is functioning under some nominal conditions co. Since the test will be carried out under some severe operating conditions, we rewrite the expression for the $R(t)$ in the form

$$R = R(t, \varepsilon_0) = P\{\xi(\varepsilon_0) > t\}, \tag{3.78}$$

where $\xi(\varepsilon_0)$ is a random period of trouble-free time under the nominal mode. Here, and further on, the notion of a mode is interpreted as the set of parameters characterizing conditions and type in which the device is functional. The formulation and solution of this problem can be solved subject to certain assumptions given below:

1) During the testing the scheme of step-loading is realized. This means that we are given some longest testing time T and the segment $[0, T]$ is divided into $m+1$ nonintersected segments $\mu_j = [s_j, s_j + 1)$, $j = 0, 1, \ldots, m$. This partition is performed on the stage of preliminary investigating tests. Each testing article is functions in the nominal mode ε_0

independently from the others. After this, if the failure doesn't occur, a switching occurs onto some more severe mode ε_1 and so on. Each interval $\mu_j$is associated with its own mode ε_j. It is very important that the choice of indicated modes lacks uniqueness.

We may only each successive mode is more severe than the previous one. For the description of this fact we introduce the notation $\varepsilon_j \succ \varepsilon_{j-1}$. It is assumed that the tests may finish as failures or as standstills, which in turn may be random or determined after the time T. Bearing in mind the technical characteristics of the tests, we can reduce them to the NC-plan, resulting in the sample $\tau = \{t^*, t\}$, where

$$t^* = (t_1^*, t_2^*, \ldots, t_d^*), \quad t^* = (t_1, t_2, \ldots, t_k), \quad d + k = n.$$

2) The failure rate function $\lambda(t)$is assumed to be piecewise constant so that $\lambda(t) = \lambda_j =$ const. for $t \in \mu_j$ $(j = 1, 2, \ldots, m)$. In other words, the failure rate function depends on the testing mode: $\lambda(t)\lambda(\varepsilon(t))$.

Suppose that more severe testing conditions uniquely imply the increasing of failure rate, i.e., the condition $\varepsilon_j \succ \varepsilon_{j-1}$implies $\lambda(\varepsilon_j) \geqslant \lambda(\varepsilon_{j-1})$ or $\lambda_j \geqslant \lambda_{j-1}$ $(j = 1, 2, \ldots, m)$.

3) The prior distribution $h(r_0)$ for TTF at some instant to is known before the testing. Further on we will mainly use, as basic, a uniform prior distribution of the parameter $R_0 = R_0(t_0, \varepsilon_0)$ in the interval $[R_\ell, R_u]$.

The assumptions we have formulated above let us solve the problem of estimation of the index $R = R(t, \varepsilon_0)$ in a classical Bayes setting. We introduce the parameterization in terms of the vector $\lambda = (\lambda_0, \lambda_1, \ldots, \lambda_m)$, whose number of components is the same as the number of modes. We apply the standard Bayes procedure for the problem solution step by step: a prior distribution density $h(\lambda)$ of the given vector, obtaining of the likelihood function $\ell(\lambda \mid \tau)$ and posterior distribution $\hbar(\lambda \mid \tau)$, obtaining of the estimates $\hat{R}^*$, $\sigma_{\hat{R}^*}$, $\underline{R}_\gamma^*$, with the help of it.

We seek the density of a prior distribution $h(A)$ in the form

$$h(\lambda) = h_0(\lambda_0)h_1(\lambda_1 \mid \lambda_0)\cdots h_m(\lambda_m \mid \lambda_0, \ldots, \lambda_{m-1}), \tag{3.79}$$

where $h_j(\lambda_j \mid \lambda_0, \ldots, \lambda_{j-1})$ is the conditional prior probability of the parameter λ_j under the condition $|\lambda_0, \lambda_1, \ldots, \lambda_{j-1}$. We define the marginal prior p.d.f. by use of a uniform prior distribution of the index $R_0 \in [R_\ell, R_u]$ and dependence $R_0 = \exp(-\lambda_0 t_0)$;

$$h_0(\lambda_0) = \frac{t_0}{R_u - R_\ell} \mathrm{e}^{-\lambda_0 t_0}, \quad \lambda_0' \leqslant \lambda_0 \leqslant \lambda_0'', \tag{3.80}$$

where $\lambda_0' = -\ln R_u / t_0$, $\lambda_0'' = -\ln R_\ell / t_0$.

The conditional prior p.d.f. $h(\lambda_j \mid \lambda_0, \ldots, \lambda_{j-1})$ is defined so that each multiplier of a prior p.d.f. (3.79) belongs to the same family of densities, namely, to the truncated potential family. This assumption is similar to another one having a more distinct physical nature: a TTF at the moment t_0 for the mode ε_j doesn't exceed a TTF at the same moment for the mode ε_{j-1}, i.e., $R(t_0,\varepsilon_j) \in [0, R(t_0,\varepsilon_{j-1})]$ for all $j = 1,2,\ldots,m$. Besides, the index $R(t_0,\varepsilon_j)$ is distributed uniformly in the mentioned interval. Using this assumption it is easy to obtain

$$h_j(\lambda_j \mid \lambda_0,\ldots,\lambda_{j-1}) = t_0 \exp[-(\lambda_j - \lambda_{j-1})t_0],$$

$$\lambda_j \geqslant \lambda_{j-1}, \quad j = 1,2,\ldots,m. \tag{3.81}$$

Substituting the expressions (3.80) and (3.81) into (3.79), after evident transformations we obtain

$$h(\lambda) = \frac{t_0^{m+1}}{R_u - R_\ell}\, e^{-\lambda_m t_0}, \quad \lambda \in D, \tag{3.82}$$

where domain D is defined by the chain of inequalities $\lambda_0' \leqslant \lambda_0 \leqslant \lambda_0''$, $\lambda_0 \leqslant \lambda_1,\ldots,\lambda_{m-1} \leqslant \lambda_m$. As follows from (3.82), a prior p.d.f. depends explicitly only on λ_m. However, $h(\lambda)$ is a function of all parameters because this dependence is expressed by the form of the domain D.

To find the likelihood function $\ell(\lambda \mid \tau)$, we use (3.21), rewritten in terms of intensity function $\lambda(t)$ and resource function $\Lambda(t)$. Using the function

$$p(t) = \begin{cases} 1, & t \in \mu_j = [s_{j-1}, s_j), \\ 0, & t \notin \mu_j, \end{cases}$$

for $\lambda(t)$ we find

$$\lambda(t) = \sum_{j=1}^{m} \lambda_j \rho_j(t) \tag{3.83}$$

After integration of the intensity function, we obtain

$$\Lambda(t) = \sum_{j=0}^{m} \rho_j(t) \left[\sum_{r=0}^{j-1} \lambda_r \Delta_r + \lambda_j (t - s_j) \right] \tag{3.84}$$

Substitution of (3.83) and (3.84) into (3.21) yields

$$\ell(\lambda \mid \tau) = c(\tau) \prod_{j=0}^{m} \rho_j(t_i^*)\lambda_j \times \exp\left\{ -\sum_{i=1}^{n}\sum_{j=0}^{m} \rho_j(\tau_i) \left[\sum_{r=0}^{j-1} \lambda_r \Delta_r + \lambda_j(\tau_i - s_j) \right] \right\}. \tag{3.85}$$

We proceed to rewrite the expression (3.85) in a more suitable form andderive the sufficient statistics.

Let m_j be the number of elements of the sample τ belonging to the interval μ_j. We denote these elements by $\tau_i^{(j)}$, $i = 1,2,\ldots,m_j$. Next we'll substitute $\tau_i^{(j)}$ successively into (3.84) and perform the summation over all indices i for all m segments. It yields

$$\sum_{i=1}^{n}\sum_{j=0}^{m} \rho_j(\tau_i) \left[\sum_{r=0}^{j-1} \lambda_r \Delta_r + \lambda_j(\tau_i - s_j) \right] = \sum_{j=0}^{m} \lambda_j k_j, \tag{3.86}$$

where

$$k_j = n_j\Delta_j + \sum_{i=1}^{m_j}\left(\tau_i^{(j)} - s_j\right),$$

$$n_j = m_{j+1} + m_{j+2} + \cdots + m_m,$$

$$j = 1,2,\ldots,m-1, \quad n_m = 0, \quad \Delta_j = s_{j+1} - s_j.$$

The quantity n_j determines the number of sample articles which don't fail after the testing in the mode j. The statistic k_j has the sense of a full lifetime during the testing in the mode j.

Analogously, if one denotes by d_j the number of failures observed during the testing in the mode j, then

$$\prod_{j=1}^{d}\left[\sum_{j=0}^{m}\rho_j(t_i^*)\lambda_j\right] = \prod_{j=0}^{m}\lambda_j^{d_j}.$$

With the help of (3.86) and (3.87) we can rewrite the likelihood function (3.85) in the following form:

$$\ell(\lambda \mid \tau) = c(\tau)\prod_{j=0}^{n}\lambda_j^{d_j}\exp\left(-\sum_{j=0}^{m}\lambda_j k_j\right). \tag{3.87}$$

As can be seen from (3.88), the sufficient statistic for this case is formed by the quantities $d_1, d_2, \ldots, d_m, k_1, k_2, \ldots, k_m$.

In accordance with the Bayes theorem for the posterior p.d.f. of the vector λ, we have

$$\hbar(\lambda \mid \tau) \sim \prod_{j=0}^{m}\lambda_j^{d_j}\exp\left[-\sum_{j=0}^{m-1}\lambda_j k_j + \lambda_m(k_m + t_0)\right], \quad \lambda \in D. \tag{3.88}$$

Since the desired index $R = R(t,\varepsilon_0)$ depends only on λ_0, for the obtaining of Bayes estimates of the index R we need to know the marginal posterior p.d.f. $\hbar(\lambda_0 \mid \tau)$. To this end, we'll integrate the relation (3.89) over the parameters $\lambda_1, \lambda_2, \ldots, \lambda_m$, where the integration domain is determined by the domain D,

$$\hbar_0(\lambda_0 \mid \tau) \sim \int_{\lambda_0}^{\infty}\int_{\lambda_1}^{\infty}\cdots\int_{\lambda_{m-1}}^{\infty}\hbar(\lambda \mid \tau)\,d\lambda_1\,d\lambda_2\cdots d\lambda_m.$$

Having performed the integration and some ambiguous transformations, we can obtain the following (the most simple) expression for $\hbar_0(\lambda_0 \mid \tau)$:

$$\hbar(\lambda_0 \mid \tau) \sim \lambda_0^{d_0} = S_m(\lambda_0)\exp\left[-\lambda_0(X_0 + t_0)\right], \tag{3.89}$$

where

$$S_m(\lambda_0) = \sum_{i_m=0}^{D_m-N_m}\cdots\sum_{i_1=0}^{D_1-N_1}\lambda_0^{D_1-N_0}\prod_{j=1}^{m}\frac{(D_j-N_j)^{(i_j)}}{(X_j+t_0)^{i_j+1}},$$

and

$$X_j = \sum_{i=0}^{m} k_i \sum_{i=0}^{j-1} k_i, \quad S_j = d - \sum_{i=0}^{j-1} d_i, \quad N_j = n - \sum_{i=0}^{j-1} i_\ell,$$

where the symbol $k^{(\ell)}$denotes the operation $k!/(k-1)!$. We find the estimates $\hat{R}^*$ and $\sigma_{\hat{R}^*}$ from the condition $R = \exp(-\lambda(\varepsilon_0)t) = \exp(-\lambda_0 t)$ using the quadratic loss function. We are starting from the expressions

$$\hat{R}^* = \int_{\lambda_0'}^{\lambda_0''} e^{-\lambda_0 t} \hbar_0(\lambda_0 \mid \tau) d\lambda_0,$$

$$\sigma_{\hat{R}^*}^2 = \int_{\lambda_0'}^{\lambda_0''} e^{-\lambda_0 t} \hbar_0(\lambda_0 \mid \tau) d\lambda_0 - \hat{R}^{*2},$$

where $\lambda_0' = -\ln R_u/t_0$, $\lambda_0'' = -\ln R_\ell/t_0$.

The final expressions for $\hat{R}^*$ and $\sigma_{\hat{R}^*}$ may be written with the help of the function of the reduced argument $v = t/t_0$ as

$$H_{\mathrm{ml}}(v) = \sum_{i_m=0}^{D_m-N_m} (m+1) \to \cdots \sum_{i_0=0}^{D_0-N_0} \frac{(D_0-N_0)^{(i_0)}}{(\omega_0+\ell v+1)^{i_0+1}} \prod_{s=1}^{m} \frac{(D_s-N_s)^{(i_s)}}{(\omega_s+1)^{i_s+1}}$$
$$\times \left(R_u^{\omega_0+\ell v+1} |\ln R_u|^{d-i} - R_\ell^{\omega_0+\ell v+1} |\ln R_\ell|^{d-i} \right), \quad \ell = 0, 1, 2, \tag{3.90}$$

where $\omega_s = X_s/t_0$, $i = i_0 + i_1 + \cdots + i_m$.

Now

$$\hat{R}^* = \frac{H_{m1}(v)}{H_{m_o}(v)}, \quad \sigma_{\hat{R}^*}^2 = \frac{H_{m12(v)}}{H_{m0(v)}} - \hat{R}^{*2}. \tag{3.91}$$

We need to solve the following equation with respect to x in order to find the lower Bayes γ confidence limit

$$\int_{\lambda_0'}^{x} \hbar_0(\lambda_0 \mid \tau) d\lambda_0 = \gamma,$$

after then $\underline{R}_\gamma^* = \exp(-xt)$. The equation for $\underline{R}_\gamma^*$ takes on the form

$$\sum_{i_m=0}^{D_m-N_m} (m+1) \to \cdots \sum_{i_0=0}^{D_0-N_0} \prod_{s=0}^{m} \frac{(D_s-N_s)^{(i_s)}}{(\omega_s+1)^{i_s+1}}$$
$$\times \left(R_u^{\omega_0+1} |\ln R_u|^{d-i} - R_\gamma^{\frac{\omega_0+1}{v}} \left| \ln \underline{R}_\gamma^{*\frac{1}{v}} \right|^{d-i} \right) - \gamma H_{m0}(v) = 0 \tag{3.92}$$

As follows from the relations (3.91)–(3.93), the set of failures $d_0, d_1, \ldots, d_m$, observed in the time intervals with unchangeable mode and dimensionless parameters $\omega_0, \omega_1, \ldots, \omega_m$, generates the sufficient Bayes statistic. The parameter ω_j has a nature of respective (with respect to t_0) operating time intesting which was fixed in the intervals $\mu_j, \mu_j+1, \ldots, \mu_m$.

Consider the reduction of the formulas (3.91)–(3.93) to the "destruction" method [122] which is a particular case of the step-loading method. It is characterized by two modes: nominal and severe. In the expressions (3.91)–(3.93) we have to put $m = 1$. The algorithm takes on a simpler form, in particular, the function $H_{1\ell}(v)$ is written as

$$H_{1\ell}(v) = \sum_{i=0}^{d_1}\sum_{j=0}^{d-i} \frac{(d-i)^{(j)}}{(\omega_0+\ell v+1)^{j+1}} \cdot \frac{d_1^{(i)}}{(\omega_1+1)^{i+1}} \times \left(R_u^{\omega+\ell v+1}\left|\ln R_u\right|^{d-i-j} - R_\ell^{\omega_0+\ell v+1}\left|\ln R_\ell\right|^{d-i-j}\right). \tag{3.93}$$

The equation for $\underline{R}_\gamma^*$ for $m = 1$ is also substantially simplified:

$$\sum_{i=0}^{d_1}\sum_{j=0}^{d-i} \frac{(d-i)^{(j)}}{(\omega_0+\ell)^{j+1}} \cdot \frac{d_1^{(i)}}{(\omega_1+1)^{i+1}} \times \left(R_u^{\omega_0+1}\left|\ln R_u\right|^{d-i-j} - \underline{R}_\gamma^{*\frac{\omega_0+1}{v}}\left|\ln \underline{R}_\gamma^{*\frac{1}{v}}\right|^{d-i-j}\right) - \gamma H_{10}(v) = 0. \tag{3.94}$$

Example 3.5. Consider the case of having 10 devices which are being tested. It is a priori known that the TTF of each device during the period of 100 hours is not less than 0.8. We have to estimate a TTF of the article being in a nominal functioning period of 140 hours. The tests are carried out by the "destruction" scheme. The mode switches after 100 hours of functioning. The limit testing time is 160 hours. The following operating times have been observed (in hours): 135, 142, 148, 135, 140, 150, 139, 144, 148, and 136, where each testing has ended by failure. The special computation algorithm based on formulas (3.92), (3.93), and (3.94) has been used. The estimates we have obtained are the following: $\hat{R}^* = 0.9055$, $\sigma_{\hat{R}^*} = 0.07054$, $\underline{R}_{0.9}^* = 0.8379$.

Chapter 4

Nonparametric Bayes Estimation

4.1 Nonparametric Bayes estimates, based on Dirichlet processes

For a long time there were a lot of unsuccessful efforts directed toward the solution of many nonparametric problems with the help of the Bayes approach. This can be explained mainly by difficulties a researcher encounter, when he attempts to find a suitable prior distribution, determined on a sample space. Such a distribution in nonparametric problems is chosen in the form of a set of probability distributions on the given sample space. The first work in this field where some progress has been achieved belongs to Ferguson [80]. Ferguson formulated the requirements which must be imposed on a prior distribution:

1) The support of a prior distribution must be large with respect to some suitable topology of a space of probability distributions, defined on the sample space;
2) The posterior distribution under the given sample of observations from the real distribution of probabilities must have as simple a form as possible.

These properties are contradictory, bearing in mind the fact that each of them can be found from each other. In the work [80] a class of prior distributions was proposed, named *Dirichlet processes*, which not only possess the first property but also satisfy the second one. Exactly such a choice was offered, because a prior distribution of a random probability measure appears to be also a Dirichlet process. Another argument in favor of using the Dirichlet distribution in practical applications is explained by the fact that this distribution is a good approximation of many parametric probability distributions. Special attention is paid to this question in the works by Dalal [51] and Hall [52]. This distribution appears also in problems dealing with order statistics [266]. In the Bayes parametric theory it is used as a conjugate with the sampling likelihood kernel for the parameters of a multinomial distribution [63]. Below we give the definition of the Dirichlet distribution and formulate (from a practical point-of-view) some of its important properties.

4.1.1 *Definition of the Dirichlet process*

Denote by $\Gamma(\alpha,\beta)$ a gamma probability distribution with the shape parameter $\alpha \geqslant 0$ and scalar parameter $\beta > 0$. For $\alpha > 0$ this distribution has the probability density

$$F(z;\alpha,\beta) = \frac{1}{\Gamma(\alpha)\beta^{\alpha}} e^{-z/\beta} z^{\alpha-1} I_{(0,\infty)}(z), \tag{4.1}$$

where $I_S(z)$ is the indicator function of the set S identically equal to unity for all $z \in S$ and equal to zero otherwise.

Let $z_1, z_2, \ldots, z_K$ be independent random variables, $z_j \sim \Gamma(\alpha_j, 1)$ where $\alpha_j \geqslant 0$ for all j and $\alpha_j > 0$ for some j. The Dirichlet distribution with the parameters $\alpha_1, \alpha_2, \ldots, \alpha_K$, denoted further on by $D(\alpha_1, \alpha_2, \ldots, \alpha_K)$, is determined as the distribution of the variables $Y_1, Y_2, \ldots, Y_K$, defined in the following way:

$$Y_j = z_j \Big/ \sum_{i=1}^{k} z_i, \quad j = 1, 2, \ldots, k.$$

Note that if some $\alpha_j = 0$, then the corresponding Y_j also degenerates to zero. Provided that $\alpha_j > 0$ for all j, $(k-1)$-dimensional distribution of the variables $Y_1, \ldots, Y_{k-1}$ is absolutely continuous with probability density

$$f(y_1,\ldots,y_K;\alpha_1,\ldots,\alpha_K) = \frac{\Gamma(\alpha_1+\cdots+\alpha_K)}{\Gamma(\alpha_1)\cdots\Gamma(\alpha_K)} \prod_{j=1}^{k-1} y_j^{\alpha_j-1} \left(1 - \sum_{j=1}^{k-1} y_j\right)^{\alpha_K-1} I_S(y_1,\ldots,y_{k-1}), \tag{4.2}$$

where S is the following set:

$$\left\{ (y_1,\ldots,y_{k-1}) : \ y_j \geqslant 0, \ \sum_{j=1}^{k-1} y_j \leqslant 1 \right\}.$$

For $k = 2$, the expression (4.2) is transformed into the beta probability distribution which will be denoted by $Be(\alpha_1, \alpha_2)$.

The use of the Dirichlet distribution is based on the following properties:

Property 4.1. *If* $(Y_1,\ldots,Y_K) \sim D$ *and* $r_1, r_2, \ldots, r_\ell$ *are some integer numbers, satisfying the inequality* $0 < r_1 < r_2 < \cdots < r_\ell = k$, *then*

$$\left(\sum_{i=1}^{r_1} Y_i, \sum_{i=r+1}^{r_2} Y_i, \ldots, \sum_{i=r_{\ell-1}+1}^{r_\ell} Y_i \right) \sim D\left(\sum_{i=1}^{r_1} \alpha_i, \sum_{i=r_1+1}^{r_2} \alpha_i, \ldots, \sum_{i=r_{\ell-1}+1}^{r_\ell} \alpha_i \right).$$

Property 4.2. *If a prior probability distribution of the variables* $Y_1,\ldots,Y_K$ *is* $D(\alpha_1,\ldots,\alpha_K)$ *and if* $P\{X = j \mid Y_1,\ldots,Y_K\} = Y_j$ *is almost surely for* $j = 1, 2, \ldots, k$, *then the posterior probability distribution of the variables* $Y_1,\ldots,Y_K$ *for* $X = j$ *is the Dirichlet distribution* $D\left(\alpha_1^{(j)},\ldots,\alpha_K^{(j)}\right)$, *where* $\alpha_i^{(j)} = \alpha_i$ *as* $i \neq j$ *and* $\alpha_i^{(j+1)} = \alpha_i + 1$ *as* $i = j$.

Further, we need the following moments of the Dirichlet distribution:

$$E[Y_i] = \frac{\alpha_i}{\alpha},$$
$$E\left[Y_i^2\right] = \frac{\alpha_i(\alpha_i+1)}{\alpha(\alpha+1)},$$

and

$$E[Y_i] = \frac{\alpha_i \alpha_j}{\alpha(\alpha+1)}, \quad i \neq j,$$

where $\alpha = \sum_{i=1}^{k} \alpha_i$.

Now we shall give the definition of the Dirichlet process. Let Ω be a sample space and $\mathscr{L}$ be a σ-algebra of this space. The probability measure P, defined on $(\Omega, \mathscr{L})$, we consider to be random in the Bayes sense and later will be called a *stochastic process*. Note that, in contrast to the parametric Bayes estimation, it is not assumed that the measure P belongs to some parametric family. The nonparametric Bayes approach, in essence, may be construed as follows: for any finite partition from the space Ω, we should determine some capasive prior distribution on the parametric space which is determined by this partition.

In this sense, a measurable partition of the space Ω is a sequence of sets $(B_1, B_2, \ldots, B_K)$ such that $B_i \in \mathscr{L}$ for all i, $B_i \cap B_j \neq \emptyset$ for all $i \neq j$ and, finally, $\bigcup_{i=1}^{k} B_i = \Omega$. The probabilities $P\{B_1\}, P\{B_2\}, \ldots, P\{B_K\}$ are random; the problem is to choose a prior distribution for these probabilities for any $k > 1$.

Definition 4.1. Let α be a nonnegative finitely-additive measure on $(\Omega, \mathscr{L})$. The random measure P on $(\Omega, \mathscr{L})$ is called a *Dirichlet process* on $(\Omega, \mathscr{L})$ with the parameter α if for each $k = 1, 2, \ldots$, and measurable partition $(B_1, \ldots, B_K)$ of the set Ω, the distribution of the random variables $P\{B_1\}, \ldots, P\{B_K\}$ is a Dirichlet distribution $D(\alpha(B_1), \ldots, \alpha(B_K))$.

In the work [80] with the help of the uniqueness property of the Dirichlet process the fulfilment of Kolmogorov consistency conditions were proven. It is easy to check that the properties of the random probability measure P are closely connected with those of the process parameter α. In particular,if $\alpha(A) = 0$, then $P\{A\} = 0$ with probability equal to one. Similarly, if $\alpha(A) > 0$ then $P\{A\} > 0$ with probability equal to unity. Besides,

$$E[P\{A\}] = \frac{\alpha(A)}{\alpha(\Omega)}. \tag{4.3}$$

To use the Dirichlet process, we have to find its posterior distribution, i.e. the conditional distribution of the Dirichlet process under the given sample. At first we introduce a notion of a sample from a random probability distribution.

Definition 4.2. Suppose P is a random probability measure on $(\Omega, \mathscr{L})$. A set $X_1, \ldots, X_n$ is called a sample of size n from P, if for any $m = 1, 2, \ldots$ and measurable sets $A_1, \ldots, A_m, C_1, \ldots, C_n$;

$$P\{X_1 \in C_1, \ldots, X_n \in C_n \mid P\{A_m\}, P\{C_1\}, \ldots, P\{C_n\}\} = \prod_{j=1}^{n} P\{C_j\} \tag{4.4}$$

almost surely. See Ferguson [80].

In other words, $X_1, \ldots, X_n$ is a sample of size n from the distribution P, if for the data $P\{C_1\}, \ldots, P\{C_n\}$ the events $\{X_1 \in C_1\}, \ldots, \{X_n \in C_n\}$ are independent from the other events of the process as well as mutually independent, so that $P\{X_j \in C_j \mid P\{C_1\}, \ldots, P\{C_n\}\} + P\{C_j\}$ for all $j = 1, 2, \ldots, n$. This definition determines a joint distribution of the variables $X_1, \ldots, X_n, P\{A_1\}, \ldots, P\{A_m\}$ as soon as we are given a distribution for the process, therefore

$$P\{X_1 \in C_1, \ldots, X_n \in C_n, P\{A_1\} \leqslant y_1, \ldots, P\{A_m\} \leqslant y_m\}$$

can be obtained by integration of the expression (4.4) with respect to the joint distribution $P\{A_1\}, \ldots, P\{A_m\}$, $P\{C_1\}, \ldots, P\{C_n\}$ over the set $[0, y_1] \times \cdots \times [0, y_m] \times \cdots \times [0, 1]$. Directly from the given definition and properties of the Dirichlet process two important statements follow:

1) If X is a sample of unit size from the Dirichlet process on $(\Omega, \mathscr{L})$ with the parameter α, then for $A \in \mathscr{L}$ we have

$$P\{X \in A\} = \alpha(A)/\alpha(\Omega).$$

2) Under the same assumptions, for any measurable partition $B_1, \ldots, B_K$ of the space Ω we have

$$P\{X \in A,\ P\{B_1\} \leqslant y_1, \ldots, P\{B_K\} \leqslant y_K\} = \sum_{j=1}^{k} \frac{\alpha(B_j \cap A)}{\alpha(\Omega)} D\left(y_1, \ldots, y_K; \alpha_1^{(j)}, \ldots, \alpha_K^{(j)}\right),$$

where $D\left(y_1, \ldots, y_K; \alpha_1^{(j)}, \ldots, \alpha_K^{(j)}\right)$ is a Dirichlet distribution function, $\alpha_i^{(j)} = \alpha(B_i)$ if $i \neq j$ and $\alpha_i^{(j)} = \alpha(B_j) + 1$ if $i = j$. Now we are ready to prove, using these statements, the theorem of a posterior distribution of the Dirichlet process which shows that the posterior distribution has the same form as the prior one, with the parameters depending on the sample. Note, if δ_X is a measure on $(\Omega, \mathscr{L})$, assigning a unit mass to the point X, i.e., $\delta_X(A) = 1$ for $X \in A$ and $\delta_X(A) = 0$ for $X \notin A$, then the following statement is valid.

Theorem 4.1. *Let P be a Dirichlet process on $(\Omega, \mathcal{L})$ with the parameter α and $X_1, \ldots, X_n$ is a sample of volume n from P. Then the conditional distribution of the process P under the given sample is a Dirichlet process with the parameter $\alpha + \sum_{i=1}^{n} \delta_{X_i}$.*

Theorem 4.1.1 is the main result of the work [80] which enables us to solve some practical problems. This theorem gives us a method of obtaining the Bayes decision rule firstly when there is no sample available ($n = 0$), n and secondly, by further reduction, replacing the parameter α by $\alpha + \sum_{i=1}^{n} \delta_{X_i}$, when we have a sample $X_1, \ldots, X_n$.

4.2 Some nonparametric estimators

We give below a number of examples illustrating the use of the Dirichlet process. As a sample space, we choose the real axis $\mathbf{R}^1$ or some part of it, for example, a positive semi axis $\mathbf{R}^+ = [0, \infty)$. $\mathcal{L}$ is used as σ-algebra of all Borel sets. For the solution of practical problems, one has to define at first the metric α which reflects a priori information about the model we have learned. Throughout what follows, a is a finite nonnegative σ-additive metric on $(\mathbf{R}^1, B)$ or on $(\mathbf{R}^+, B)$.

Example 4.1 (The estimate of a cumulative distribution function and TTF). Suppose at first that we have to estimate a c.d.f of a random variable $F(t) = P\{(-\infty, t)\}$ with a quadratic loss function. If P is a Dirichlet process, then $F(t) \sim Be(\alpha(-\infty, t])$, $(\alpha((t, \infty))$ for each t. The Bayes risk for the problem without a sample is minimized by a choice of such an estimate $\hat{F}^*(t)$ for each t that the quantity $E\left[\left(F(t) - \hat{F}(t)\right)^2\right]$ is minimal. This is accomplished if one chooses as $\hat{F}^*$ the quantity $E[F(t)]$. Thus, the Bayes decision rule for the problem without a sample is

$$\hat{F}^*(t) = F_0(t) = E\left[F(t)\right].$$

In accordance with (4.3),

$$F_0(t) = \frac{\alpha\left((-\infty, t]\right)}{\alpha(\mathbf{R}^1)}. \tag{4.5}$$

The expression (4.5) with the help of the earlier chosen metric a gives us a priori information about the form of the unknown distribution $F(t)$.

Starting with Theorem 4.1.1, analogous to the relation (4.5) for the sample of volume n, we have the following decision rule:

$$\begin{aligned} \hat{F}^*(t \mid x_1, \ldots, x_n) &= \frac{\alpha((-\infty, t]) + \sum_{i=1}^{n} \delta_{x_i}((-\infty t])}{\alpha(\mathbf{R}^1) + n} \\ &= p_n F_0(t) + (1 - p_n) F_n(t \mid x_1, \ldots, x_n), \end{aligned} \tag{4.6}$$

where

$$p_n = \frac{\alpha(\mathbf{R}^1)}{\alpha(\mathbf{R}^1)+n}$$

$$F_n(t \mid x_1,\ldots,x_n) = \frac{1}{n}\sum_{i=1}^{n} \delta_{x_i}((-\infty,t])$$

is the empirical distribution function.

Therefore, the Bayes decision rule (4.6) is a blend of a priori information about the form of $F(t)$ and the empirical distribution function with the corresponding weights p_n and $(1-p_n)$. If $\alpha(\mathbf{R}^1)$ is large, in comparison with n, then the observations are given a small weight. Provided that $\alpha(\mathbf{R}^1)$ is small in comparison with n, then a small weight is given to a prior conjecture about the form of $F(t)$). $\alpha(\mathbf{R}^1)$ can be interpreted as a correctness measure of a prior conjecture about the form of $F(t)$ expressed as a number of the units of measurement. It should be noted that whatever a true distribution function may be, the Bayes estimate (4.6) converges to it almost surely. Thisfollows from the fact that $p_n \to 0$ as $n \to \infty$.

Suppose now that we have to estimate the probability of a time-to-failure $R(t) = 1-F(t)$ at some time t dealing with the outcomes of independent tests with the fixed failure time. All arguments mentioned above remain valid, if one replaces $\mathbf{R}^1$ by $\mathbf{R}^+$since $t \in [0,\infty)$. As a result we obtain

$$\hat{R}^*(t) = p_n R_0(t) + (1+o_n)\left[1-\frac{m(t)}{n}\right], \tag{4.7}$$

where $R_0(t)$ is a priori information about TTF, $m(t)$ is the number of objects failed by time t.

As can be seen from formula (4.7), the value of the Bayes estimate is strongly subjected to $\alpha(\mathbf{R}^+)$. If, for example, one assumes that a mean time to first failure follows a priori the exponential distribution with the parameter λ and puts

$$\alpha((0,t]) = \mathrm{e}^{-\lambda t},$$

hence $\alpha(\mathbf{R}^+) = 1$, and, consequently

$$\hat{R}^*(t) = \frac{1}{n+1}\mathrm{e}^{-\lambda t} + \frac{n}{n+1}\left[1-\frac{m(t)}{n}\right].$$

It is interesting to note that in the case of failure in one trial, the a priori TTF estimate should be reduced twice; in case of two failures in two trials-three times, etc. Clearly, the significance of a prior estimate is very small in this case.

Example 4.2 (The Bayes estimate of quantiles). A quantile of a distribution $F(t) = P\{(-\infty,t]\}$ of the probability q, denoted by t_q, is introduced with the help of a probability measure P in the following manner:

$$P\{(-\infty,t_q)\} \leqslant q \leqslant P\{(-\infty,t_q]\}.$$

It is easy to verify that for $0 < q < 1$ a q-quantile is unique with the probability equal to unity. Thus, t_q is a well-defined random variable. Ferguson [80], considered the problem of estimating t_q with a loss function

$$L(t_q,\hat{t}_q) = \begin{cases} p\,(t_q-\hat{t}_q), & t_q \geqslant \hat{t}_q \\ (1-p)\,(\hat{t}_q-t_q), & t_q < \hat{t}_q \end{cases}, \tag{4.8}$$

for some p $(0 < p < 1)$. The variable p plays the role of a weight coefficient. In particular, for $p = \frac{1}{2}$ we have $L(t_q,\hat{t}_q) = \frac{1}{2}\left|t_q-\hat{t}_q\right|$. Due to this circumstance a loss function of the form (4.8) can be interpreted as a generalization of the broadly used loss function having a type of absolute error. The distribution of the random variable t_q can be found from the condition $F(t) \sim Be(\alpha((-\infty,t]),\, \alpha((t,\infty)))$. We have

$$P\{t_q \leqslant t\} = P\{F(t) > q\} = \int_q^1 \frac{\Gamma(A)}{\Gamma(ua)\Gamma((1-u)a)} z^{ua-1}(1-z)^{(1-u)a-1}dz, \tag{4.9}$$

where

$$a = \alpha(\mathbf{R}^1) \quad \text{and} \quad u = \frac{\alpha((-\infty,t])}{\alpha(\mathbf{R}^1)} = F_0(t).$$

According to Ferguson [80], any p-quantile of the distribution t_q is a Bayes estimate of t_q with a loss function of the form (4.8). In order to find a p-quantile of the distribution of the random variable t_q, the expression (4.9) must be equated to p and solved with respect to t:

$$\int_q^1 \frac{\Gamma(A)}{\Gamma(ua)\Gamma((1-u)a)} z^{ua-1}(1-z)^{(1-u)a-1}dz = p. \tag{4.10}$$

Consider the relation (4.10) as an equation with respect to u and denote by $u(p,q,\alpha(\mathbf{R}^1))$ the unique root of this equation. Then the Bayes estimate t_q^* in the problem without a sample is determined with the help of the equation

$$u\left(p,q,\alpha(\mathbf{R}^1)\right) = \frac{\alpha\left((-\infty,t_q^*]\right)}{\alpha(\mathbf{R}^1)} \tag{4.11}$$

or

$$u\left(p,q,\alpha(\mathbf{R}^1)\right) = F_0\left(t_q^*\right).$$

Thus, the Bayes estimate of the quantile t_q in absence of a sample is a quantile of the distribution $F_0(t)$ of the probability $u(p,q,\alpha(\mathbf{R}^1))$ obtained by itself from the equation (4.10).

For the sample $x_1,\dots,x_n$ the Bayes estimate t_q^* in accordance with (4.11) is determined from the equation

$$u\left(p,q,\alpha(\mathbf{R}^1)+n\right)=\frac{\alpha\left((-\infty,t_q^*]\right)+\sum_{i=1}^n\delta_{x_i}\left((-\infty,t_q^*]\right)}{\alpha(\mathbf{R}^1)+n},$$

i.e., in the given case t_q^* is a quantile of the probability $u(p,q,\alpha(\mathbf{R}^1)+n)$ of the distribution $\hat{F}_n^*(t\mid x_1,\dots,x_n)$ defined by the expression (4.6). For the practical use of the given scheme it is desirable to have tables for the function $u(p,q,\alpha)$ which may be obtained from the tables of the incomplete beta-function.

The developments mentioned above have very serious limitations: the quantity P, considered as a Dirichlet stochastic process, is discrete with probability one. This can be explained as follows: dealing with samples from the Dirichlet process one can expect the appearance of the observation which exactly equals each other. In the proposed examples the possibility of sample elements coinciding doesn't play an intrinsic role. At the same time there exists a problem in which this fact is of great importance. One such problem is described by Ferguson. The problem is to verify the hypothesis H_0, giving the fact that a distribution on $[0,1]$ is uniform. If one chooses as an alternate hypothesis the Dirichlet process with the parameter α, of having a uniform distribution on $[0,1]$, and given a sample of volume $n\geqslant 2$, then the unique nontrivial nonrandomized Bayes decision rule requires us to reject the hypothesis H_0 if and only if two or more observations are equal to each other. In validity it is not something like the verifying of the hypothesis that the distribution is continuous against the alternative hypothesis that it is discrete.

4.2.1 *Further development of the Ferguson theory*

The work by Ferguson cited above has initiated numerous investigations having both a theoretical and applied influence in the field of nonparametric Bayes estimates which uses prior Dirichlet processes. The most interesting theoretical work touching upon this field belongs to Yamato [269]. He considers the relationship between the nonparametric Bayes estimates, based on the Dirichlet process, with U-statistics [266]. Zaks [272] introduced the concept of the estimable parameter. A parameter $\theta(P)$ is called estimable if it has an unbiased estimate, i.e, if there exists such a statistic $\alpha(x_1,\dots,x_n)$ such that

$$\theta(P)=\int_{\Omega^n}a(x_1,\dots,x_n)\prod_{i=1}^n dP(x_i),$$

where $\Omega^n=\Omega\times\cdots\times\Omega$. Degree of the estimable functional $\theta(P)$ is called the minimum size of a sample for which there exists an unbiased estimate of this functional. It is clear that the mean, considered as parameter, has first degree, and the variance second degree. Ferguson [80] deals as a rule, with first degree and, sometimes, with second degree parameters. Yamato [269] obtained nonparametric Bayes estimates of the parameters having the second and third degree. Investigation of the dependence between the Bayes estimates and U-statistics is not fortuitous. The point is that U-statistics in the class of unbiased estimates of the parameter $\theta(P)$ with the given volume of a sample possesses the minimal variance. Denote by θ_k the k-degree parameter which admits an estimate in the sense of [272]. The main result of the work [269] lies in the following. Suppose that $x_1,\ldots,x_n$ is a sample from the distribution $F \sim D(\alpha)$, where α is a finite nonnegative measure on $(\Omega,\mathscr{L})$. Then the Bayes estimate of the parameter

$$\theta_3 = \iiint a_3(x,y,z)dF(x)dF(y)dF(z),$$

where $a(\cdot)$ is a measurable real function, symmetric with respect to the arguments x, y, z and possessing an absolute moment of the first order, is defined by the expression

$$\hat{\theta}_3^* = \frac{[\alpha(\Omega)+n]^2}{[\alpha(\Omega)+n+1][\alpha(\Omega)+n+2]} \iiint a_3(x,y,z)dF_n^*(x)dF_n^*(y)dF_n^*(z)$$

$$+\frac{3[\alpha(\Omega)+n]}{[\alpha(\Omega)+n+1][\alpha(\Omega)+n+2]} \iint a_3(x,x,y)dF_n^*(x)dF_n^*(y)$$

$$+\frac{2}{[\alpha(\Omega)+n+1][\alpha(\Omega)+n+2]} \int a_3(x,x,x)dF_n^*(x) \tag{4.12}$$

where

$$F_n^*(\cdot) = p_nF_0(\cdot)+(1-p_n)F_n(\cdot), \quad p_n = \frac{\alpha(\Omega)}{\alpha(\Omega+n)},$$

$F_0(\cdot)$ and $F_n(\cdot)$ are correspondingly a prior and empirical distribution functions. For the estimable functional of the second degree,

$$\theta_2 = \iint a_2(x,y)dF(x)dF(y),$$

under the same assumptions, the following Bayes estimate is obtained:

$$\hat{\theta}_2^* = \frac{\alpha(\Omega)+n}{\alpha(\Omega)+n+1}\Bigg[p_n^2 \iint a_2(x,y)dF_0(x)dF_0(y)$$

$$+\frac{2}{n}p_n(1-p_n)\sum_{i=1}^{n}\int a_2(x,x_i)dF_0(x)+\frac{1}{n^2}(1-p_n)^2\sum_{i=1}^{n}\sum_{j=1}^{n}a_2(x_i,x_j)$$

$$+\frac{1}{\alpha(\Omega)+n+1}\left[p_n\int a_2(x,x)dF_0(x)\frac{1}{n}(1-p_n)\sum_{i=1}^{n}a_2(x_i,x_i)\right]\Bigg] \tag{4.13}$$

As can be seen from the expressions (4.12) and (4.13), the values of the estimates $\hat{\theta}_2^*$ and $\hat{\theta}_3^*$ with a fixed sample $x_1,\ldots,x_n$ are determined by a choice of a prior measure α. The last, as was mentioned above, is uniquely determined in the case when the value $\alpha(\Omega)$ is given and there exists a priori information about the distribution function $F_0(x)$. It is interesting to learn the behavior of the estimates as $\alpha \to 0$. This case, it seems, can be considered in the absence of a priori information. The functions $a_k(x,y,\ldots)$ are vanishing if at least two arguments are equal. Under these conditions the Bayes estimates $\hat{\theta}_2^*$ and $\hat{\theta}_3^*$ have, as $\alpha \to 0$, the form

$$\hat{\theta}_{02}^* = \frac{2}{n(n+1)} \sum_{1 \leqslant i<j \leqslant n}\sum a_2(x_i,x_j), \tag{4.14}$$

and

$$\hat{\theta}_{03}^* = \frac{6}{n(n+1)(n+2)} \sum_{1 \leqslant i<j<k \leqslant n}\sum a_3(x_i,x_j,x_k). \tag{4.15}$$

The Bayes estimates we have obtained are similar to U-statistics for which there are well-known results, that is,

$$U_2 = \frac{2}{n(n-1)} \sum_{1 \leqslant i<j \leqslant n}\sum a_2(x_i,x_j),$$

and

$$U_3 = \frac{6}{n(n-1)(n-2)} \sum_{1 \leqslant i<j<k \leqslant n}\sum a_3(x_i,x_j,x_k).$$

Thus, we have the following finite relations for the Bayes estimates k and U-statistics:

$$\hat{\theta}_{02}^* = \frac{n-1}{n+1} U_2 \quad \text{and} \quad \hat{\theta}_{03}^* = \frac{(n-1)(n-2)}{(n+1)(n+2)} U_3.$$

Using these relationships we may conclude that $\hat{\theta}_{0k}^*$ converges to U_k as $n \to \infty$.

Consider two examples of nonparametric Bayes estimates for parameters admitting the second order estimate.

Example 4.3 (Estimate of the square of the mean, m^2, for an unknown distribution F). If one puts $a_2(x,y) = xy$, we obtain $\theta_2 = m^2$. From the expression (4.13) immediately follows

$$\begin{aligned}\hat{m}^{*2} =& \frac{\alpha(\mathbf{R}^1)+n}{\alpha(\mathbf{R}^1)+n+1}\left[p_n \int x dF_0(x) + (1-p)\bar{x}_n\right]^2 \\ &+ \frac{1}{\alpha(\mathbf{R}^1)+n+1}\left[p_n \int x^2 dF_0(x) + (1-p)\bar{x}_n^2\right],\end{aligned}$$

where $\bar{x}_n = \frac{1}{n}\sum_{i=1}^{n} x_i$. It is interesting to note that the corresponding U-statistic has form

$$U_2 = \frac{1}{n(n-1)} \sum_{1 \leqslant i<j \leqslant n}\sum x_i x_j = \frac{n}{n-1}(\bar{x}_n)^2 + \frac{1}{n-1}\bar{x}_n^{2}.$$

Example 4.4 (Estimate of the variance of the distribution F). For $a_2(x,y) = (x-y)^2/2$ we have $\theta_2 = \sigma^2$, where s is mean-squared value of the distribution F. From the expressions (4.13) and (4.14) one obtains

$$\hat{\sigma}^{2*} = \frac{\alpha(\mathbf{R}^1)+n}{\alpha(\mathbf{R}^1)+n+1}\left\{p_n\left[\int x^2 dF_0(x) - \left(\int x dF_0(x)\right)^2\right]\right.$$

$$\left. + \frac{1}{n}(1-p_n)\sum_{i=1}^{n}(x_i-\bar{x}_n)^2 + p_n(1-p_n)\left(\int x dF_0(x) - x_n\right)^2\right\}. \tag{4.16}$$

As $\alpha \to 0$, we have

$$\hat{\sigma}_0^{2*} = \frac{1}{n+1}\sum_{i=1}^{n}(x_i-\bar{x}_n)^2. \tag{4.17}$$

The estimate (4.16) coincides with the estimate of the variance obtained by Ferguson [80]. The U-statistic, corresponding to the Bayes estimate (4.17), is a well-known unbiased estimate of the variance

$$U_2 = \frac{1}{n-1}\sum_{i=1}^{n}(x_i-\bar{x}_n)^2.$$

Further development of [80] can be found in the work by Susarla and Van Ryzin [246] in which a nonparametric Bayes TTF estimate $R(t) = 1 - F(t)$ is obtained for $F(t) \sim D(\alpha)$ for censored data. Let, as in Chapter 3, t_i^* be failure moments ($i = 1, 2, \ldots, n$), and t_i be censoring moments. Besides, during the experiment it is observed the minimal of mentioned quantities: $\tau_i = \min\{t_i^*, t_i\}$. The sufficient statistic can be represented as a union of two vectors (τ, δ), where $\delta = (\delta_1, \ldots, \delta_n)$, and $\delta_i = 1$ if $t_i^* \leqslant t_i$, i.e., the failure is observed, and $\delta_i = 0$ otherwise. It is assumed that failure times and censoring times are mutually independent. Note that all Bayes decision rules are independent of the order of elements in the sample representation. Therefore, we can present a sample so that its first d elements $\tau_1, \ldots, \tau_d$ arethe failure times and the last k elements $\tau_{(d+1)}, \ldots, \tau_{(n)}$ are censoring times. We denote, at last, by $\tau_{(d+1)}, \ldots, \tau_{(m)}$ the different one from other elements of the set of the censoring moments $\tau_{d+1}, \ldots, \tau_n$, and by λ_j is the number of censoring times equal to t τ_j. As a parameter of a prior Dirichlet process for the considered case is chosen a positive finite measure on $(\mathbf{R}^+, \mathrm{B})$, where $\mathbf{R}^+ = [0, \infty)$, and B is σ-algebra of all Borel sets on $\mathbf{R}^+$. The expression for the posterior moments of a random variable $R(t) = 1 - F(t)$ is obtained by following the work of Ferguson [80]. For $t \in \left[\tau_{(\ell)}, \tau_{(\ell+1)}\right]$, $\ell = d, \ldots, m$ and $\tau_{(d)} = 0$, $\tau_{m+1} = \infty$, we have

$$E\left[R(t))^p \mid (\tau,\delta)\right] = \prod_{s=0}^{p-1}\left\{\frac{\alpha([t,\infty)) + s + N^+(t)}{\alpha(\mathbf{R}^+) + s + n}\prod_{j=d+1}^{\ell}\frac{\alpha\left(\left[\tau_{(j)},\infty\right)\right) + s + N(\tau_j)}{\alpha([\tau_j,\infty)) + s + N(\tau_j) - \lambda_j}\right\},$$

where $N_{(u)}$ is the number of elements of the sample τ exceeding or equal u, $N^+(u)$ is the number of elements which are strictly greater than u. Besides, as $t < \tau_{(k+1)}$ the inner product in the expression (4.18) is equal to one. The expression (4.18) enables us to write, without any difficulties, the pointwise TTF estimate $\hat{R}^*(t) = E\left[R(t) \mid (\tau,\delta)\right]$ and the posterior variance $E\left(R^2(t) \mid (\tau,\delta)\right] - \hat{R}^{*2}(t)$. In particular, for $t \in \left[\tau_{(\ell)}, \tau_{(\ell+1)}\right]$

$$\hat{R}^*(t) = \frac{\alpha([t,\infty)) + N^+(t)}{\alpha(\mathbf{R}^+) + n} \prod_{j=d+1}^{\ell} \frac{\alpha\left(\left[t_{(j)},\infty\right)\right) + N^+\left(t_{(j)}\right)}{\alpha\left(\left[t_{(j)},\infty\right)\right) + N^+\left(t_{(j)}\right) - \lambda_j} \tag{4.18}$$

We compare the Bayes estimate (4.19) with the corresponding Kaplan-Meier estimate [121]

$$\hat{R}(t) = \prod_{j \in I_0(t)} \frac{n-j}{n-j+1} \tag{4.19}$$

where $I_0(t)$ is the set on indices of the variational row $\tau_1' \leqslant \tau_2' \leqslant \cdots \leqslant \tau_n'$ composed of the sample τ, such that $\tau_i' \leqslant t$ and τ_i' is failure time. The comparison of the estimates (4.19) and (4.20) shows that the Bayes estimates is more preferable. First, the Kaplan-Meier estimate uses only information about the number of censoring times contained between the failure times. The Bayes estimate is all information contained in the sufficient statistic (τ,δ). Secondly, although both estimates (4.19) and (4.20) are piecewise- smooth and have finite increments at the failure points, the Bayes estimate in the time between failures is a decreasing function (because of the continuity of a prior measure α), the estimate (4.20) equal to some constant. Finally, if the last element of the variational row τ_n' is a censoring time, in the interval $[\tau_n', \infty)$ the estimate (4.20) is undefined.

The limit passing in the expression (4.19) as $\alpha \to 0$ (that corresponds to a priori information) transforms it into the Kaplan-Meier estimate. In the case when such a coincidence is possible, the Kaplan–Meier estimate is written as

$$R(t) = \begin{cases} \dfrac{N^+(t)}{n} \displaystyle\prod_{i \in I_0(t)} \left[\frac{N^+(\tau_i) + \lambda_i}{N^+(\tau_i)}\right]^{\delta_i}, & t < \tau_n', \\ 0, & t \geqslant \tau_n', \end{cases} \tag{4.20}$$

where $I_0(t)$ is the set of the first indices among the repeating elements of the sample τ, satisfying the condition $\tau_i \leqslant t$. The formulas (4.20) and (4.21) give the same estimates as $\lambda_i = 1$ for all i, but the latter one is more general.

The properties of nonparametric estimates having the type (4.18) for samples of large volume are investigated by Susarla and Van Ryzin in [245-246]. We briefly formulate the main results in these works. Both these estimate are mean squared point wisely consistent of order $o\left(n^{-1}\right)$ and strictly consistent of order $o(n^{-1/2}/\ln n)$. In addition to this, both estimates are asymptotically normal with the same variance. Hence, from the point-of-view of the theory of large samples, we may conclude that nonparametric Bayes estimates, based on the Dirichlet process and Kaplan–Meier estimate, are equivalent.

The comparison of these estimates for small size samples was done by Rai, Susarla and Van Ryzin [209]. Their work is interesting from the methodological point-of-view. It proposes one method of practical use of nonparametric Bayes estimates, based on the Dirichlet process. The choice of a prior measure $\alpha(\cdot)$ plays the intrinsic role in this method. Once it was made, it remains only to apply formula (4.18). Let us introduce a real-valued function $\alpha(x) = \alpha([x,\infty))$. Then a priori information on TTF in accordance with (4.5) takes on the form

$$R_0(t) = \alpha(t)/\alpha(0) = \alpha(t)/\beta, \text{ where } \beta = \alpha(0), \tag{4.21}$$

and the Bayes estimate of TTF, $\hat{R}^*(t)$ for the quadratic loss function under absence of censoring is rewritten as

$$\hat{R}^*(t) = \frac{\beta}{\beta+n} R_0(t) + \frac{n}{\beta+n}\hat{R}_n(t), \tag{4.22}$$

where $\hat{R}_n$ is the cumulative TTF estimate, based on the sample of n independent observations. Unfortunately, we cannot write the estimate of the type (4.23), substituting, for example, the Kaplan–Meier estimate instead of $\hat{R}_n(t)$. Nevertheless, for the choice of a prior measure $\alpha(\cdot)$ it is advisable touse its interpretation, defined by the expression (4.22). Suppose, in accordance with a priori information, that the random mean functioning time is subjected to the exponential law with the parameter μ. Then, in view of (4.22) one has

$$\alpha(t) = \beta \exp\left(-\frac{t}{\mu}\right). \tag{4.23}$$

In the work [209] an estimate, which is based on the given measure α, is called reduced nonparametric Bayes estimate. Instead of exponential prior distribution for $F_0(t)$, we might just as well have used the Weibull distribution, gamma-distribution, etc., and obtain the estimate which is more "narrow" as a result of the imposed restriction. In the work [209] the parameter μ is estimated not with the help of a priori information but statistically: instead of m one substitutes into the function (4.24) its maximum likelihood estimate $\hat{\mu} = \sum_{i=1}^{n} \tau_i/d$, where d is the number of noncensored observations. Then, with the help of (4.19) the Bayes TTF estimate may be written as

$$\hat{R}^*(t) = \frac{\beta\exp\left(-\frac{t}{\mu}\right) + N^+(t)}{\beta+n} \prod_{i\in I_0} \left[\frac{\beta\exp\left(-\frac{t_i}{\mu}\right) + N^+(\tau_i) + \lambda_i}{\beta\exp\left(-\frac{t_i}{\mu}\right) + N^+(\tau_i)}\right]^{\delta_i}. \tag{4.24}$$

It should be noted that the estimate (4.25) is not, strictly speaking, a Bayes estimate. It should rather be called an empirical Bayes estimate because the parameter of a prior distribution μ is estimated with the help of empirical data.

In applying the estimate (4.25), an open problem is the value of β. In [209] the authors considered the mean-squared error of (4.23), that is,

$$E\left[\left(\hat{R}^*(t)-R(t)\right)^2\right]=\left(\frac{\beta}{\beta+n}\right)^2(R_0(t)-R(t))^2+\frac{b}{(\beta+n)^2}R(t)\,(1-R(t)). \qquad (4.25)$$

The first term in (4.26) determines the square of the bias, caused in the Bayes estimate by a priori information about the TTF; the second one is a variance of the unbiased estimate$\hat{R}(t)$. While n increases, the mean-squared error decreases, where

$$\lim_{n\to\infty}\left(n^{-1}\beta(n)\right)=0,$$

and thus, $\beta(n)$ satisfies the condition $\beta(n)=O(n^{\alpha})$, for $\alpha<1$. The authors of [209] make the following necessary assumption that both terms of the squared error (4.26) have the same order of smallness of n^{-1}. This is achieved when $\beta=c\sqrt{n}$, where c is some constant value which may depend on the current value of t. In practical calculations of [209] the value $c=1$ is assigned.

Comparison of Bayes estimates with those of Kaplan-Meier for small samples has been studied [209] subject to the following criteria:

a) As a criterion of comparison we choose a parametric estimate;
b) We use two forms of modeling: exponential modeling, corresponding to the chosen prior measure (4.24) and beta modeling, which contradicts it.
c) Modeling is carried out for different values of a theoretical mean μ, and different percentages of censoring.

In Table 4.1 and Table 4.2 we give TTF values averaging over 200 samples. The table data enables us to draw the following conclusion: the Bayes estimate is better than the Kaplan-Meier estimate; moreover, this fact remains valid not only for the case when empirical data are in full accordance with a prior distribution, but also in the situation when they are contradicted. The deviation between the Kaplan–Meier and Bayes estimates increases with the increasing of the censoring percentage; moreover, while the first one removes from the parametric, the second estimate approaches to them. Application of a prior measure, based on more flexible distributions, for example on the Weibull distribution leads, most probably, to a better estimate, although with increasing computational complexity.

The estimate analogous to (4.19) was found by Zehniwirth [273]. It is called a linear Bayes estimate and may be interpreted as a Kaplan-Meier estimate, constructed by blending a priori and experimental data.

Table 4.1 Comparison of TTF estimates under modeling of the exponential distribution.

Estimate	Censoring Percentage	$n=10$		$n=30$	
		$\mu=1$	$\mu=5$	$\mu=1$	$\mu=5$
Parametric Bayes Kaplan–Meier	0	0.113 0.175 0.203	0.252 0.391 0.454	0.071 0.108 0.118	0.158 0.242 0.264
Parametric Bayes Kaplan–Meier	25	0.141 0.194 0.236	0.315 0.434 0.529	0.092 0.119 0.139	0.183 0.266 0.311
Parametric Bayes Kaplan–Meier	50	0.171 0.198 0.275	0.383 0.444 0.615	0.094 0.117 0.198	0.211 0.261 0.442
Parametric Bayes Kaplan–Meier	75	0.209 0.223 0.412	0.467 0.499 0.919	0.116 0.126 0.380	0.260 0.283 0.847

From a practical point-of-view, an important nonparametric Bayes estimate was found by Cambell and Hollander [36]. They considered the problem of defining a predicted interval containing the given number of future observations which is formulated as follows. Let $x_1,\ldots,x_n$ be the initial sample from $F \sim D(\alpha)$, and $y_1,\ldots,y_n$ be the sample of future observations.

According to the definition of the statistic given in [36], $a_1(x_1,\ldots,x_n)$ and $a_2(x_1,\ldots,x_n)$ form 100% predicted interval (a_1,a_2) for M from N future observations, if the probability $P_{M,N}$ of the event that at least M of N observations get into (a_1,a_2) equals γ. The probability γ is called a prediction coefficient. A difference of a_1 and a_2 from tolerant limits is that the last ones assume that we have to consider the whole set of future observations. For the case $a_2=\infty$ we deal with a unilateral prediction interval.

A good illustration for the considered problem may be the following technical example. A manufacturer of some technical device has a sample of values of the leading parameter $x_1,x_2,\ldots,x_5$ for the set containing five such devices. The set of three such devices is put into operation. It is necessary to find the lower value of the leading parameter, guaranteed with a probability 0.9, which can be achieved for all three devices. In the given case, $n=5$, $N=3$, $M=3$, $\gamma=0.9$.

The solution for this problem is based on the following idea, traditional for Dirichlet processes: first we solve the problem in absence of empirical data; thereupon, using the property of conjugacy of the Dirichlet distribution, the solution is generalized for the case when $n>0$. The resulting calculations, used for the solution of the problem, are derived from the following theoretical result of the work [36]. Suppose that for some future observations

Table 4.2 Comparison of TTF estimates under modeling of a gamma distribution.

Estimate	Censoring Percentage	$n = 10$		$n = 30$	
		$\mu = 1$	$\mu = 5$	$\mu = 1$	$\mu = 5$
		0.158	0.535	0.133	0.296
Parametric Bayes Kaplan–Meier	0	0.156	0.348	0.092	0.205
		0.181	0.403	0.1	0.223
		0.167	0.373	0.135	0.301
Parametric Bayes Kaplan–Meier	25	0.167	0.372	0.101	0.225
		0.201	0.449	0.113	0.253
		0.182	0.408	0.145	0.324
Parametric Bayes Kaplan–Meier	50	0.184	0.412	0.117	0.262
		0.232	0.518	0.145	0.324
		0.188	0.423	0.139	0.313
Parametric Bayes Kaplan–Meier	75	0.191	0.427	0.121	0.272
		0.315	0.701	0.266	0.592

$y_1,\ldots,y_n$ random variables $I = I_X$, $J = J_{xy}$, $K = K_y$ denote, correspondingly, the number of the sample elements not exceeding, greater than x but less or equal to y, and, finally, greater than y. In [36] it is proved that the quantities I,J,K obey the composite Dirichlet distribution which may be written in the notations, introduced above, as

$$P\{(I,J,K) = (i,j,k)\} = \frac{N!}{(N-i)!(N-j)!(N-k)} \times \frac{\alpha((-\infty,x])^{[i]}\alpha((x,y])^{[j]}\alpha((y,\infty))^{[k]}}{\alpha(\mathbf{R}^1)^{[N]}} \tag{4.26}$$

where $c^{[m]} = c(c+1)\cdots(c+m-1)$, and $c^{[0]} = 1$, $c[0] = 1$.

Consider at first the case of construction of a unilateral predicted 100% interval (a_1,∞). To this end we put $k = 0$ and $y = \infty$. It gives us a bivariate random variable (I,J) whose marginal distribution J has the form

$$P\{J = j\} = \frac{N!}{(N-J)!j!} \cdot \frac{\alpha((-\infty,x])^{[N-j]}\alpha((x,\infty))^{[j]}}{\alpha(\mathbf{R}^1)^{[N]}}. \tag{4.27}$$

The expression (4.28) determines the probability of the event that exactly j elements of the sample $y_1,\ldots,y_n$ are exceeding or equal to x. Consequently, the probability $P_{M,N}$ is written as a sum $P_{M,N} = P\{J = M\} + P\{J = M+1\} + \cdots + P\{J = N\}$. After this, for the obtaining of α_1 in the absence of a sample, it is necessary to solve the equation

$$\sum_{j=M}^{n} \frac{N!}{(N-j)!\,j!} \cdot \frac{\alpha((-\infty,x])^{[N-j]}\alpha((x,\infty))^{[j]}}{\alpha(\mathbf{R}^1)^{[N]}} = \gamma. \tag{4.28}$$

Here $\alpha(\cdot)$ has the sense of a prior measure, connected with a priori information about the c.d.f. $F_0(x)$ by the relation $\alpha((-\infty x]) = \beta F_0(x)$, where $\beta = \alpha(\mathbf{R}^1)$ has the sense of a weight significance of a prior distribution. In absence of data the estimate a_1, as follows from (4.29), is invariant with respect to the choice of. In the case when a sample $x_1,\ldots,x_n$

is given, one should replace $\alpha(\cdot)$ in (4.29) by

$$\alpha'(A) = \alpha(A) + \sum_{i=1}^{n} \delta_{x_i}(A),$$

where $\delta_{x_i=1}$, if $x_i \in A$, otherwise $\delta_{x_i} = 0$. To find a bilateral 100% predicted interval (a_1, a_2) we act analogously. In particular, the following equation holds:

$$\sum_{j=M}^{n} \frac{N!}{(N-j)!j!} \cdot \frac{\alpha'((x,y])^{[j]}\alpha'\left(\mathbf{R}^1 - (x,y]\right)^{[N-j]}}{\alpha(\mathbf{R}^1)+n} = \gamma. \tag{4.29}$$

Moreover, among the values of $a_1 = x$, $a_2 = y$ we choose such two numbers, for which the interval length is minimal. The conclusion of the work [36] gives numerous examples illustrating the stability of the obtained estimates.

In the work [53], Dalal and Phadia use a prior Dirichlet processes for the solution of the problem of estimating the relationship between random variables and verifying the corresponding statistical hypotheses. They consider a bivariate distribution $F(x,y)$ which is assumed to be a probabilitymeasure, subjected to a prior Dirichlet distribution $D(\alpha)$ in addition, a is nonzero measure on $(\mathbf{R}^2, \mathscr{L})$. As a measure of dependence, a consistency coefficient Δ is used:

$$\Delta = \Delta_F = P_F\{(X-X')(Y-Y') > 0\} + \frac{1}{2}P_F\{(X-X')(Y-Y') = 0\} \tag{4.30}$$

where (X,Y) and (X',Y') are two independent observations from $F(x,y)$. The coefficient Δ is connected with the often used τ-parameter of Kenndal by the relation $\Delta = (\tau+1)/2$. The form of (4.31) assumes that random variables X and Y are not necessarily continuous. The problem of obtaining the Bayes estimate Δ^* was solved in [53] in accordance with the Ferguson theory [80]. Suppose t and U are two sets in $\mathbf{R}^2$ such $T = \{(x,y,x',y') : (x-x')(y-y') > 0\}$, $U = \{(x,y,x',y') : (x-x')(y-y') = 0\}$. There upon we write (4.31) as

$$\Delta = \int \left(I_T + \frac{1}{2}I_u\right) d\left[F(x,y)F(x',y')\right],$$

where I_T and I_u are the indicator functions of sets. Having chosen a quadratic loss function, we obtain the following Bayes estimate of the parameter Δ:

$$\Delta^* = \int \left(I_T + \frac{1}{2}I_u\right) dE[F(x,y)F(x',y')]. \tag{4.31}$$

The expected value E is defined with respect to a prior distribution $D(\alpha)$. In particular, in absence of the testing data,

$$E[F(x,y)F(x',y')] = \frac{1}{\beta+1}F_0'(x,x',y,y') + \frac{\beta}{\beta+1}F_0(x,y)F_0(x',y'), \tag{4.32}$$

where $F_0'(x,x',y,y') = F_0\big(\min(x,x'),\min(y,y')\big)$, F_0, as previously, has the sense of a priori information about the bivariate distribution function, and $\beta = \alpha(\mathbf{R}^2)$.

Substitution of the relation (4.33) into (4.32) allows us to write the following Bayes estimate of in the absence of empirical data:

$$\Delta^* = \frac{\beta}{\beta+1}\Delta_{F_0} + \frac{1}{2(\beta+1)}, \tag{4.33}$$

where Δ_{F_0} is computed with the help of the formula (4.31) for the distribution F_0. If it is found that the quantities X, Y are a priori independent, $\Delta_{F_0} = 1/2$, and (4.34) implies $\Delta^* = 1/2$. In the case of existence of experimental data $(x_1,y_1),\ldots,(x_n,y_n)$ the expected value of (4.32) should be defined by the Dirichlet prior distribution with the parameter

$$\alpha' = \alpha + \sum_{i=1}^{n} \delta_{(x_i,y_i)} = (\beta+n)P^*.$$

Here P^* is the posterior measure for which the bivariate distribution function has the form

$$F^*(x,y) = p_n F_0(x,y) + 1(1-p_n)\hat{F}_n(x,y),$$

where $\hat{F}_n(x,y)$ is the empirical distribution function, based on the sample (x_1,y_1),...,(x_n,y_n), and $p_n = \beta/(\beta+n)$. The resulting expression for the Bayes estimate is written in the following form:

$$\Delta^* = \frac{\beta+n}{\beta+n+1}\left[p_n^2\Delta_{F_0} + 2p_n(1-p_n)\Delta\big(F_0,\hat{F}_n\big) + (1-p_n)^2\Delta_{\hat{F}_n}\right] + \frac{1}{2}\cdot\frac{1}{\beta+n+1}, \tag{4.34}$$

where

$$\Delta_{\hat{F}_n} = \frac{1}{n^2}\sum_{i=1}^{n}\sum_{j=1}^{n}\left\{I\left[(x_i-x_j)(y_i-y_j)>0\right] + \frac{1}{2}I\left[(x_i-x_j)(y_i-y_j)=0\right]\right\},$$

$$\Delta\big(F_0,\hat{F}_n\big) = \frac{1}{n}\sum_{i=1}^{n} P_{F_0}\left\{(X-x_i)(Y-y_j)>0\right\} + \frac{1}{2}P_{F_0}\left\{(X-x_i)(Y-y_j)=0\right\}.$$

If we choose for F_0 a bivariate normal distribution $N_2(\mu_1,\mu_2,\sigma_1,\sigma_2,\rho)$, then, for $\mu_1=\mu_2=0$, and $\sigma_1=\sigma_2=1$, in accordance with [53], we obtain

$$\Delta_{F_0} = \frac{1}{2} + \frac{1}{\pi\sin\rho}. \tag{4.35}$$

Next, if one denotes by $\Phi(x,y)$ a function of the bivariate normal distribution $N_2(0,0,1,1,\rho)$ and $\bar{\Phi}(x,y) = 1-\Phi(x,\infty)-\Phi(\infty,y)-\Phi(x,y)$, it yields

$$\Delta\big(F_0\hat{F}_n\big) = \frac{1}{n}\left[\sum_{i=1}^{n}\left(\Phi\left(\frac{x_i-\mu_1}{\sigma_1},\frac{y_i-\mu_2}{\sigma_2}\right) + \bar{\Phi}\left(\frac{x_i-\mu_1}{\sigma_1},\frac{y_i-\mu_2}{\sigma_2}\right)\right)\right] \tag{4.36}$$

The obtained relations allow us to find the estimate of Δ^* for the chosen value β.

Note, that as $n \to \infty$, the Bayes estimate (4.35) approaches the sample size one. At the same time, for $\beta = 0$ (i.e., we have no a priori information), the expression (4.35) gives the usual nonparametric estimate of the coefficient Δ.

In one of his works Ferguson [82] develops the theory based on Dirichlet processes in conformity to the successive estimation. In particular, he proposes procedures for obtaining nonparametric Bayes estimates of the cumulative distribution function and the mean. The essence of these procedures lies in the following. To each single trial is assigned some positive number c, interpreted as cost and having the same dimension as that of the loss function. The loss function has a quadratic form and is written as

$$\ell\left(F,\hat{F}\right) = \int_{\mathbf{R}^1} \left[F(x) - \hat{F}(x)\right]^2 dW(x),$$

where $W(x)$ is a weight function on $\mathbf{R}^1$. After each testing, a statistician has to make a decision: whether he has to continue testing or to stop and choose the necessary estimate. As a criterion for making decisions, we use the total losses caused by the general procedure of estimating. These losses are added, on one hand, to the expected value of the loss function (Bayes risk), that is,

$$G_n = \frac{1}{\beta+n+1} \int_{\mathbf{R}^1} \hat{F}_n^*(x)\left[1 - \hat{F}_n^*(x)\right] dW(x),$$

where $\hat{F}_n^*(x)$ is a nonparametric Bayes estimate, based on a Dirichlet process (see the expression (4.6)), $\beta = \alpha(\mathbf{R}^1)$. On the other hand, the cost of testing should be added to the total losses.

Let, for example, in absence of a sample ($n = 0$), a Bayes estimate $\hat{F}^* = F_0$ and losses be

$$G_0 = \frac{1}{\beta+1} \int F_0\left(1 - F_0\right)(x) dW. \tag{4.37}$$

If we carry out one testing, that is, we will obtain the value x_1, the total conditional losses (under the condition x_1) will be

$$c + \frac{1}{\beta+2} \int \left[F_1^*(1 - F_1^*)\right] dW,$$

and their expected value will be equal:

$$c + \frac{1}{\beta+2} E\left[\int F_1^*(1 - F_1^*) dW\right] = c + \frac{1}{(\beta+2)^2} \int F_0(1 - F_0) dW. \tag{4.38}$$

Here we used the relation $E[F_1] = F_0$. For making the decision about the necessity of conducting the first testing, we have to compare the two quantities (4.38) and (4.39). If the first quantity is not greater than the second one, i.e., we have the inequality

$$\int F_0\left(1 - F_0\right) dW \leqslant c(\beta+1)^2, \tag{4.39}$$

it is not necessary to carry out the first testing (in accordance with a criterion of total losses) and the estimate $\hat{F}^*$ should be chosen as a priori information about the distribution function F_0.

In the general case for decision making after conducting n tests, one has to use another similar inequality

$$\hat{F}_n^* \left(1-\hat{F}_n^*\right) dW \leqslant c(\beta+n+1).$$

This method is called the one-step procedure. Ferguson [82] has generalized this method for the case of multi-step procedures.

Several authors have taken a different approach than Ferguson in using the Dirichlet distribution. As an example, we touch upon the works by Lochner and Basu [153–155]. These works have practical usefulness, connected with a test of the hypothesis about a cumulative distribution function $F(x)$ belonging to the class S_0 including failure rate distributions.

With a given sample of a device $\tau = (\tau_1,\ldots,\tau_n) = (\mathbf{t}^*,\mathbf{t})$, where $\mathbf{t}^* = (t_1^*,\ldots,t_d^*)$ is the vector of failure times, $\mathbf{t} = (t_1,\ldots,t_k)$ is a vector of times of nonrandom censoring. For some value t, coinciding with one of the censoring times, we construct the set of values $0 = x_0 < x_1 < x_2 < \cdots < x_m = T$ so that each value x_i coincides with one of the moments of censoring The test statistic is of the form $z = (s_1,\ldots,s_m,r_1,\ldots,r_m)$, where s_j is the number of devices failed during the time $(x_{j-1},x_j]$, $j = 1,2,\ldots,m, r_j$ is the number of devices which tested successfully by the time x_j $(j = 1,\ldots,m-1)$, and r_m is the number of devices failed by the time x_m or having a failure after x_m. Let $p = (p_1,\ldots,p_m)$ be a vector consisting of increments of the distribution function, $p_j = F(X_j) - F(x_{j-1})$. As is proved in [153], z is a sufficient statistic for p.

Further, we assume that p has a prior Dirichlet distribution with a density

$$h(P) \sim p_1^{\nu_1-1}\cdots p_m^{\nu_m-1}(1-p_1-\cdots-p_m)^{\nu_{m+1}-1} \tag{4.40}$$

on the set

$$\rho = \left\{p: 0 \leqslant p_j \leqslant 1,\ j = 1,\ldots,m,\ \sum_{j=1}^{m} p_j \leqslant 1\right\}.$$

The numbers $\nu_1,\nu_2,\ldots,\nu_m,\nu_{m+1}$ are parameters of a prior distribution. Consider a vector $u = (u_1,\ldots,u_m)$ such that $u_1 = (1-p_1)$ and

$$u_j = \frac{1-p_1-\cdots-p_j}{1-p_1-\cdots-p_{j-1}}, \qquad j = 2,\ldots,m.$$

The quantities u_j are linked with a failure rate function of the device in the interval $(t,t+\Delta)$:

$$\lambda(t,\Delta) = \frac{F(t+\Delta)-F(t)}{\Delta[1-F(t)]}$$

by the relation

$$u_j = 1 - \lambda\,\frac{x_{j-1}, x_j - x_{j-1}}{x_j - x_{j-1}}.$$

It follows from (4.41) that $u_1, u_2, \ldots, u_m$ are a priori independent and subject to the beta-distribution with the probability density

$$h_j(u_j \mid v) \sim u_j^{w_j-1}(1-u_j)^{v_j-1}, \quad v = (v_1, \ldots, v_{m+1}),$$

where $w_j = v_{j+1} + \cdots + v_{m+1}$. Moreover, it follows from the property of conjugacy of a Dirichlet distribution that the distribution for which

$$h_j(u_j \mid z, v) u_j^{\alpha_j-1}(1-u_j)^{\beta_j-1} \tag{4.41}$$

where $\alpha_j = \sum_{i=j+1}^{m}(s_i + r_i + v_i) + r_j + v_{m+1}$, $\beta_j = s_j + v_j$ appears to be also posterior for u_j. Since F is a random probability measure, the event $F(t) \in S_0$ is random. The following upper estimate is found in [154] for the probability $P\{F(t) \in S_0 \mid z, v\}$:

$$P\{F(t) \in S_0 \mid z, v\} < P\{u_1 < u_2 < \cdots < u_m \mid z, v\}.$$

With the help of (4.42) we can obtain

$$P\{u_1 < u_2 < \cdots < u_m \mid z, v\} = \int_0^1 \int_0^{u_1} \cdots \int_0^{u_{m-1}} \prod_{j=1}^{m} \frac{u_j^{\alpha_j-1}(1-u_j)^{\beta_j-1}}{\beta(\alpha_j, \beta_j)} du_m \cdots du_1; \tag{4.42}$$

in addition, the finite analytical expression for integer β_j is obtained in [155]. For large m the probability (4.43) is almost near to $P\{F(t) \in S_0 \mid z, v\}$. The procedure of estimating the fact that $F(t)$ belongs to the class of failure rate distributions S_0 is easily constructed starting from (4.43).

In addition to the mentioned procedure, we can estimate, with the help of a prior density, the probabilities of future events. Let ξ be a failure time for the future testing or for the operation time. Then

$$P\{x_{i-1} < \xi \leqslant x_i \mid z, v\} = \gamma_1 \gamma_2 \cdots \gamma_{i-1}(1-\gamma_i), \tag{4.43}$$

where $\gamma_j = \alpha_j/(\alpha_j + \beta_j)$, and hence

$$P\{\xi \leqslant x_i \mid z, v\} = \sum_{j=1}^{i} \gamma_1 \gamma_2 \cdots \gamma_{i-1}(1-\gamma_i) = 1 - \prod_{j=1}^{i} \gamma_j \tag{4.44}$$

Relations (4.44) and (4.45) allow us to find the estimate of any reliability indices.

In the work [45] you can find a comparatively easy way of using the Ferguson scheme. The authors use as a priori information the empirical distribution function, constructed on some hypothetical sample $\mathbf{t}_h^* = \left(t_{h_1}^*, t_{h_2}^*, \ldots, t_{h_m}^*\right)$ of the failure times. As a measure of significance of the prior information, $\beta = \alpha(\mathbf{R}^1)$ is chosen the number $m+1$. If $\mathbf{t}^* = (t_1^*, \ldots, t_n^*)$ is a sample of failure times, then the nonparametric Bayes estimate $\hat{F}^*(t)$ of the distribution function $F(t)$ in accordance with (4.6) has the form

$$\hat{F}^*(t) = \begin{cases} 0 & \text{if } t < 0, \\ \dfrac{k}{s+1} & \text{if } t_k \leqslant t < t_{k+1} \ (k = 0, 1, \ldots, s), \\ 1 & \text{if } t_{s+1} \leqslant t, \end{cases} \tag{4.45}$$

where $\{t_1, \ldots, t_s\}$ is the sample in ascending order $\{\mathbf{t}_h^*, \mathbf{t}\}$. The generalization of this result is given in [45] for the case of censored samples.

4.3 Nonparametric Bayes estimates in which Dirichlet processes are not used

4.3.1 *Neutral to the right processes*

One of the general representations of stochastic processes which cannot be reduced to Dirichlet processes are the so-called neutral to the right processes initiated by Doksum [67]. A neutral to the right process, or NR-process, is introduced by Doksum in the form of a random probability measure $F(t)$ on $\mathbf{R}^1$ such that, for any t_1 and t_2 $(t_1 < t_2)$ the relation $[1 - F(t_2)]/[1 - F(t_1)]$ is independent of F for any $t \leqslant t_1$. A NR-process can be expressed with the help of a process called a process with independent increments.

The mentioned processes are introduced and investigated by Levy [138]. In accordance with his definition, Y is called a *stochastic function with independent increments*, if its increments $Y_{st} = Y_t - Y_s$ on intersected segments $[s,t)$ are independent. A process with independent increments is called a *family of such stochastic functions*, determined on some sample space with the same increments ([138], p. 561). By means of Y_t a NR-process is determined in the following way [67].

Definition 4.3 (NR-process). A stochastic distribution function is said to be *NR-process*, if it can be represented in the form

$$F(t) = 1 - \mathrm{e}^{-Y_t}, \tag{4.46}$$

where Y_t is a process with independent increments, besides, Y_t is nondecreasing and continuous to the right and

$$\lim_{t \to \infty} Y_t = \infty \ \text{a.s.}, \qquad \lim_{t \to -\infty} Y_t = 0 \ \text{a.s.}$$

In accordance with the theory of Lent, the stochastic process Y_t has no more than a countable number of discontinuity points $t_1, t_2, \ldots,$ The random variables $S_1, S_2, \ldots,$ determine the jumps at the points $t_1, t_2, \ldots$, respectively. The process Z_t, defined as the difference and sum of the jumps

$$Z_t = Y_t - \sum_j S_j I_{[t_j,\infty)}(t),$$

where I_B is set indicator function, is also a nondecreasing a.s. process with independent increments. Moreover, Z_t does not contain the points of discontinuity and, therefore, has infinitely dividable distribution, satisfying the expression

$$\ln E\left[\mathrm{e}^{-\theta Z_t}\right] = -\theta b(t) + \int_0^\infty \left(\mathrm{e}^{-\theta} - 1\right) dN_t(z),$$

where $b(t)$ is a nondecreasing continuous function which tends to zero as $t \to -\infty$, N_t is a continuous Levy's metric [138].

The main result of [67] is that, if $x_1, \ldots, x_n$ is a sample of censored values of a random variable of the distribution $F(t)$ which, in essence, is an NR-process, then the posterior distribution $F(t)$ is also neutral to the right. Suppose that X is a univariate sample from $F(t)$. Then the posterior distribution $F(t)$ for $X = x$ is neutral to the right. The posterior increment of the process $Y(t)$ for $t > x$ coincides with a prior one, and a prior distribution of increments of the process Y_t to the left of x can be obtained by multiplying the prior distribution by e^{-y}. Thus, if $h(y)$ is a prior distribution density of the increment $Y = Y_t - Y_s$ for $s < t < x$, then the posterior distribution density $\hbar(y)$ for $X = x$ has the form

$$\hbar(y \mid x) \sim \mathrm{e}^{-y} h(y).$$

To find the posterior distribution of the process increment at the point x, Doksum [67] introduces the process $Y_t^- = \lim_{s \to t-0} Y_s$, which is continuous to the left a.s. and also has independent increments. With the help of this process, the jump at the point may be written as $S = Y_x - Y_x^-$. In spite of the simplicity of the representation of S, we cannot write the posterior distribution of the jump at the point x for each case. Its density we denote by $\hbar_X(s \mid x)$. If x is a point of discontinuity fixed a priori with a p.d.f. of a jump $h_X(s)$, then $\hbar_X(s \mid x) \sim (1 - \mathrm{e}^s) h_X(s)$.

The work by Ferguson and Phadia [83] is devoted to the generalization of the work by Doksum for the case of censored samples and touches upon question of construction of the general theory of NR-processes. The censoring, considered in [83], has the following difficulties: 1) the times of censoring are not random; 2) the authors distinguish two types of nonrandom censoring: including the censoring, satisfying the condition that $X \geqslant x$, and excluding censoring for which $X > x$. The posterior distribution $F(t)$ for the given types of censoring is determined from the following theorem [83].

Theorem 4.2. *Let $F(t)$ be a NR-random distribution function, x be a random sample of volume 1, x is a real number. Then*

a) *the posterior distribution F under the condition $X > x$ is neutral to the right, the posterior distribution of increments of the process Y_t to the right of x coincides with a prior one, and $Y = Y_t - Y_s$ for $s \leqslant t \leqslant x$ satisfies the relation $\hbar(y \mid x) \sim e^{-y}h(y)$;*
b) *the posterior distribution F under the condition $X \geqslant x$ is neutral to the right, the posterior distribution of the process Y_t to the right of x or at the point x coincides with a prior one, and $Y = Y_t - Y_s$ for $s < t < x$ satisfies the relation $\hbar(y \mid x) \sim e^{-y}h(y)$.*

The case of a censored sample will be simpler in view of Theorem 4.2.1, since it doesn't require individual consideration of a prior distribution of the jump.
The Bayes estimate of $F(t)$ is sought for the quadratic loss function andappears to be a mean value of $F(t)$. In accordance with definition (4.47),

$$F^*(t) = E[F(t)] = 1 - E\left[e^{-Y_t}\right] = 1 - M_t(1), \tag{4.47}$$

where $M_t(1)$ is the value of a moment-generating function $M_t(\theta) = E\left[e^{-\theta Y_t}\right]$ at the point $\theta = 1$. Now, suppose that $x_1,\ldots,x_n$ is a sample and $u_1,\ldots,u_k$ is a sequence of elements of a sample distinct from one another, ordered so that $u_1 < u_2 < \cdots < u_k$. Denote by $\delta_1,\ldots,\delta_k$ the numbers of noncensored observations, by $v_1,\ldots,v_k$ which are the numbers of exceptionally censored values, and $\mu_1,\ldots,\mu_k$ are the numbers of inclusively censored values of a sample. The family of vectors $u = (u_1,\ldots,u_k)$, $\delta = (\delta_1,\ldots,\delta_k)$, $v = (v_1,\ldots,v_k)$ and $\mu = (\mu_1,\ldots,\mu_k)$ generate a testing statistic denoted by k. The quantity

$$\omega_j = \sum_{i=j+1}^{k} (\delta_i + v_i + \mu_i)$$

denotes the number of elements of the initial sample, exceeding u_j, and $j(t)$ is the number of elements u_i of the ordered sample which are less than or equal to t. We will also use the following notations: $M_t^-(\theta) = \lim_{s\to t_0} M_s(\theta)$ moment-generating function Y_t^-, $h_u(s)$ and $\hbar u(s \mid u)$, respectively, the prior and the posterior p.d.f. of the jump $S = Y_t - Y_t^-$ at the point u under the condition $X = u$. The main result of the work [83] is the expression for the posterior moment-generating function of the process Y_t:

$$M_t(\theta \mid K) = \frac{M_t\left(\theta + \omega_{j(t)}\right)}{M_t\left(\omega_{j(t)}\right)} + \prod_{i=1}^{j(t)} \left[\frac{M_{u_i}^-(\theta + \omega_{i-1})}{M_{u_i}^-(\omega_{i-1})}\right] \cdot \frac{C_{u_i}(\theta + \omega_i + v_i, \delta_i)}{C_{u_i}(\omega_i + v_i, \delta)} \cdot \frac{M_{u_i}(\omega_i)}{M_{u_i}(\theta + \omega_i)}. \tag{4.48}$$

The function $C_u(\alpha, \beta)$ in (4.49) is defined as

(i) if u is a priori fixed point of discontinuity of the process Y_t, then

$$C_u(\alpha,\beta) = \int_0^{\infty} e^{\alpha s}\left(1-e^{-s}\right)^{\beta}\hbar_u(s)ds;$$

(ii) if u is not a priori fixed point of discontinuity, then

$$C_u(\alpha,\beta) = \int_0^{\infty} e^{-\alpha s}\left(1-e^{-s}\right)^{\beta-1}\hbar(s \mid u)ds$$

for $\beta \geqslant 1$ and $C = 0$ for $\beta = 0$.

The expression (4.49) enables us to find the Bayes estimate of $F(t)$ and the estimate of any of its linear transformations. Let us write, in addition, the expression for the Bayes TTF estimate $R(t) = 1 - F(t)$, assuming that $t \in \mathbf{R}^+$. To simplify the expression of $M_t(1)$, we introduce (see [83]) the functions

$$m_t(\omega) = \frac{M_t(\omega+1)}{M_t(\omega)} \quad \text{and} \quad r_u(\alpha,\beta) = \frac{C_u(\alpha+1,\beta)}{C_u(\alpha,\beta)}.$$

Then

$$\hat{R}^*(t) = E[R(t) \mid K] = M_t(1 \mid K) = m_t(\omega_j(t)) \prod_{i=1}^{j(t)} \frac{m_{u_i}(\omega_i - 1)}{m_{u_i}(\omega_i)} \tau_{u_i}(\omega_i - v_i, \delta_i). \tag{4.49}$$

Obtaining a prior density of the jump $h_u(s)$ at the point u for a single observation $h_u(s)$ represents a significant difficulty for evaluation of the estimate (4.50). There is a subclass of NR-processes for which the problem solution is simplified. As an example we consider the so-called uniform processes, having the property that the increment of the process $Y_t = -\ln(1 - F(t))$ has the Levy's function, which is independent of t. This means that moment generating function of the process $Y(t)$ has the form

$$M_t(\theta) = \exp\left[\gamma(t)\int_0^{\infty}\left(e^{-\theta z} - 1\right)dN(z)\right], \tag{4.50}$$

where $N(\cdot)$ is the Levy's metric on $(0,\infty)$, for which

$$\int_0^{\infty} z(1+2)^{-1}dN(z) < \infty,$$

and $\gamma(t)$ is a nondecreasing function, where $\lim_{t\to-\infty}\gamma(t) = 0$, $\lim_{t\to\infty}\gamma(t) = \infty$.
For the uniform NR-process, a prior p.d.f. of the jump of the process $Y(t)$ at the point x, under the condition that one observation $X = x$ appears, is independent of the value x and can be represented in the form

$$\hbar(s \mid x)ds \sim \left(-e^{-z}\right)dN(s). \tag{4.51}$$

We can easily write with the help of (4.52) under the given Levy's metric the Bayes TTF estimate of $R^*(t)$. If one introduces the function

$$\phi(\alpha,\beta,N) = \begin{cases} \int_0^{\infty} e^{\alpha z}(1-e^{-z})^{\beta}dN(z), & \beta \geqslant 1, \\ 1, & \beta = 0, \end{cases} \tag{4.52}$$

then the functions $C_u(\alpha,\beta)$, $m_t(\Omega)$, $r_u(\alpha,\beta)$, appearing in (4.50), may be rewritten in the form:

$$C_u(\alpha,\beta) = \begin{cases} \dfrac{\phi(\alpha,\beta,N)}{\phi(0,1,N)} & \beta \geqslant 1, \\ 1, & \beta = 0, \end{cases}$$

$$m_t(\Omega) = \exp\left[-\gamma(t)\phi(\omega,1,N)\right], \tag{4.53}$$

and

$$r_u(\alpha,\beta) = \frac{\phi(\alpha+1,\beta,N)}{\phi(\alpha,\beta,N)}, \tag{4.54}$$

We give below some examples of nonparametric Bayes estimates for two special types of NR-processes.

Example 4.5 (Gamma-process). If independent increments of the process Y_t are-distributed, the process Y_t is called a gamma process. A moment-generating function of a gamma-process can be written in one of the following three ways:

$$\begin{aligned} M_t(\theta) &= \frac{\tau^{\gamma(t)}}{\Gamma(\gamma(t))}\int_0^\infty e^{-\theta y}\cdots e^{-ry}\cdots y^{\gamma(t-1)}dy \\ &= \left(\frac{\tau}{\tau+\theta}\right)^{\gamma(t)} = \exp\left[\gamma(t)\int_0^\infty (e^{-\theta z}-1)e^{-\tau z}z^{-1}dz\right]. \end{aligned} \tag{4.55}$$

A gamma process has a parameter of a $\gamma(t)$ and a parameter of the inverse scale (or intensity) τ independent of t. Using (4.51) and (4.56) for the Levy's metric, we can write

$$dN(z) = e^{-\tau z}z^{-1}dz.$$

Thus, for the gamma-process the function (4.53) takes the form

$$\phi(\alpha,\beta,n) \equiv \phi_\Gamma(\alpha,\beta) = \begin{cases} \displaystyle\int_0^\infty e^{-\alpha z}(1-e^{-z})^\beta z^{-1}dz, & \beta \geqslant 1, \\ 1, & \beta = 0. \end{cases} \tag{4.56}$$

Since β is integer, $\phi_\Gamma(\alpha,\beta)$ can be written in its final form using the binomial formula, and after integration becomes

$$\phi_\Gamma(\alpha,\beta)\sum_{i=0}^{\beta-1}\binom{\beta-1}{i}(-1)^i\ln\left(\frac{\alpha+i+1}{\alpha+i}\right). \tag{4.57}$$

With the help of (4.50) we can obtain the Bayes estimate of TTF for a prior uniform gamma-process:

$$\hat{R}^*(t) = \left(\frac{\omega_{j(t)}+\tau}{\omega_{j(t)}+\tau+1}\right)^{\gamma(t)}\prod_{i=1}^{j(t)}\left\{\left[\frac{(\omega_{i-1}+\tau)(\omega_i+\tau+1)}{(\omega_{i-1}+\tau+1)(\omega_i+\tau)}\right]^{\gamma(u_i)}\frac{\phi_\Gamma(\omega_i+v_i+\tau+1,\delta_i)}{\phi_\Gamma(\omega_i+v_i+\tau,\delta_i)}\right\}. \tag{4.58}$$

It is interesting that the Dirichlet processes, considered above, $\alpha(\mathbf{R}^1)$ has a simple form, and a metric $\alpha(\cdot)$ is represented with the help of the a priori representation of the cumulative distribution function. In [83] Ferguson and Phadia investigate an analogous question for the gamma-processes. Suppose $R_0(t)$ is the a priori information about TTF $R(t)$. In accordance with (4.56), the parameters τ and $\gamma(t)$ must satisfy the condition $\tau/(\tau+1)^{\gamma(t)} = R_0(t)$. Hence it follows, that for any t, lying in the domain of definition of the function $\gamma(t)$, with a fixed τ, is

$$\gamma(t) = \frac{\ln R_0(t)}{\ln[\tau/(\tau+1)]}. \tag{4.59}$$

The parameter τ may be interpreted as a measure of certainty of a priori information. To understand this interpretation it suffices to consider $\hat{R}^*(t)$ for a single censored observation. For $n = 1$ and using (4.49) we obtain

$$\hat{R}^*(t) = E[R(t) \mid X = x] = \begin{cases} R_0(t)^{\ell(\tau)}, & t < x, \\ R_0(t)R_0(x)^{\ell(\tau)-1}\ell(\tau), & t \geqslant x, \end{cases} \tag{4.60}$$

where

$$\ell(\tau) = \frac{\ln[(\tau+2)/(\tau+1)]}{\ln[(\tau+1)/\tau]}.$$

The function $\ell(\tau)$ is monotonic, where, as $\tau \to \infty$ we have $\ell(\tau) \to 0$, and as $\tau \to \infty$, $\ell(\tau) \to 1$. As seen from (4.60), for large τ, $\ell(\tau)$ is near to 1, and the estimate $\hat{R}^*(t)$ is near to $R_0(t)$. For small τ, a prior form of TTF $R_0(t)$ is changed substantially. To this end, it is interesting to consider the behavior of the estimate as $\tau \to 0$, i.e., when we have no a priori information. Recall that a Bayes estimate based on Dirichlet processes under similar conditions tends to the estimate of maximum likelihood. In [83] this question is investigated in conformity with a noncensored sample for $v_i = 0$, $\delta_i = 1$, and $\omega_i = n - i$ for all $i = 1, 2, \ldots, n$. The parameter $\gamma(t)$ is chosen in accordance with (4.60). From the expression (4.61) putting $\tau \to 0$ one has

$$E[R(t) \mid K] \to \frac{\ln[(n+1)n]}{\ln[(n-j(t)+1)/(n-j(t))]}. \tag{4.61}$$

This limit coincides with the maximum likelihood estimate.

Example 4.6 (A simple uniform process). This process was artificially chosen by Ferguson to avoid the shortage of a gamma-process. A moment-generating function for the considered process has the form

$$M_t(\theta) = \exp\left[\gamma(t)\int_0^\infty (\mathrm{e}^{-\theta z}-1)\mathrm{e}^{-\tau z}(1-\mathrm{e}^{-z})^{-1}dz\right]. \tag{4.62}$$

The Levy's metric is written as

$$dN(z) = \mathrm{e}^{-\tau z}\left(1-\mathrm{e}^{-z}\right)^{-1} dz. \tag{4.63}$$

A priori information for TTF $R_0(t)$ allows us to write

$$\gamma(t) = -\tau \ln R_0(t), \tag{4.64}$$

where the parameter τ as before, can be interpreted as the degree of certainty in the prior information as given above, has a sense of certainty in a prior information. Using (4.65), we obtain the final expression of TTF given by

$$\hat{R}^*(t) = E[R(t) \mid K] = \left[R_0(t)\right]^{\frac{\tau}{\omega_{j(t)}+\tau}} \prod_{i=1}^{j(t)} \left\{ \left[R_0(u_i)\right]^{-\frac{\tau(\omega_{i-1}-\omega_i)}{(\omega_{i-1}+\tau)(\omega_i+\tau)}} \cdot \frac{\omega_i+\nu_i+\tau}{\omega_i+\nu_i+\delta_i+\tau} \right\}. \tag{4.65}$$

As $t \to 0$

$$\hat{R}^*(t) = \begin{cases} \displaystyle\prod_{i=1}^{j(t)} \frac{\omega_i+\nu_i}{\omega_i+\nu_i+\delta_i}, & t < u_K, \\ \displaystyle\frac{R_0(t)}{R_0(u_K)} \prod_{i=1}^{k} \frac{\omega_i+\nu_i}{\omega_i+\nu_i+\delta_i}, & t \geqslant u_K, \end{cases} \tag{4.66}$$

coinciding with the maximum likelihood estimate. In particular, if the including censoring is absent; the estimate (4.67) is a Kaplan–Meier estimate.

The work by Kalbfleisch [118], touching upon the Bayes analysis of the Koks reliability model, contains important results devoted to the practical use of NR-processes. The model is represented by the relation

$$R(t) = P\{\xi > t \mid z\} = \exp\left[-\Delta(t)\exp(z\beta)\right], \tag{4.67}$$

where $z = (z_1, z_2, \ldots, z_n)$ is a vector of parameters of the system, $\beta = (\beta_1, \beta_2, \ldots, \beta_p)'$ is a vector of regression coefficients, and $\Lambda(t)$ is a resource function as defined earlier. The problem is to estimate TTF of the form (4.68), starting from some a priori information about the distribution of the random variable ξ and results of the experiment, $(t_1, z^{(1)}), (t_2, z^{(2)}), \ldots, (t_n, z^{(n)})$, where $z^{(j)}$ is a realization of the vector z in the j-th test. The problem is solved in the following manner:

(i) Starting with the a priori information, one chooses a prior estimate of the resource function $\Lambda_0(t)$;

(ii) For the chosen estimate of $\Lambda_0(t)$, one finds the estimates of the regression coefficients of the model (4.68);

(iii) Given vector β the posterior estimate of the resource function $\Lambda^*(t)$ is found.

The final expression for the TTF estimate is found by substitution of $\Lambda(t)$ and the estimates of the regression coefficients into (4.68).

To obtain the Bayes estimate of the resource function, we assume that $\Lambda(t)$ is a stochastic process which we can study with the help of the following model. The positive semi-axis is divided into k nonintersecting segments $[\alpha_0, \alpha_1)$, $[\alpha_1, \alpha_2), \ldots, [\alpha_{k-1}, \alpha_k)$, where $\alpha_0 = 0$, $\alpha_k = \infty$. For each segment one introduces a conditional probability

$$q_i = P\{\xi \in [\alpha_{i-1}, \alpha_i) \mid \xi \geqslant \alpha_{i-1}\Lambda\}, \tag{4.68}$$

if $P\{\xi \geqslant \alpha_{i-1} \mid \Lambda\} > 0$, and otherwise $q_i = 1$. It follows from (4.69) that $\Lambda(\alpha_0) = 0$ and

$$\Lambda(\alpha_i) = \sum_{j=1}^{i} -\ln(1-q_j) = \sum_{j=1}^{i} r_j, \quad i = 1, \ldots, k.$$

It is assumed further that $\Lambda(t)$ is a nondecreasing process with independent increments. Under this assumption we conclude that random variables $q_1, \ldots, q_k$ have independent prior distributions, and the stochastic process generated by $q_1, \ldots, q_k$ is NR-process. In order to describe the stochastic process $\Lambda(t)$, it is necessary to determine the distribution for the increments $\tau_i = -\ln(1-q_i)$, $i = 1, 2, \ldots, k$. In the work [118] it is assumed that $\tau_1, \ldots, \tau_k$ have independent gamma-distributions

$$\tau_i \sim \Gamma(\alpha_i - \alpha_{i-1}, c), \tag{4.69}$$

where c is some constant, and parameters α_i are determined with the help of a resource function chosen in a specific way. The parameters c and $\Lambda_0(t)$have the following simple interpretation. If one considers a partition $(0,t)$, $[t,\infty)$, then from (4.70) it follows that $\Lambda(t) \sim \Gamma(c\Lambda_0(t), c)$ and $E[\Lambda(t)] = \Lambda_0(0)$, $D[\Lambda(t)] = \Lambda_0(t)/c$. Thus, $\Lambda_0(t)$ has, in essence, a priori information about the resource function and c is a quantity characterizing the degree of significance of this a priori information.

The estimates of the regression coefficients are found with the help of the maximum likelihood method using the following scheme. For the sample $(t_1, z^{(1)}), \ldots, (t_n, z^{(n)})$, the distribution is written as

$$P\{\xi_1 \geqslant t_1, \ldots, \xi_n \geqslant t_n \mid \beta, \underset{\sim}{z}, \Lambda\} = \exp\left\{-\sum_{i=1}^{n} \Lambda(t_i) \exp\left(z^{(i)}\beta\right)\right\}, \tag{4.70}$$

which is conditional with respect to the stochastic process $\Lambda(t)$. We denote by $\underset{\sim}{z}$ a $p \times n$-dimensional matrix with the outcomes of n tests. Clearly, for obtaining an estimate on β we require that the distribution (4.71) be independent of $\Lambda(t)$. This is achieved with the assumption that

$$r_i = \Lambda(t_i) - \Lambda(t_{i-1}) \sim \Gamma(c\Lambda_0(t_i) - c\Lambda_0(t_{i-1}), c), \quad i = 1, 2, \ldots, n+1,$$

where, without loss of generality, $t_1 \leqslant t_2 \leqslant \cdots \leqslant t_n$ and $t_0 = 0$, $t_{n+1} = \infty$. Here we use t_i instead of α_i and apply the above reasoning. Since $\Lambda(t_i) = \sum_{j=1}^{i} r_j$, the distribution (4.71) is rewritten in the following form:

$$P\left\{\xi_1 \geqslant t_1, \ldots, \xi_n \geqslant t_n \mid \beta, \underset{\sim}{z}, r_1, \ldots, r_{n+1}\right\} = \exp\left(-\sum_{j=1}^{n} r_j A_j\right), \tag{4.71}$$

where

$$A_j = \sum_{\ell=j}^{n} \exp\left(z^{\ell}\beta\right), \quad j = 1, 2, \ldots, n.$$

Integration of (4.71) over multivariate gamma-distribution (4.72) yields

$$P\left\{\xi_1 \geqslant t_1, \ldots, \xi_n \geqslant t_n \mid \beta, \underset{\sim}{z}\right\} = \exp\left(-\sum_{j=1}^{n} cB_j\Lambda_0(t_j)\right), \tag{4.72}$$

where

$$B_j = -\ln\left[1 - \exp\left(z^{(j)}\beta\right)/(c + A_j)\right].$$

The expression (4.73) is valid for any $\Lambda_0(t)$, discrete or continuous. If we assume that $\Lambda_0(t)$ is continuous and there are no samples of coinciding elements, then, by differentiation of (4.73), we may obtain a p.d.f., interpreted as a likelihood function $\ell(\beta)$. In the final form the function $\ell(\beta)$ is represented by the expression [118]

$$\ell(\beta) = c^n \exp\left[-\sum_{j=1}^{n} cB_j\Lambda_0(t_j)\right] \prod_{i=1}^{n} \lambda_0(t_i)B_i \tag{4.73}$$

where $\lambda_0(t) = \lambda'(t)$.

Further, the maximum likelihood estimate β_*, obtained by minimization of the function (4.74), is used for obtaining a prior Bayes estimate $\Lambda^*(t)$. This estimate is defined in [118] with the help of the property of conjugacy of a gamma-distribution, according to which the quantities $r_1, r_2, \ldots, r_k$ have as independent prior the gamma-distributions. We consider first the case of the univariate sample; thereafter, we shall give the generalization for the case of arbitrary n. The final result of [118] is contained in the following theorem.

Theorem 4.3. *If a sample $\tau = (t_1, t_2, \ldots, t_n)$ does not contain the same values and $t_1 < t_2 < \cdots < t_n$, then for $t \in [t_{i-1}, t_i)$ the posterior distribution $\Lambda(t)$ coincides with the distribution of the sum of the random variables*

$$X_1 + U_1 + \cdots + X_{i-1} + U_{i-1} + \delta_i,$$

where

$$X_j \sim \Gamma\left[c\Lambda_0(t_{j-1}) - c\Lambda_0(t_j), c + A_j\right],$$
$$\delta_i \sim \Gamma\left[c\Lambda_0(t_{j-1}) - c\Lambda_0(t_{j-1}), c + A_i\right],$$

and

$$U_j \sim U(c+A_j, c+A_{j+1}).$$

The last distribution $U(a,b)$ has the following density function:

$$f(u) = \frac{\exp(-bu)-\exp(-au)}{u\ln(a/b)}.$$

If one uses a quadratic loss function for obtaining a prior estimate of the resource function, the resulting expression will be

$$\hat{\Lambda}^*(t) = E\left[\Lambda(t) \mid \tau, \underset{\sim}{z}, \beta_*\right] \sum_{j=1}^{i-1} (E(X_j)+E(U_j))+E(\delta_j),$$

where $E(X_j)$ and $E(\Delta_i)$ are the expected values of the random variables having, respectively, gamma-distributions, and for $E(U_j)$ the following relation holds:

$$E(U_j) = \frac{\exp\left(z^{(j)}\beta\right)}{(c+A_j)(c+A_{j+1})} \ln\frac{c+A_{j+1}}{c+A_j}.$$

For small c that corresponds to the case of absence of a priori information, the values $E(X_j)$ and $E(\Delta_i)$ are near zero, and $\hat{\Lambda}^*(t)$ is almost like a maximum likelihood estimate.

Generalized gamma-processes

Dykstra and Loud [70] solve a problem of estimating TTF by an alternative construction of gamma-processes which are not neutral to the right. A prior distribution, proposed in [70], is absolutely-continuous and cannot, therefore, be reduced to prior distributions by Ferguson and Doksum, as mentioned above.

The method of construction of nonparametric Bayes estimate of TTF they have proposed is based on the so-called *generalized gamma-processes (GG-processes),* defined in the following manner. Suppose the parameters of the gamma-distribution $\Gamma(\alpha,\beta)$ with density

$$g(t;\alpha,\beta) = t^{\alpha-1}\exp\left(\frac{t}{\beta}\right)\frac{I_{(0,\infty)}(t)}{\Gamma(\alpha)\beta^{\alpha}}$$

are functions of t. In addition, $\alpha(t) > 0$ ($t \geqslant 0$) is a nondecreasing left continuous real-valued function, having a left-hand limit at the point 0. By $Z(t)$ we denote a gamma-process having independent increments with respect to $\alpha(t)$. For any two points the increment $Z(t)-Z(s)$ is independent of the process increment on the other interval, nonintersecting with $[s,t]$, and obeys a gamma-distribution $\Gamma(\alpha(t)-\alpha(s),1)$. In addition to this, $Z(0)=0$. Ferguson [80] proves the existence of such a process.

Definition 4.4 (Definition of GG-process). Let a process $Z(t)$ have nondecreasing continuous left-continuous sample trajectories. Then a stochastic process

$$\lambda(t) = \int_0^t \beta(x)\, dZ(x), \tag{4.74}$$

where $\beta(x)$ is a positive right-continuous real-valued function, having a right-hand limit at the point $x = 0$ and integration carried out over the sample trajectories, is called a generalized gamma-process $\Gamma(\alpha(\cdot), \beta(\cdot))$.

The stochastic process (4.75) may be used to describe a random failure rate function. With the help of (4.75) one can write a random cumulative distribution function in the form

$$F(t) = 1 - \exp\left[-\int_0^t \lambda(x)dx\right]. \tag{4.75}$$

We compare this construction with the theory of NR-processes by Ferguson and Doksum. In accordance with the c.d.f., $F(t)$ is neutral to the right if $\Lambda(t)$ has independent increments. It is easy to see that the intensity function (4.75) is a process with independent increments, consequently $\Lambda(t)$ doesn'thave independent increments, and $F(t)$ is not NR-process.
It is proved in [70] that the characteristic function for $\lambda(t)$ in some neighborhood of the origin has the form

$$\psi_{\lambda(t)}(\theta) = \exp\left\{-\int_0^t \ln\left[1 - i\beta(s)\theta\right] d\alpha(s)\right\},$$

hence the following formulas are valid for a mean value and variance:

$$E[\lambda(t)] = \int_0^t \beta(s)d\alpha(s), \quad D[\lambda(t)] = \int_0^t \beta^2(s)d\alpha(s). \tag{4.76}$$

Using the representation of a failure rate with the help of GG-process, one can write the conditional distribution of a sample of size n in the form

$$P\{\xi_1 \geqslant t_1, \ldots, \xi_n \geqslant t_n \mid \lambda(t)\} = \prod_{i=1}^{n} \exp\left[-\int_0^t \lambda(t)dt\right]. \tag{4.77}$$

We can obtain, using (4.78), a prior distribution of a random intensity $\lambda(t)$ for a given sample. Note that since the process $Z(t)$ has nondecreasing realizations, $\lambda(t)$, due to (4.75), is nondecreasing almost surely. Therefore, a priori information about the cumulative distribution function $F(t)$ should be sought in the class of non-failure rate distributions S_0.
A prior distribution for $\lambda(t)$ can be identified if the functions $\alpha(t)$ and $\beta(t)$ are given. These functions are determined by the expression (4.77) under the condition that both have a nondecreasing expected value $\mu(t)$ and a variance $\sigma^2(t)$ are given. The function $\mu(t)$, in essence, has a priori information about $\lambda(t)$, and the variance $\sigma(t)$ characterizes a measure

of uncertainty with respect to the value of a failure rate at each point t. Let us rewrite the relations (4.77) in the form

$$\mu(t) = \int_0^t \beta(s)\alpha'(s)ds, \quad \sigma^2(t) = \int_0^t \beta^2(s)\alpha'(s)ds,$$

and hence,

$$\beta(t) = \frac{d\sigma^2(t)}{dt} \Big/ \frac{d\mu(t)}{dt} \tag{4.78}$$

and

$$\frac{d\alpha(t)}{dt} = \left[\frac{d\mu(t)}{dt}\right]^2 \Big/ \frac{d\sigma^2(t)}{dt}. \tag{4.79}$$

The expressions (4.79) and (4.80) let us write a prior distribution $\Gamma(\alpha(t), \beta(t))$.

The following statements are proved in [70] for a prior distribution of a stochastic process $\lambda(t)$:

(i) If $\tau = (t_1, t_2, \ldots, t_k)$ is a completely censored sample, then $\Gamma(\alpha(\cdot), \beta(\cdot))$ appears to be a prior distribution $\lambda(t)$ under the given sample τ. where

$$\hat{\beta}(t) = \frac{\beta(t)}{1 + \beta(t) \sum_{i=1}^{k} (t_i - t)\chi(t_i - t)}. \tag{4.80}$$

(ii) If $\tau = (t_1^*, t_2^*, \ldots, t_d^*)$ is a noncensored sample, the a posteriori distribution $\lambda(t)$ under the given sample τ is a mix of generalized gamma-processes:

$$P\{\lambda(t \in B \mid \tau)\} = \frac{\int_0^{t_d^*} \cdots \int_0^{t_1^*} \prod_{i=1}^{d} \hat{\beta}(z_i) F\left(B; \Gamma\left(\alpha + \sum_{i=1}^{d} I_{z_i,\infty} \hat{\beta}(z_i)\right)\right) \prod_{i=1}^{d} d\left[\alpha + \sum_{j=i+1}^{d} I_{z_j,\infty}\right](z_i)}{\int_0^{t_d^*} \cdots \int_0^{t_1^*} \prod_{i=1}^{d} \hat{\beta}(z_i) \sum_{i=1}^{d} d\left[\alpha + \sum_{j=i+1}^{d} I_{z_j,\infty}\right](z_i)} \tag{4.81}$$

where $F(B;Q)$ denotes the probability of the event B for the stochastic process, distributed by the law Q, and integration is carried out from z_1 to z_2.

If one uses a quadratic loss function, then the posterior estimate of the failure rate $\lambda(t)$ is defined in the form of the posterior mean value. For the case when we deal with a completely censored sample, $\hat{\lambda}^*(t)$ appears to be a mean value corresponding to the distribution

$\Gamma(\alpha(t), \hat{\beta}(t))$, where $\hat{\beta}(t)$ is computed with the help of (4.81). For a noncensored sample, $\hat{\lambda}^*(t)$ is a mean value of the variable distributed by the law (4.82) and can be written as

$$\hat{\lambda}^*(t) = \frac{\int_0^{t_d^*} \cdots \int_0^{t_1^*} \int_0^{t} \prod_{i=0}^{d} d\left[\alpha + \sum_{j=i=1}^{d} I_{z_j,\infty}\right](z_i)}{\int_0^{t_d^*} \cdots \int_0^{t_1^*} \prod_{i=1}^{d} \hat{\beta}(z_i) \sum_{i=1}^{d} d\left[\alpha + \sum_{j=i+1}^{d} I_{z_j},\infty\right](z_i)}. \tag{4.82}$$

The censored data may be added if one computes $\hat{\lambda}^*(t)$ with the help of (4.83) and the estimate $\hat{\beta}$ calculated by the formula (4.81) both for censored and noncensored data.

Other approaches

We shall consider an interesting approach for the construction of a nonparametric Bayes TTF estimate proposed by Padgett and Wei [183] and not connected with the Ferguson approach. A prior distribution is defined with the help of a step stochastic process for a failure rate $\lambda(t)$: the function $\lambda(t)$ represents, by itself, a step process with constant jumps, equal to ε, at the points $T_1, T_2, \ldots$, which are the moments of the events of a Poisson process with intensity v. Such a representation of $\lambda(t)$ is connected with real physical interpretation: at random moments $T_1, T_2, \ldots$, a technical device is subjected to a negative effect, which increases the failure rate by a positive quantity ε, and jumps occur in accordance with a Poisson process. By virtue of our assumptions, one can write the expressions for the intensity function $\lambda(t)$ and resource function $\Lambda(t)$ in the following form

$$\lambda(t) = \varepsilon N(t) \tag{4.83}$$

and

$$\Lambda(t) = \varepsilon \sum_{i=1}^{N(t)} (t - T_i), \tag{4.84}$$

where $N(t)$ is the number of Poisson events that have appeared by the moment t. Thus, a prior distribution is defined with the help of the stochastic process $\lambda(t)$ on the parametric space θ determined by the set of all nondecreasing intensity functions. There are no additional assumptions about $F(t)$, except $F(t) \in S_0$. The process $R(t)$ is written with the help of $\lambda(t)$ as

$$R(t) = 1 - F(t) = \exp\left[-\int_0^t \lambda(x)dx\right] = \exp\left[-\varepsilon \sum_{i=1}^{N(t)} (t - T_i)\right]. \tag{4.85}$$

Note that the relation (4.86), under the chosen specification of $\lambda(t)$, gives the continuous representation for $F(t)$ consequently, the considered approach cannot be reduced to Ferguson and Doksum methods. In addition to this, we observe that the representation of a priori information has a simple, handy form: to find a prior process we need to know only two numbers: the height of a jump ε and the parameter of the intensity of a Poisson process ν.
The posterior probability measure $P_n(B)$ for $B \in \theta$ is defined by the Bayes theorem, written in the following form

$$P_n(B) = \frac{\int_B \ell(\varepsilon, \nu, \tau) dP_0}{\int_\Theta \ell(\varepsilon, \nu, \tau) dP_0}, \tag{4.86}$$

where $\ell(\varepsilon, \nu, \tau)$ is a likelihood function, generated by a sample τ. If τ is a noncensored sample, $\tau = (t_1^*, \ldots, t_d^*, t_1, \ldots, t_k)$, then for the likelihood function the following expression holds:

$$\ell(\varepsilon, \nu; \tau) = \prod_{i=1}^{d} \varepsilon N(t_i^*) \prod_{i=1}^{n} \exp\left[-\varepsilon \sum_{j=1}^{N(\tau_i)} (\tau_i - T_j)\right]. \tag{4.87}$$

If one uses a quadratic loss function, then the posterior mean value $\hat{R}^*(t)$, corresponding to the distribution (4.87), is the Bayes estimate and

$$\hat{R}^*(t) = E[R(t) \mid \tau] = \frac{\int_\Theta R(t) \ell(\varepsilon, \nu; \tau) dP_0}{\int_\Theta \ell(\varepsilon, \nu; \tau) dP_0} \tag{4.88}$$

in which $R(t)$ is defined by the expression (4.86), and $\ell(\varepsilon, \nu; \tau)$ is defined by the expression (4.88). The integrals appearing in (4.89) express, in essence, a fact of averaging of corresponding integrands over all possible values $N(\tau_1), \ldots, N(\tau_n)$, $T_1, \ldots, T_{N(\tau_n)}$. For example,

$$\int_\Theta \ell(\varepsilon, \nu; \tau) dP_0 = \int_\Theta \prod_{i=1}^{d} [\varepsilon N(t_i^*)] \exp\left[-\varepsilon \sum_{i=1}^{n} \sum_{j=1}^{N(\tau_i)} \varepsilon(\tau_i - T_j)\right]$$
$$\times dP\left\{N(\tau_1), \ldots, N(\tau_n), T_1, \ldots, T_{N(\tau_n)}\right\}. \tag{4.89}$$

To solve integrals of the type (4.90) requires special numerical algorithms. In [183] the authors represent one such algorithm. The problem may be solved only with computer tools. The numerical example demonstrates the possibility of practical use of the estimate (4.89) and its satisfactory quality.
An interesting nonparametric solution is given by Proschan and Singpurwalla [198-199]. They considered the problem of estimating the failure rate of a technical device using the results of forced tests and a priori information of a special form. It is assumed that a device is tested in k regimes, and each regime is associated with its own failure rate function $\lambda_j(t)$, where

$$\lambda_1(t) > \lambda_2(t) > \cdots > \lambda_k(t) > \lambda(t) \tag{4.90}$$

and $\lambda(t)$ is a failure rate corresponding to the device functioning in a normal regime. For obtaining Bayes estimates, the authors use the following stochastic process.

Let $N_j(t)$ be the number of devices being tested in j-regime at the moment t. The interval $[0,L]$ of possible testing periods is divided by the points $s_1, s_2, \ldots$, into equal subintervals of length Δ so that the number of all intervals $m = L/\Delta$. Also, let $n_{j,i}$ be the number of devices tested in a j-regime during the i-period; $d_{j,i}$ is the corresponding number of failures; $p_{j,i}$ is the probability of observing a failure for the device tested in j-regime during the i-period. The stochastic process we will use later is determined by the mean intensity in the interval $[s_i, s_i+\Delta]$:

$$\mu_{j,i} = \frac{p_{j,i}}{1 - \sum\limits_{\ell=1}^{i-1} p_{\ell,i}}, \qquad i = 1,2,\ldots,m; \;\; j = 1,2,\ldots,k, \tag{4.91}$$

which is a conditional probability of a failure by the time $s_i+\Delta$ under the condition that by the time s_i the device is functioning. It is assumed that each $\mu_{j,i}$ satisfies a beta-distribution $Be(\alpha,\beta_j)$ with a density given by

$$H_{j,i}(P) = h_{j,i}(p;\alpha,\beta_j) \sim p^{\alpha-1}(1-p)^{\beta_j-1};$$

moreover, the random variables $\mu_{j,i}$ are mutually independent. The set of all $\mu_{j,i}$ generates a Poisson process, defined on the parametric space, satisfying condition (4.91). The parameters α, $\beta_1, \beta_2, \ldots, \beta_k$ contain a priori information. To satisfy (4.91) it is necessary that $\mu_{j-1,i} > \mu_{i,i}$ almost surely for all $j = 2,3,\ldots,k$. This has been proven in [199] under the condition that $\beta_1 < \cdots < \beta_k$. This inequality symbolizes the difference in severity of testing.

The procedure for obtaining posterior distributions of conditional probabilities $\mu_{j,i}$ is based on the property of conjugacy of a beta-distribution in conformity to a specific sample plan which assumes that censoring is absent. It is proved in [198] that the posterior distribution of $\mu_{j,i}$ is a beta distribution for a given $N_{j,i}$ and $d_{j,i}$

$$\hbar_{j,i}(p \mid N,d) = \frac{\Gamma(\alpha^*_{j,i}+\beta^*_{j,i})}{\Gamma(\alpha^*_{j,i})\Gamma(\beta^*_{j,i})} p^{\alpha^*_{j,i-1}}(1-p)^{\beta^*_{j,i-1}}, \tag{4.92}$$

where $\alpha^*_{j,i} = \alpha + d^*_{j,i}$, $\beta^*_{j,i} = \beta_j + N_{j,i} - d_{j,i}$.

Now, if one uses a quadratic loss function to obtain the Bayes estimate $\mu_{j,i}$, this estimate takes on the form of the posterior mean value, corresponding to the distribution (4.93):

$$\mu^*_{j,i} = \frac{\alpha + d_{j,i}}{\alpha + \beta_j + N_{j,i}}. \tag{4.93}$$

The proposed approach characterizes, as a whole, the clearness of a logical construction and simplicity of the numerical algorithm. At the same time, we don't know, unfortunately, in what way the parameters α and β_i ($i = 1,\ldots,m$) should be chosen.

4.4 The nonparametric Bayes approach of quantile estimation for increasing failure rate

Obtaining statistical conclusions about the value of a quantile x of the level p for failure rate distributions is a matter of great interest in reliability theory:

$$x_p = \inf\{x : F(x) \geqslant p\} \tag{4.94}$$

In this section we'll consider a problem of obtaining the Bayes estimate for x_p assuming that $F(x)$ belongs to the class of failure rate distributions S_0. It is shown in [14] that for the approximation of failure rate c.d.f., it is customary to use a two-parametric family E_0 of exponential cumulative distribution functions of the following form:

$$F(t;\theta) = \chi(t-\mu)\left[1-\exp\left(-\frac{t-\mu}{m_0}\right)\right], \tag{4.95}$$

where μ is absolutely guaranteed time to-failure, $(\mu+m_0)$, a mean TTF, $\theta = (\mu+m_0)$. For this family, a p-level quantile has the form

$$x_p = \mu + m_0\Lambda_p, \quad \text{with } \Lambda_p = \ln\frac{1}{1-p}. \tag{4.96}$$

In the present case Belyaev [14], uses a Bayes estimate of the quantile x_p, obtained for the nonparametric family E_0, for the construction of the estimate of a similar quantile for $F(t) \in S_0$. It is carried out by the specification of a transformation $u_p : F \to F_0$ ($F \in S_0$, $F_0 \in E_0$) and by the foundation of a lower bound of a prior probability of the statement $\{x_p \geqslant x\}$ over all possible transformations u_p. The Bayes estimate x_p is constructed with the help of a sample $\tau = (t_1^*,\ldots,t_d^*,t_1,\ldots,t_k)$, obtained after the realization of the NC-plan. For the likelihood function $\ell(\theta \mid \tau) = \ell(\mu,m_0 \mid \tau)$ we use the expression (3.22), and in accordance with it,

$$\ell(\mu,m_0 \mid \tau) = c(\tau)\prod_{i=1}^{d}\chi(t_i^*-\mu)\frac{1}{m_0^d}\exp\left[-\frac{1}{m_0}\int_{\mu}^{\infty}N(t)dt\right],$$

where $N(t)$ is the number of devices tested at the time t, $c(\tau)$ is independent of μ, m_0. This expression may be simplified if one takes into account the relations

$$\prod_{i=1}^{d}\chi(t_i^*-\mu) = \chi(t_{(1)}^*-\mu),$$

where $t_{(1)}^* = \min(t_1^*,t_2^*,\ldots,t_d^*)$, and

$$\int_{\mu}^{\infty}N(t)dt = \int_{t_{(1)}}^{\infty}N(t)dt + \int_{\mu}^{t_{(1)}}N(t)dt = s(t_{(1)}^*) + s(\mu,t_{(1)}^*),$$

where, the statistics $s(t_{(1)}^*)$ and $s(\mu,t_{(1)}^*)$ have the total operating times during the testing period which lasts after the first failure $t_{(1)}^*$ has occurred during the interval $[\mu,t_{(1)}^*]$. If there are no failures, one should put $t^*_{(1)}$ equal to the period of testing t. The resulting expression for the likelihood function is

$$\ell(\theta \mid \tau) = c(\tau)\chi\left(t^*_{(1)} - \mu\right)\frac{1}{m_0^d}\exp\left[-\frac{s\left(t^*_{(1)}\right) + s\left(\mu, t^*_{(1)}\right)}{m_0}\right]. \tag{4.97}$$

A prior p.d.f. of the vector of parameters $\theta = (\mu, m_0)$ is represented in the form

$$h(\mu, m_0) = h(m_0)h(\mu \mid m_0), \tag{4.98}$$

where $h(m_0)$ is a prior p.d.f. of the parameter m_0, $h(\mu \mid m_0)$ is a priori conditional p.d.f. of the parameter μ under the condition the parameter m_0. If one uses a prior p.d.f. $h(\mu, m_0)$, conjugated with a likelihood kernel, then an expression for $h(m_0)$ and $h(\mu, m_0)$ takes on the form

$$h(m_0) = \frac{\left[1 - \exp\left(-\frac{ct_0}{m_0}\right)\right] s_0^{d_0-2}\exp\left(\frac{s_0}{m_0}\right)}{(d_0-3)!\left[1 - \left(\frac{s_0}{ct_0+s_0}\right)^{d_0-2}\right] m_0^{d_0-1}}, \tag{4.99}$$

and

$$h(\mu \mid m_0) = \frac{c\chi(t_0 - \mu)\exp\left[-\frac{c(t_0-\mu)}{m_0}\right]}{1 - \exp\left(-c\frac{t_0}{m_0}\right) m_0}. \tag{4.100}$$

A prior density, defined by the expressions (4.99)–(4.101), depends on four parameters: c, t_0, d_0, s_0. Applying the Bayes theorem and relations (4.98)–(4.101), we can obtain the multipliers of the posterior distribution density corresponding to $h(m_0)$ and $h(\mu \mid m_0)$:

$$\hbar(m_0, \tau) = \frac{\left\{1 - \exp\left[-\frac{s_1(0,r)}{m_0}\right]\right\} s_2(r)^{d_0+d-2}\exp\left[-\frac{s_2(r)}{m_0}\right]}{(d_0+d-3)!\left\{1 - \left[\frac{s_2(r)}{s_0(r)}\right]^{d_0+d-2}\right\} m_0^{d_0+d-1}} \tag{4.101}$$

and

$$\hbar(\mu \mid m_0, \tau) = \frac{c + N(\mu)}{m_0} \cdot \frac{\chi(r-\mu)\exp\left[-\frac{s_1(\mu,r)}{m_0}\right]}{1 - \exp\left[-\frac{s_1(0,r)}{m_0}\right]}, \tag{4.102}$$

where

$$r = \min\left\{t^*_{(1)}, t_0\right\}, \quad s_1(\mu, r) = \int_\mu^r [c + N(t)]dt,$$

$$s_2(r) = s_0 + s_1(r), \qquad s_1(r) \quad = c(t_0 - r) + s(r).$$

with help of (4.102) and (4.103) the posterior density of the vector of parameters $\theta = (\mu, m_0)$ is found analogously to a prior one (see (4.99)):

$$\hbar(\mu, m_0 \mid \tau) = \hbar(m_0 \mid \tau)\hbar(\mu \mid m_0, r).$$

If $F(t)$ is represented by the expression (4.96), then while the data is accumulated, the posterior distribution is concentrated in the neighborhood of the true values of the parameters μ, m_0. Accumulation of data corresponds to the union of testing outcomes over the set of tests, containing k NC-plans, as k increases infinitely.

With the help of a prior p.d.f. (4.100) and (4.101), a prior density of the quantile $x_p = \mu + m_0\Lambda_p$ is expressed in the following form:

$$h_p(x_p) = \int_G h(m_p \mid m_0)h(m_0)dm_0$$
$$= \frac{c(1-p)s_0^{d_0-2}(d_0-2)}{\left[1-\left(\frac{s_0}{s_0+ct}\right)^{d_0-2}\right]s_3^{d_0-1}} \left\{\ell_{d_0-2}\left(\Lambda_p\frac{s_3}{x_p}\right) - \chi(x_p-t_0)L_{d_0-2}\left(\Lambda_p\frac{s_3}{x_p-t_0}\right)\right\},$$

where $m_p = x_p - m_0\Lambda_p$, $s_3 = s_0 + c(t_0 - x_p)$, the integration interval $G = ((x_p - x_0)/\Lambda_p)^+$, x_p/Λ_p, and a^+ denotes that $a^+ = a$, if the symbol $a > 0$, $a^+ = 0$, if $a \leqslant 0$, $L_d(x) = \sum_{k=0}^{d} x^k e^{-x}/k!$.

For the posterior p.d.f. $\hbar_p(x_p \mid \tau)$ of the quantile values with the help of (4.102) and (4.103) one obtains analogously

$$\hbar_p(x_p \mid \tau) = K\int_{G'} \frac{c+N(m_p)}{m_0^{d_0+d}} \exp\left[-\frac{s_0+s_1(m_p)}{m_0}\right] dm_0, \tag{4.103}$$

where

$$K = \frac{s_2(r)^{d_0+d-2}}{\left\{1-\left[\frac{s_2(r)}{s_2(0)}\right]^{d_0+d-2}\right\}(d_0+d-3)!},$$

and the interval over which we integrate is

$$G' = \left[((x_p - r)/\Lambda_p)^+,\ x_p/\Lambda_p\right].$$

For practical convenience, we use the posterior p.d.f. (4.104) to represent the integral (4.104) in the finite form. To this end we present the following scheme: consider a variational raw $t_{(1)}, \ldots, t_{(\ell)}$, consisting of the values of censoring times which precede r. The time $t_{(i)}$ is associated with the finite increment of the integrand in (4.104). The set G' is divided into a sequence of intervals

$$\Delta_\ell = \left[\left(\frac{x_p - r}{\Lambda_p}\right)^+,\ \left(\frac{x_p - t_{(1)}}{\Lambda_p}\right)^+\right],$$

$$\Delta_i = \left[\left(\frac{x_p - t_{(i+1)}}{\Lambda_p}\right)^+,\ \left(\frac{x_p - t_{(i)}}{\Lambda_p}\right)^+\right], \quad i = 1, 2, \ldots, \ell - 1,$$

with

$$\Delta_0 = \left[\left(\frac{x_p - t_{(1)}}{\Lambda_p} \right)^+, \frac{x_p}{\Lambda_p} \right].$$

In the intervals Δ_i $(i = 0, 1, \ldots, \ell)$, the function $N(m_p)$ is constant. Suppose that at the censoring time $t_{(i)}$, N devices are taken out. Then $N_i = N - n_1 - \cdots - n_i$ is the number of devices which are still being tested after $t_{(i)}$. The constant values of the function $N(m_p)$ in the intervals Δ_i are written in the following form:

$$N(m_p) = \begin{cases} N & \text{if } m_0 \in \Delta_0, \\ N_i & \text{if } m_i \in \Delta_i, \end{cases}$$

whence it easily follows

$$s_1(m_p) = \begin{cases} (c+N)\big(t_{(1)} - m_p\big) + s_1\big(t_{(1)}\big), & m_0 \in \Delta_0, \\ (c+N_i)\big(t_{(i+1)} - m_p\big) + s_1\big(t_{(i+1)}\big), & m_0 \in \Delta_i, \quad i = 1, \ldots, \ell - 1, \\ (c+N_\ell)(r - m_p) + s_1(r), & m_0 \in \Delta_\ell. \end{cases}$$

The last expression lets us write

$$\begin{aligned} J(\Delta_i) &= \int_{m_0 \in \Delta_i} \frac{c + N(m_p)}{m_0^{d_0+d}} \exp\left[-\frac{s_0 + s_1(m_p)}{m_0} \right] dm_0 \\ &= c_i \left\{ \chi\big(x_p - t_{(i)}\big) L_{d_0+d-2}\left(\Lambda_p \frac{s_0(c+N_i)\big(t_{(i+1)} - x_p\big) + s_1\big(t_{(i+1)}\big)}{x_p - t_{(i+1)}} \right) \right\} \\ & \qquad i = 1, 2, \ldots, \ell - 1, \end{aligned} \tag{4.104}$$

where

$$c_i = \frac{(d_0 + d - 2)!(c + N_i)(1 - p)^{c+N_i}}{\big[s_0 + (c + N_i)\big(t_{(i+1)} - x_p\big) + s_1\big(t_{(i+1)}\big)\big]^{d_0+d-1}} \tag{4.105}$$

The integrals $J(\Delta_0)$ and $J(\Delta_\ell)$ are computed by the same formulas (4.105) and (4.106) in which one should put $N_i = N$, $t_{(i)} = 0$ for the first integral, and $N_i = N_\ell$, $t_{(i+1)} = r$ for the second one. The resulting expression for the posterior quantile $\hbar(x_p \mid \tau)$ takes on the form of a sum

$$\hbar_p(x_p \mid \tau) = \sum_{i=0}^{\ell} KJ(\Delta_i). \tag{4.106}$$

The number of terms in (4.107) may be less than $\ell + 1$, since some of the intervals Δ_i degenerate into a point.

The case corresponding to the situation when censoring is not carried out until the moment r ($t_{(1)} \geqslant r$) is the most simple for calculations. In this case the sum (4.107) consists of only one term, corresponding to $i = 0$. The posterior density of the quantile values has the form

$$\hbar_p(x_p \mid \tau) = W\left\{ L_{d_0+d-2}\left(\Lambda_p \frac{s_0 + (c+N)(r-x_0) + s_1(r)}{x_p}\right) - \chi(x_p - r)L_{d_0+d-2}\left(\Lambda_p \frac{s_0 + (c+N)(r-x_0) + s_1(r)}{x_p - r}\right)\right\} \quad (4.107)$$

where

$$W = \frac{s_2(r)^{d_0+d-2}(c+N)(1-p)^{c+N}(d_0+d-2)!}{\left[1-\frac{s_2(r)}{s_2(0)}\right]^{d_0+d-2}\left[s_0+(c+N)(r-x_p)+s_1(r)\right]^{d_0+d-1}}.$$

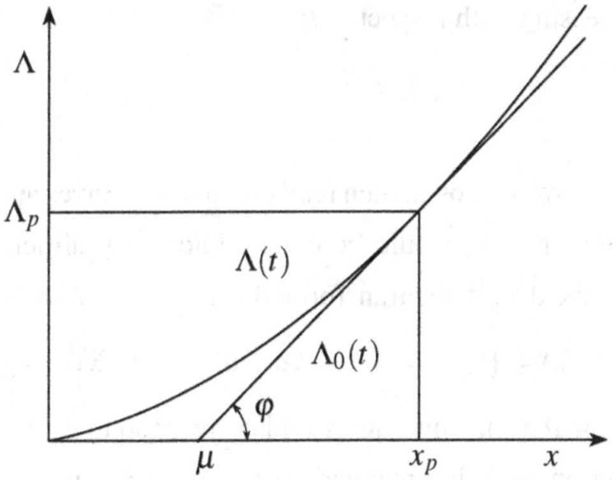

Fig. 4.1 Approximation of the resource function

The formula (4.108) may be used in tests which are conducted by the plans $[N, U, R]$, $[N, U, T]$, when N articles are being tested during the given time t, where the censoring is not carried out until the time t.

Consider now an approach which enables us to use the above cited results for the condition when $F(t)$ belongs to the class of failure rate distributions S_0. The problem is to make a statistical conclusion about the value of the quantile x_p with the help of a sample τ obtained while one is conductinga test by the NC-plan. To use the Bayes approach, we have to define a prior distribution on the class S_0 of all failure rate distribution functions. The method described below lets us, in some sense, bypass the difficulties of representation of a prior distribution.

Any c.d.f., $F(t) \in E_0$ is a failure rate, since $E_0 \in S_0$. Let us define the map $u_p : F(t) \to F_0(t)$, where $F(t) \in S_0$, $F_0(t) \in E_0$. To do this, we put $F_0(t) = F(t)$, if $F(t) \in E_0$. Provided that $F(t) \notin E_0$ we assign to it c.d.f., $F_0(t) \in E_0$, with

$$F_0(t) = 1 - \exp(-\Lambda_0(t)), \quad \Lambda_0(t) = \max\{0, \Lambda_p + \lambda_p(t - x_p)\}. \quad (4.108)$$

Here $\lambda_p = \tan\phi$ the minimal possible value of the slope of the tangent of the slope ϕ . to the graph of the resource function $\Lambda(t) = -\ln[1-F(t)]$at the point (x_p, Λ_p). The graph of the resource function $\Lambda_0(t)$ is a polygon line, containing the segment $[0,\mu]$ and the ray of the straight line outgoing from the point $(\mu,0)$ at the angle ϕ (Fig. 4.1). We can associate the map $u_p : F \to F_0$ with the function $u_p(t)$, such that

$$F(t) = F_0(u_p(t)).$$

As follows from (4.109) the function $u_p(t)$ possesses the following properties:

(i) $u_p(t)$ is nondecreasing with respect to t;

(ii) $u_p(t) \geqslant t, \forall t > 0$;

(iii) $x_p = u_p(x_p)$.

If the function $t' = u_p(t)$ were known, then realization of the Bayes approach to the problem of estimating of the quantile x_p would be done without any difficulties. To do this one should use, instead of the data τ, the transformed data

$$\tau(u_p) = \{v_i,\ i = 1,2,\dots,d;\ \omega_j,\ j = 1,2,\dots,k\}, \tag{4.109}$$

where $v_i = u_p(t_i^*)$, $\omega_j = u_p(t_j)$. This data would correspond to c.d.f. $F_0(t) \in E_0$.
Any prior distribution on So being mapped by $u_p : F \to F_0$ turns into the corresponding prior distribution on E_0. To simplify calculations, this distribution can be approximated by the distributions with p.d.f., represented by (4.100) and (4.101). Furthermore, we may use the calculations performed for the posterior p.d.f. $\hbar_p(x_p \mid \tau(u_p))$, since the values of the quantile x_p are the same for $F(t)$ and $F(t_0)$. We may find, using the posterior p.d.f. $\hbar_p(x_p \mid \tau(u_p))$, the posterior probability of the event $x_p \geqslant x$. This probability equals

$$P\{x_p \geqslant x \mid \tau(u_p)\} = \int_X^\infty \hbar_p(x_p \mid \tau(u_p))dx_p. \tag{4.110}$$

We cannot solve the problem defined above using only (4.111) because we don't know the mapping $u_p : F \to F_0$ which transforms the data T into the form (4.110). It is possible, however, to find the lower bound

$$P_0\{x_p \geqslant x \mid \tau\} = \inf P\{x_p \geqslant x \mid \tau(u_p)\}, \tag{4.111}$$

where inf is taken over the possible functions $u_p(t)$ possessing the properties (i)–(iii). It can be achieved by searching through all possible data $\tau(u_p)$ whose components v_i and ω_j satisfy the inequalities

$$v_i \geqslant t_i^*, \quad i = 1,2,\dots,d,$$

$$\omega_j \geqslant t_j, \quad j = 1,2,\dots,k.$$

Table 4.3 The lower estimate of the posterior probability of the statement $\{x_{0.01} \geqslant x\}$ [14].

x, h	65	90	100	110	120	130	140	150
$P\{x_p \geqslant x \mid \tau\}$	0.992	0.985	0.922	0.872	0.794	0.679	0.479	0.255
$P_0\{x_p \geqslant x \mid \tau\}$	0.991	0.956	0.921	0.855	0.741	0.527	0.232	0.064

The finding of inf in the problem (4.111) can be simplified substantially if censoring is not carried out until the first failure, $\ell = 0$. In this case, we compute $\hbar_p(x_p \mid \tau(u_p))$ using formula (4.108), and then inf in (4.111) is obtained by substituting $s_1(r)$ in (4.108) by $s \geqslant s_1(r)$.

The method of reducing a nonparametric problem to a parametric one, as described above, is called a method of concentration, since it is based on the idea of concentration of the prior distribution in the set $E_0 \subset S_0$.

We give a numerical example corresponding to the case $\ell = 0$ [14]. During the test a sample is obtained, containing 20 failure times, represented by the following ranked data set:

$$\{108.4, 120.8, 161.3, 172.4, 176.3, 177.3, 190.8, 267.8, 320.0, 331.5,$$

$$334.6, 337.1, 352.4, 371.1, 440.8, 467.9, 480.8, 508.9, 567.4, 569.9\} \text{ hours.}$$

In Table 4.3 we present the results of the calculations performed in accordance with the method of concentrations: the first row consists of the values of the posterior probability of the statement $\{x_p \geqslant x\}$, corresponding to the given set of parameters t_0, s_0, d_0 and c under the assumption $F(t) \in E_0$; the last row contains the values $P_0\{x_p \geqslant x \mid \tau\}$ corresponding to (4.111). Decreasing of values $P_0\{x_p \geqslant x \mid \tau\}$ in comparison with $P\{x_p \geqslant x \mid \tau\}$ will be significant for large values of x. It can be caused by the replacement of the family E_0 by the broader class of failure rate c.d.f., S_0.

The methods we've described above admit different generalizations. In particular, instead of the parametric family E_0, one can use $E_1 \in S_0$, defined by the relations

$$F_1(t) = 1 - e^{-\Lambda_1(t)},$$

where

$$\Lambda_1(t) = \begin{cases} \lambda_0(t), & t \leqslant x_p, \\ \lambda_1 t - (\lambda_1 - \lambda_0)x_p, & t > x_p, \quad \lambda_0 = \dfrac{\Lambda_p}{x_p}, \end{cases}$$

which define a two-parametric family of c.d.f. The mapping $u_p : F \to F_1 \in E_1$ may be associated with the function $u_p(t)$, having the properties $u_p(t) \leqslant t$ and $x_p = u_p(x_p)$. All further arguments will be the same.

Chapter 5

Quasi-Parametric Bayes Estimates of the TTF Probability

5.1 Parametric approximations for a class of distributions with increasing failure rate

A quasiparametric Bayes estimate plays the intermediate role between the parametric and nonparametric estimates in the following sense. Let $\{\Omega, \mathscr{L}, F\}$ be a sample space, characterizing a statistical model, generated by some plan P; a probability measure F (distribution) which belongs to some class S. A quasiparametric estimate of a time to failure probability r, connected functionally with F, is constructed in the following manner. Starting with given a priori information, the probability measure is approximated with the help of $\widetilde{F} \in S_\theta$, where S_θ is a parametric family chosen in accordance with the form of representation of a priori information, where $S_\theta \in S$. The parameter q is random and the space $\{\Theta, \mathscr{E}, \mathrm{H}\}$ where $H \in \mathrm{H}$ is a prior probability measure of the parameter θ on $(\Theta, \mathscr{E})$. The estimate of the probability of a TTF is sought in the form of the Bayes estimate of the corresponding function $R = R(\theta)$, measurable on θ. A specific Bayes procedure is determined by the form of a priori information and by the chosen approximation of c.d.f., F, on the class S. These estimates are proposed and investigated in the works [218, 219]. Consider some important aspects from a practical point-of-view, cases dealing with a construction of the approximation of the unknown c.d.f., $F(t)$, on the classes of failure rate S_θ or failure rate in mean S_1 distributions [9, 10]. Throughout what follows we will use a representation of the approximation distribution function with the help of the resource function:

$$F(t) \approx \widetilde{F}(t;\theta) = 1 - \exp\left[-\widetilde{\Lambda}(t;\theta)\right] \tag{5.1}$$

assuming that $\widetilde{\Lambda}(t)$ is an approximation of the genuine resource function $\Lambda(t)$ guaranteeing that the c.d.f. $\widetilde{F}(t,\theta)$ is in the class S_θ (or S_1).

5.1.1 *The case of a univariate prior distribution*

This case characterizes the situation when an engineer possesses some information about the device reliability at the fixed moment t_0, i.e., if a prior p.d.f., $h(r)$, is given for TTF $R_{t_0} = P\{\xi > t_0\}$ on the interval R_ℓ, R_u. In this particular case $h(r)$ can be uniform, and then it suffices to find the values R_ℓ, R_u to represent all a priori information.

Suppose, at first, that R_{t_0} is fixed, i.e., the interval R_ℓ, R_u degenerates into a point. Fin such an approximation $\widetilde{\Lambda}(t)$ such that: 1) the values of c.d.f., $F(t)$ and $\widetilde{F}(t)$ coincide, 2) the approximate c.d.f., $\widetilde{F}(t)$, belongs to the class of increasing failure rate distributions. In accordance with the first condition

$$\widetilde{\Lambda}(t_0) = \Lambda(t_0). \tag{5.2}$$

$\Lambda(t_0) = -\ln[1-F(t_0)] = -\ln R_{t_0}$, and the value R_{t_0}, by the assumption, is fixed. Represent the function in the form of a two linked polygonal line, satisfying the condition (5.2) (Figure 5.1) and write the equations for the links. Since the link $\ell_1(t)$ passes through the origin, its equation will be defined by a single parameter which we denote by Λ_0. The condition (5.2) implies

$$\ell_1(t) = \lambda_0(t), \quad t \leqslant t_0, \tag{5.3}$$

where

$$\lambda_0 = \frac{\Lambda(t_0)}{t_0} = \frac{1}{t_0}\ln R_{t_0}, \tag{5.4}$$

i.e., λ_0 is defined uniquely, if R_{t_0} is given. The equation for the link $\ell_2(t)$ depends on two parameters: the parameter λ_0 mentioned above and a new parameter λ_1. Then

$$\ell_2(t) = \lambda_1 t - (\lambda_1 - \lambda_0)t_0, \quad t > t_0 \tag{5.5}$$

Taking into account (5.3) and (5.5) we can represent the approximation of the resource function in the form

$$\widetilde{\Lambda}(t) = \widetilde{\Lambda}(t;\lambda_0,\lambda_1) = \begin{cases} \lambda_0 t, & 0 \leqslant t \leqslant t_0, \\ \lambda_1 t - (\lambda_1 - \lambda_0)t_0, & t > t_0, \end{cases}$$

or, if we use the sign function,

$$\widetilde{\Lambda}(t) = \chi(t_0 - t)\lambda_0 t + \chi(t - t_0)\left[\lambda_1 t - (\lambda_1 - \lambda_0)t_0\right]. \tag{5.6}$$

Note that the parameter λ_0 (given R_{t_0}) is defined uniquely by the relation (5.4). At the same time, for λ_1 we may find only the domain of admissible values. To this end we use the assumption about the approximation of the c.d.f. $\widetilde{F}(t)$, belongs to the class S_0 :

$$\widetilde{F}(t) = \widetilde{F}(t;\lambda_0,\lambda_1) = 1 - \exp\left[-\widetilde{\Lambda}(t;\lambda_0,\lambda)\right] \in S_0 \tag{5.7}$$

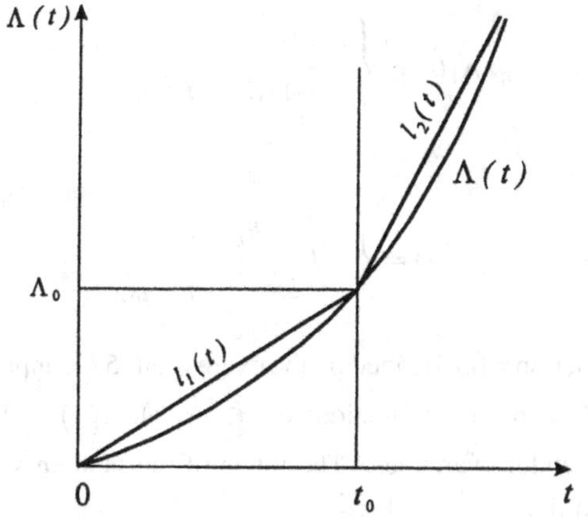

Fig. 5.1 Two-linked approximation of the resource function.

The condition (5.7) is equivalent to the statement that the resource function $\widetilde{\Lambda}(t)$ is concave [14], i.e.,

$$\widetilde{\Lambda}\left(\frac{t_1+t_2}{2}\right) \leqslant \frac{1}{2}\left[\widetilde{\Lambda}(t_1)+\widetilde{\Lambda}_2(t_2)\right] \quad \forall t_1 < t_2 \tag{5.8}$$

For the cases $t_1 < t_0$, $t_2 < t_0$ and, $t_1 > t_0$, $t_2 > t_0$ the condition (5.8) is filled for any λ_1. Let now $t_1 < t_0$, $t_2 > t_0$. For $t_1 + t_2 \leqslant 2t_0$ (for concave $\widetilde{\Lambda}(t)$) we have

$$\lambda_0(t_1+t_2) \leqslant \lambda_0 t_1 + \lambda_1 t_2 - (\lambda_1 - \lambda_0)t_0,$$

whence $\lambda_1 \geqslant \lambda_0$. For $t_1 + t_2 \geqslant 2t_0$ we obtain a similar result. Thus, the interval $[\lambda_0 \infty)$ appears to be the domain of values of the parameter λ_1 guaranteeing the fulfillment of' the condition (5.7).

The TTF value R_{t_0}, in general, is not fixed but appears to be random, in the Bayes sense, and lies in the interval $[R_\ell, R_u]$. Therefore, we will discuss not a usual approximation of a resource function, but a Bayes one in which the parameters λ_0 and λ_1 are random. The point is that the genuine resource function $\Lambda(t)$ is random and may take on one realization in some space, determined by the given a priori information. In our case this space is bounded by the curves $\Lambda_1(t)$ and $\Lambda_2(t)$ which also are random by themselves too. The fact that these curve pass respectively through the points (t_0, Λ_{02}) and (t_0, Λ_{01}), where $\Lambda_{02} = -\ln R_\ell$, $A_{01} = -\ln R_u$, is nonrandom accordingly the segment of a prior uncertainty. In the class S_0 the curves $\Lambda_1(t)$ and $\Lambda_2(t)$ are approximated by the following polygonal lines (see Fig 5.2):

$$\widetilde{\Lambda}_1(t) = \begin{cases} 0, & t \leqslant t_0, \\ -\dfrac{t}{t_0}\ln R_u, & t > t_0, \end{cases}$$

and

$$\widetilde{\Lambda}_2(t) = \begin{cases} -\dfrac{t}{t_0}\ln R_\ell, & t \leqslant t_0, \\ \infty, & t > t_0, \end{cases}$$

Thus, the resource function $\widetilde{\Lambda}(t)$, defined by the expression (5.6), approximates an arbitrary random realization of the resource function $\Lambda(t) \in \left[\widetilde{\Lambda}_1(t), \widetilde{\Lambda}_2(t)\right]$. The parameters λ_0 and λ_1 used in (5.6) are random variables. The range of the random variables λ_0 and λ_1 is defined by the inequalities

$$\lambda_0' \leqslant \lambda_0 \leqslant \lambda_0'', \quad \lambda_0 \leqslant \lambda_1 \leqslant \infty, \tag{5.9}$$

where $\lambda_0' = -\ln R_u/t_0$, $\lambda_0'' = -\ln R_\ell/t_0$, and the first inequality has been obtained from the condition $R_{t_0} \in [R_\ell, R_u]$, and the second one from the assumption $F(t) \in S_0$.

Define the domain D, having replaced in the above reasoning S_0 by a more general class S_1 of failure rate distributions. The leading property of the class S_1 is the property of the nondecreasing of the function $\eta(t) = \Lambda(t)/t$.

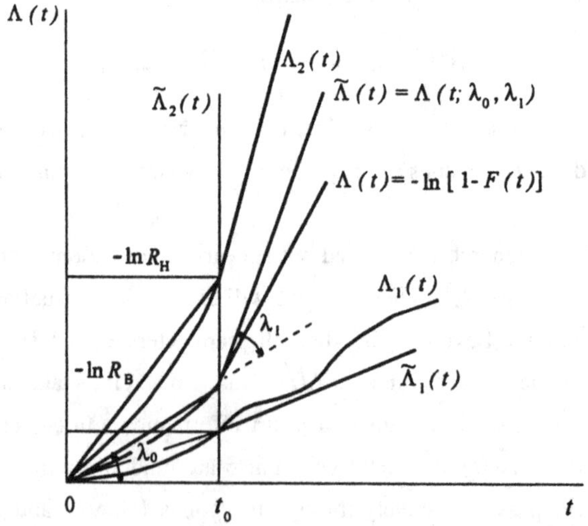

Fig. 5.2 Bayes two-linked approximation of the resource function.

(see [14]). For the resource function $\widetilde{\Lambda}(t;\lambda_0,\lambda_1)$ of the form (5.6) with $t > t_0$ we have

$$\eta(t) = \lambda_1 - (\lambda_1 - \lambda_0)\frac{t_0}{t}.$$

From the condition $\eta'(t) \geqslant$ there follows

$$(\lambda_1 - \lambda_0)\frac{t_0}{t^2} \geqslant 0,$$

whence $\lambda_1 \geqslant \lambda_0$. Therefore, the assumption $F(t) \in S_0$ gives us the same domain for the random parameters λ_0 and λ_1 of the form (5.9).

It should be noted in conclusion that approximation of the resource function by the expression (5.6) is equivalent to a rough replacement of the intensity function $\lambda(t) = \Lambda'(t)$ by the piecewise-constant function

$$\widetilde{\lambda}(t) = \widetilde{\lambda}(t;\lambda_0,\lambda_1) = \lambda_0\chi(t_0 - t) + \lambda_1\chi(t - t_0). \tag{5.10}$$

5.1.2 *Generalization of the case of a univariate prior distribution*

This can be carried out by increasing the number of links of the polygonal line used for the approximation of the resource function $\Lambda(t)$. Let us choose some number t_e so that the interval $[0,T_e]$ contains all empirical data. Next we divide the interval $[0,T_e]$ into $N+M$ intervals $\mu_j = [s_j - 1, s_j)$, $j = 1,2,\ldots,N+M$ of the same length, such that $S_N = t_0$, $s_{N+M} = T_e$. It is easy to see that the interval $[0,t_0)$ contains N intervals $\mu_1,\ \mu_2,\ldots,\mu_n$, and $[t_0,T_e)$ is M intervals $\mu_{N+1},\ldots,\mu_{N+M}$. With the help of the obtained value lattice $S_2,\ s_1,\ldots,s_{N+M}$ we will approximate the intensity function $\lambda(t)$ inside the interval $[0,T_e]$. Suppose further that:

1) The approximation of the intensity function at each point of the lattice gets on an increment. The increment value is the same for all intervals $\mu_j \in [0,t_0)$ and equals $\delta_1 \geqslant 0$. For the intervals $\mu_j \in [t_0,T_e)$ the value of a jump δ_2 differs, in general, from δ_1. The choice of different values for δ_1 and δ_2 is caused by the following circumstance: by the approach of the stated problem, δ_1 has a bounded variation induced by a segment of a prior uncertainty $[R_\ell,R_u]$. δ_2 is not subject to a similar restriction, hence, $\delta_2 \in [0,\infty)$.
2) The quantities δ_1 and δ_2 are taken as parameters of the approximation of the intensity function and play the role of the parameters λ_0 and λ_1 from the previous case.

We will distinguish between two approximations of the intensity function: an upper one $\widetilde{\lambda}(t)$ and a lower one $\underset{\sim}{\lambda}(t)$. In Fig. 5.3, $\widetilde{\lambda}(t)$ is shown by the solid line, and $\underset{\sim}{\lambda}(t)$ by the dotted line. Note that the approximations $\widetilde{\lambda}(t)$ and $\underset{\sim}{\lambda}(t)$ are named as upper and lower ones only conventionally, in view of the inequality $\widetilde{\lambda}(t) > \underset{\sim}{\lambda}(t)$. Actually it is not necessary that the double inequality $\underset{\sim}{\lambda}(t) \leqslant \lambda(t) \leqslant \widetilde{\lambda}(t)$ be fulfilled.

For the sake of simplicity we'll write

$$\widetilde{\lambda}(t) = \begin{cases} j\delta_1 & \forall t \in \mu_j, \quad j = 1, 2, \ldots, N \\ N\delta_1 + k\delta_2 & \forall t \in \mu_{N+k}, \quad k = 0, 1, \ldots, M. \end{cases} \tag{5.11}$$

In addition to this, it is clear that $\underset{\sim}{\lambda}(t) = \widetilde{\lambda}(t) - \delta_1$. To find a more handy expression, we use the function

$$\chi_j(t) = \chi(t - t_{j-1})\chi(t_j - y) = \begin{cases} 1 & \text{if } t \in \mu_j, \\ 0 & \text{if } t \notin \mu_j. \end{cases}$$

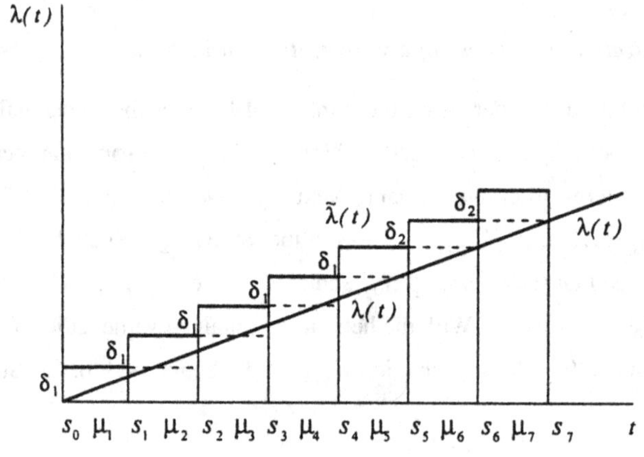

Fig. 5.3 Multiply-linked approximation of the intensity function.

After simple transformations we obtain

$$\widetilde{\lambda}(t) = \delta_1 \left[\sum_{j=1}^{n} j\chi_j(t) + N \sum_{k=1}^{m} \chi_{N+k}(t) \right] + \delta_2 \sum_{k=1}^{m} k\chi_{N+k}(t). \tag{5.12}$$

Formal integration of the intensity function (5.12) lets us find an expression for the approximate resource function $\widetilde{\Lambda}(t) = \widetilde{\Lambda}(t;\delta_1,\delta_2)$. After some complicated transformations one can obtain

$$\widetilde{\Lambda}(t;\delta_1,\delta_2) = \delta_1 \sum_{j=1}^{n} \left[K_{j-1}\Delta + j(t - s_{j-1})\right]\chi_j(t) + \sum_{j=1}^{m} \Big\{K_n\Delta_1\Delta + \left[N(j-1)\delta_1 + K_{j-1}\Delta_2\right]\Delta$$
$$+ (N\delta_1 + j_2)\big(t - s_{N+j-1}\big)\chi_{N+j}(t)\Big\}, \tag{5.13}$$

where

$$\Delta = s_{j+1} - s_j, \quad K_m = 0 + 1 + \cdots + m \quad (m = 0, 1, 2, \ldots).$$

For further approximation of the resource function, we proceed analogously:

$$\underset{\sim}{\Lambda}(t;\delta_1,\delta_2) = \delta_1 \sum_{j=2}^{n} \left[K_{j-2}\Delta + (j-1)(t - s_{j-1})\right] \chi_j(t)$$

$$+ \sum_{j=1}^{m} \left\{K_{N-1}\Delta_1\Delta + \left[(N-1)(j-1)\delta_1 + K_{j-1}\Delta_2\right]\Delta\right.$$

$$\left. + \left[(N-1)\delta_1 + j\delta_2\right]\left(t - s_{N+j-1}\right)\right\} \chi_j(t) \tag{5.14}$$

The expressions we have obtained represent, by themselves, the basis for solution of the problem of finding TTF estimates in the Bayes problem setting.

The qualitative characteristic of the Bayes approximation of the resource function, given by (5.13), is represented by Fig. 5.4. Since we don't change the form of representation of a priori information, i.e., $R_{t_0} \in [R_\ell, R_u]$ the function $\widetilde{\Lambda}(t;\delta_1,\delta_2)$ belongs to the domain bounded by the curves $\widetilde{\Lambda}_1(t)$ and $\widetilde{\Lambda}_2(t)$ introduced earlier. Define the domain d_δ formed by the possible values of the parameters δ_1 and δ_2. As before, we will start from the interval of a prior uncertainty $[R_\ell, R_u]$ and suppose that $F(t)$ belongs to the failure rate class of mean distributions.

Taking into account the chosen approximation of the resource function, we have

$$R_{t_0} = \exp\left\{-\widetilde{\Lambda}(t_0;\delta_1,\delta_2)\right\} \in [R_\ell, R_u]. \tag{5.15}$$

At the same time, (5.13) yields

$$\widetilde{\Delta}(t_0) = k_n \Delta \Delta_1. \tag{5.16}$$

Using (5.15) and (5.16), we obtain

$$R_\ell \leqslant \exp(-K_n\Delta\Delta_1) \leqslant R_u,$$

whence

$$\delta_1' \leqslant \Delta_1 \leqslant \Delta_1'',$$

where

$$\delta_1' = -\frac{1}{\Delta}\ln R_u, \quad \Delta_1'' = -\frac{1}{\Delta}\ln R_\ell, \text{ and } \Delta_1 = K_n\Delta.$$

Further, taking into account the condition

$$\frac{\partial}{\partial t}\left[\frac{\widetilde{\Lambda}(t;\delta_1,\delta_2)}{t}\right] \geqslant 0,$$

under which the c.d.f. $\widetilde{F}(t;\delta_1,\delta_2) = 1-\exp\left[-\widetilde{\Lambda}(t)\right]$ belongs to the class of distributions with increasing failure rate on the average, we obtain $\delta_2 \geqslant 0$. Thus, the range d_δ of the random parameters δ_1 and δ_2 of the approximation of the resource functions D(t) and D˜(t) has a structure

$$\delta_1' \leqslant \Delta_1 \leqslant \Delta_1'', \quad 0 \leqslant \Delta_2 < \infty \tag{5.17}$$

This completes the construction of Bayes parametric approximation of the c.d.f. on the class S_1 for a univariate prior probability distribution.

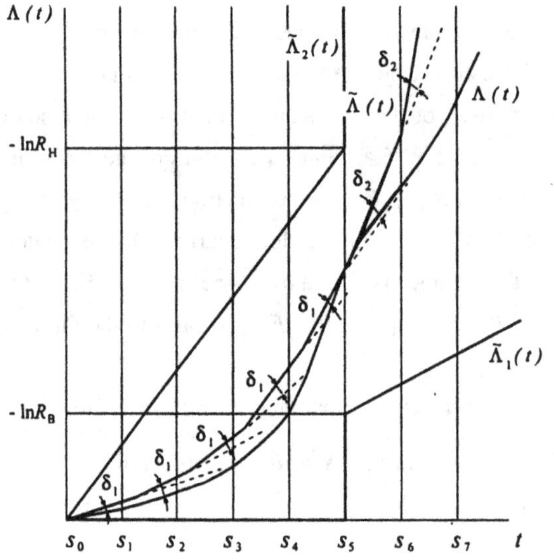

Fig. 5.4 Bayes multiply-linked approximation of the resource function.

5.1.3 *The case of a multivariate prior distribution*

This case characterizes the situation when an engineer possesses a priori information about reliability for the given set of moments $t_{10}, t_{20}, \ldots, t_{M0}$. In particular, it may occur that for each of the mentioned moments is given the interval of a prior indeterminacy $\left[R_{j\ell}, R_{ju}\right]$, $j = 1,2,\ldots,M$. We will solve the problem of construction of the parametric approximation for c.d.f. $F(t)$ in the following cases:

(1) Uncertain intervals $\left[R_{j\ell}, R_{ju}\right]$ satisfy the condition of consistency. We will distinguish two conditions of consistency: strict and nonstrict. In accordance with the first condition,

the intervals of a prior uncertainty may be partially overlapping, but $R_{j1} \leqslant R_{(j+1)\ell}$ and $R_{ju} \leqslant R_{(j+1)u}$. For the condition of strict consistency such overlapping is inadmissible, i.e., $R_{j1} \geqslant R_{(j+1)u}$. The indicated forms of representation of prior information are depicted in Fig. 5.5. and Fig. 5.6. Note that in practice we may meet both forms, depending on the methods of obtaining and using a priori information. Evidently, if the condition of nonstrict consistency is fulfilled, we should include in the statistical model additional conditions, ensuring monotonicity of the reliability function.

(2) An intensity function is approximated by a piecewise-constant function $\lambda(t)$, having finite increments $t_{10}, t_{20}, \ldots, t_{M0}$. In the capacity of model parameters one chooses constant values of the intensity function on the intervals $\left[t_{(j-1)0}, t_{j0}\right)$, $j = 1, 2, \ldots, M+1$; it is assumed also that $t_{(M+1)0} = \infty$.

In accordance with the second assumption, the approximate intensity function can be written in the form

$$\widetilde{\lambda}(t) = \sum_{j=1}^{M+1} \lambda_j \chi_j(t), \tag{5.18}$$

where $\lambda_1, \lambda_2, \ldots, m\lambda_{M+1}$ are parameters of the function (t). The approximate resource function $\widetilde{\lambda}(t)$, in view of (5.18), can be written as

$$\widetilde{\Lambda}(t) = \sum_{j=1}^{M+1} \chi_j(t) \left(\sum_{i=1}^{j-1} \lambda_i \left(t_{i0} - t_{(i-1)0}\right) + \lambda_j \left(t - t_{(j-1)0}\right) \right). \tag{5.19}$$

Find the domain of admissible values of the random parameters $\lambda_1, \lambda_2, \ldots, \lambda_{M+1}$. As it follows from the problem setting, this domain must be completely determined by the intervals of a prior uncertainty $\left[R_{j\ell}, R_{ju}\right]$, $j = 1, 2, \ldots, M$, and the approximate c.d.f. $\widetilde{F}(t) = 1 - \exp\left[-\widetilde{\Lambda}(t)\right]$ belongs to the class of failure rate mean distributions. For $t = t_{10}$, from (5.19) we obtain

$$R_{10} = \exp\left[-\widetilde{\Lambda}\left(t_{10}\right)\right] = \exp\left(-\lambda_1 t_{10}\right).$$

Thereafter, from the inequality $R_{1\ell} \leqslant R_{10} \leqslant R_{1u}$ there follows

$$-\frac{1}{t_{10}} \ln R_{1u} \leqslant \lambda_1 \leqslant -\frac{1}{t_{10}} \ln R_{1\ell}. \tag{5.20}$$

Let us now obtain an analogous inequality for any time t_{j0}. Having denoted $\Delta_j = t_{j0} - t_{(j-1)0}$, with the help of (5.19) we can write

$$R_{j0} = \exp\left[-\widetilde{\Lambda}\left(t_{j0}\right)\right] = \exp\left(\sum_{i=1}^{j} \lambda_i \Delta_i\right).$$

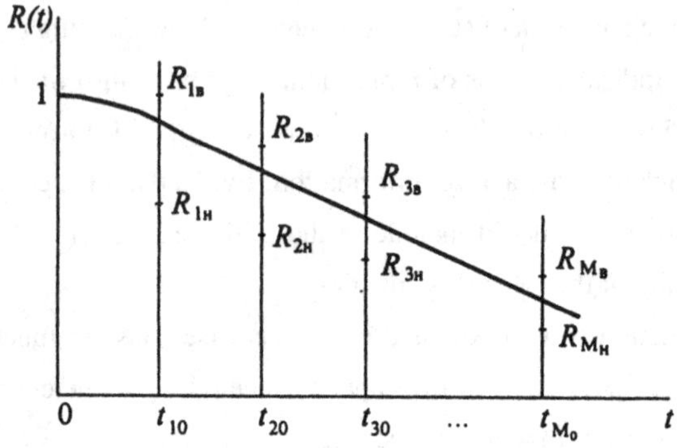

Fig. 5.5 Intervals of a prior uncertainty under the condition of fulfillment of nonstrict consistency.

Using the j-th interval of a prior uncertainty $\left[R_{j\ell}, R_{ju}\right]$, inside of which lies the value R_{j0}, we obtain

$$R_{j\ell} \leqslant \exp\left(\sum_{i=1}^{j} \lambda_i \Delta_i\right) \leqslant R_{ju}$$

whence follows the inequality for λ_j;

$$-\frac{1}{\Delta_j}\left(\ln R_{ju} + \sum_{i=1}^{j-1} \lambda_i \Delta_i\right) \leqslant \lambda_j \leqslant -\frac{1}{\Delta_j}\left(\ln R_{j\ell} + \sum_{i=1}^{j-1} \lambda_i \Delta_i\right). \tag{5.21}$$

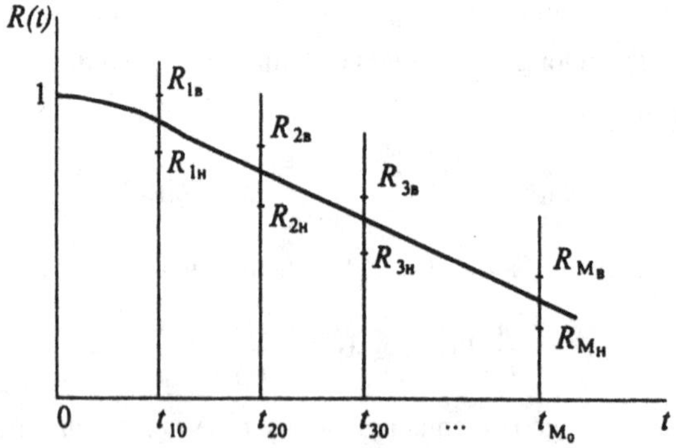

Fig. 5.6 Intervals of a prior uncertainty under the condition of fulfillment of strict consistency.

Now, we apply the condition of $\widetilde{F}(t)$ belonging to the class S_1. Introduce for $\widetilde{\Lambda}(t)$ the function $\eta(t) = \widetilde{\Lambda}(t)/t$. For an arbitrary interval $[t_{(j-1)0}, t_j]$ we obtain

$$\eta(t) = \frac{1}{t}\left[\sum_{i=1}^{j-1} \lambda_i \Delta_i + \lambda_j (t - t_{(j-1)0})\right].$$

The derivative of the function $\eta(t)$ has the form

$$\eta'(t) = \frac{1}{t^2}\left[\lambda_j t_{(j-1)0} - \sum_{i=1}^{j-1} \lambda_i \Delta_i\right],$$

and from the condition $\eta'(t) \geqslant 0$ it follows that

$$\lambda_j \geqslant \frac{\lambda_1 \Delta_1 + \lambda_2 \Delta_2 + \cdots + \lambda_{j-1}\Delta_{j-1}}{\Delta_1 + \Delta_2 + \cdots + \Delta_{j-1}}. \tag{5.22}$$

Putting together the inequalities (5.21), (5.22) and (5.20), we obtain the following domain d_λ of values of the parameters $\lambda_1, \lambda_2, \ldots, \lambda_{M+1}$ under the fulfillment of the condition of nonstrict consistency for the intervals of a prior uncertainty:

$$\begin{gathered} \lambda_i' \leqslant \lambda_i \leqslant \lambda_i'', \quad i = 1, 2, \ldots, M, \\ \lambda_{M+1}' \leqslant \lambda_{M+1} < \infty, \end{gathered} \tag{5.23}$$

where

$$\lambda_1' = -\frac{1}{\Delta_1} \ln R_{1u}, \quad \lambda_1'' = -\frac{1}{\Delta_1} \ln R_{2\ell}$$

$$\lambda_j' = \max\left\{ -\frac{1}{\Delta_1}\left(\ln R_{1u} + \sum_{i=1}^{j-1} \lambda_i \Delta_i\right), \; \frac{\sum_{i=1}^{j-1} \lambda_i \Delta_i}{\sum_{i=1}^{j-1} \Delta_i} \right\}, \quad j = 1, \ldots, M,$$

and

$$\lambda_{M+1}' = \sum_{i=1}^{m} \lambda_i \Delta_i \Big/ \sum_{i=1}^{m} \Delta_i.$$

In the case when the indeterminacy interval satisfies the condition of strict consistency $R_{j\ell} \geqslant R_{(j+1)u}$, it is easy to show that

$$-\frac{1}{\Delta_j}\left(\ln R_{ju} + \sum_{i=1}^{j-1} \lambda_i \Delta_i\right) \leqslant \sum_{i=1}^{j-1} \lambda_i \Delta_i \Big/ \sum_{i=1}^{j-1} \Delta_i.$$

Thus the common relation (5.23) for the domain d_λ has the same form, and the expression for λ_j', $j = 2, 3, \ldots, M$, changes into

$$\lambda_j' = -\frac{1}{\Delta_i}\left(\ln R_{ju} + \sum_{i=1}^{j-1} \lambda_i \Delta_i\right).$$

Note that the model of approximation of a c.d.f., considered in 5.1.3 generalizes the case of a univariate prior distribution, i.e., having put $M = 1$, we obtain all relations given in 5.1.1.

5.2 Approximation of the posterior distribution of a time to failure probability for the simplest distribution function

The solution of the problem of Bayes estimate of reliability indices under the given parametric approximation of a c.d.f. $F(t)$ follows the Bayes procedure described in Chapter 2. This procedure consists of determining the expression for the likelihood function, forming of prior distribution on the given parametric space, and obtaining the posterior distribution for the parameters of the approximate c.d.f. with the help of the Bayes theorem. In turn, the indicated posterior distribution lets us find arbitrary estimates of the required reliability index.

As it was done earlier, we begin with censored data, obtained after realization of the NC-plan. We represent these data as a vector $\tau\{\mathbf{t}^*,\mathbf{t}\}$, where $\mathbf{t}^* = (t_1^*, t_2^*, \ldots, t_d^*)$ is a vector of failure moments, $\mathbf{t} = (t_1, t_2, \ldots, t_k)$ is a vector of standstills (random and determinate). The ways of representing the posterior information depends substantially on the chosen approximation of the c.d.f. $F(t)$. Therefore, we shall consider separately each of the cases, discussed in § 5.1.

5.2.1 *The case of a univariate prior distribution*

This case is parameterized with the help of the quantities λ_0 and λ_1, which represent the failure rate in the intervals $[0, t_0)$ and $[t_0, \infty)$, respectively. To find a reliability function corresponding to this case, we will use the usual expression (3.21) for the NC-plan. Having substituted the expressions (5.6)and (5.10) into (3.21), we obtain

$$\ell(\lambda_0, \lambda_1 \mid \tau) = c(\tau) \prod_{i=1}^{d} [\chi(t_0 - t_i^*)\lambda_0 + \chi(t_i^* - t_0)\lambda_1]$$

$$\times \exp\left\{ -\sum_{i=1}^{d+k} \chi(t_0 - \tau_i)\lambda_0 \tau_i + \chi(\tau_i - t_0)\left[\lambda_1 \tau_1 + (\lambda_1 - \lambda_0) t_0\right] \right\} \tag{5.24}$$

Denote by d_0 and d_1, respectively, the number of failures observed before and after t_0 by k_0, and k_1 is the number of standstills before and after t_0. Clearly $d_0 + d_1 = d$ and $k_0 + k_1 = k$. Thus,

$$\prod_{i=1}^{d} [\chi(t_0 - t_i^*)\lambda_0 + \chi(t_i^* - t_0)\lambda_1] = \lambda_0^{d_0} \lambda_1^{d_1},$$

$$-\sum_{i=1}^{d+k} \chi(t_0 - \tau_i)\tau_i = \alpha_0, \quad \sum_{i=1}^{d+k} \chi(t_i - \tau_0)\tau_i = \alpha_1,$$

and

$$\sum_{i=1}^{d+k} \chi(t_i - \tau_0)\tau_0 = (d_1 + k_1)t_0.$$

The statistics α_0 and α_1 can be interpreted as the operating times before and after the time, t_0, respectively. Substituting the obtained relations into (5.24), we can rewrite the likelihood function $\ell(\lambda_0, \lambda_1 \mid \tau)$ in a shorter form, that is,

$$\ell(\lambda_0, \lambda_1 \mid \tau) = c(\tau)\lambda_0^{d_0}\lambda_1^{d_1} \exp\{-[\lambda_0(\alpha_0 + n_1 t_0) + \lambda_1(\alpha_1 + n_1 t_0)]\}, \tag{5.25}$$

where $n_1 = d_1 + k_1$.

Now, we shall prove that the function $\ell(\lambda_0, \lambda_1 \mid \tau)$ has a bounded variation in the domain D defined by the relation (5.9). To this end, it suffices to prove that the expression in the square brackets is not less than zero. This follows easily from the inequality

$$\alpha_1 = \sum_{i=1}^{d+k} \chi(t_i - t_0)\tau_i \geqslant (d_1 + k_1)t_0 = n_1 t_0.$$

As can be seen from the relation (5.25), the quantities d_0, d_1, k_0, k_1, where $k_0 = \alpha_0 + n_1 t_0$, $k_1 = \alpha_1 + n_1 t_0$, generate the minimal sufficient statistic. The resulting expression for the likelihood function is written in the form

$$\ell(\lambda_0, \lambda_1 \mid \tau) = c(\tau)\lambda_0^{d_0}\lambda_1^{d_1} \exp[-(\lambda_0 k_0 + \lambda_1 k_1)]. \tag{5.26}$$

Let us now consider the problem of choosing the prior probability distribution. One of the most frequently applied methods is to choose a prior which is conjugate to the maximum-likelihood kernel. Appealing to (5.26), the prior density $h_p(\lambda_0, \lambda_1)$ in this case can be written as

$$h_p(\lambda_0, \lambda_1) = \frac{1}{\beta}\lambda_0^{c_0}\lambda_1^{c_1} e^{-(\lambda_0\alpha_0 + \lambda_1 c_1)} \tag{5.27}$$

where β is a normalizing factor. Now the kernel of the posterior p.d.f., in accordance with the Bayes theorem, takes the form

$$\hbar_p(\lambda_0, \lambda \mid \tau_1) \sim \lambda_0^{c_0+d_0}\lambda_1^{c_1+d_1} \exp\{-[(\alpha_0 + k_0)\lambda_0 + (\alpha_1 + k_1)\lambda_1]\}, \quad (\lambda_0, \lambda_1) \in D.$$

Verification of the possible application of the conjugated prior distributions has been done in Chapter 2. The main difficulty in the practical use is that one cannot choose the prior p.d.f. parameters in a sufficiently justified way. Here, we deal with four such parameters: c_0, c_1, α_0, α_1, but one cannot givea method for assigning their values.

There is an alternative method for the choice of a prior distribution, partially used in Chapter 3. In determining a prior p.d.f. $h(\lambda_0, \lambda_1)$, one uses only the segment of a prior uncertainty $[R_\ell, R_u]$ and the assumption of uniformity of the TTF distribution R_{t_0}:

$$h(r) = \begin{cases} \dfrac{1}{R_u - R_\ell}, & R_\ell \leqslant r \leqslant R_u, \\ 0, & r < R_\ell, \quad r > R_u. \end{cases} \tag{5.28}$$

We seek a prior p.d.f. $h(\lambda_0,\lambda_1)$ in the form

$$h(\lambda_0,\lambda_1)=h_0(\lambda_0)h_1(\lambda_1\mid\lambda_0). \tag{5.29}$$

At first we define a marginal p.d.f. $h_0(\lambda_0)$. Taking into account the dependence $R_{t_0}=\exp(-\lambda_0 t_0)$, we obtain

$$\begin{aligned}h_0(\lambda_0)&=h\left(R_{t_0}(\lambda_0)\right)\left|R'_{t_0}(\lambda_0)\right|\\&=\frac{t_0}{R_u-R_T}\mathrm{e}^{-\lambda_0 t_0},\quad \lambda_0'\leqslant\lambda_0\leqslant\lambda_0''\end{aligned} \tag{5.30}$$

Since the parameters λ_0 and λ_1 have the same meaning, we define the conditional p.d.f. $h_1(\lambda_1,\lambda_0)$ analogous to (5.30), i.e., we will assume that $h_1(\lambda_1,\lambda_0)$ belongs to the parametric family of truncated exponential distributions. Suppose, conditionally, that some value of λ_1 is associated with a totally defined TTF value at the time t_0;

$$R_1=\exp(-\lambda_1 t_0). \tag{5.31}$$

Since $\lambda_1\in[\lambda_0,\infty)$, we obtain $R_1\in[R_{1\ell},R_{1u}]$; moreover,

$$R_{1\ell}=\lim_{\lambda_1}\mathrm{e}^{-\lambda_1 t_0}=0\quad\text{and}\quad R_{1u}=\mathrm{e}^{-\lambda_0 t_0}. \tag{5.32}$$

Taking into account the relations (5.31) and (5.32), analogous to (5.30), one obtains

$$h_1(\lambda_1\mid\lambda_0)=\frac{t_0}{R_u-R_\ell}\mathrm{e}^{-\lambda_1 t_0},\quad \lambda_0\leqslant\lambda_1<\infty.$$

and finally

$$h_1(\lambda_1\mid\lambda_0)=t_0\mathrm{e}^{-(\lambda_1-\lambda_0)t_0},\qquad \lambda_0\leqslant\lambda_1<\infty. \tag{5.33}$$

Next we substitute the expressions (5.30) and (5.33) into (5.29) and write the finite relation for a prior p.d.f. of the parameters λ_0 and λ_1 :

$$h(\lambda_0,\lambda_1)=\frac{t_0^2}{R_u-R_\ell}\mathrm{e}^{-\lambda_1 t_0},\quad (\lambda_0,\lambda_1)\in D. \tag{5.34}$$

There is no explicit dependence on the parameter λ_0. However, the form p.d.f. appears to be a joint probability density function of the parameters λ_0 and λ_1, since the dependence on λ_0 is expressed by the form of D. It should be noted that the obtained p.d.f. $h(\lambda_0,\lambda_1)$ is a partial case of theconjugated prior p.d.f. $h_p(\lambda_0,\lambda_1)$, represented by the expression (5.27) with the parameters $c_0=c_1=\alpha_0=0$, $\alpha_1=t_0$; the above given arguments may be considered as a method to justify the choice of the parameters of the conjugated prior distribution.

Using a prior density (5.34) and the likelihood function (5.26) and taking into account the Bayes theorem, we write the kernel of the desired posterior p.d.f.

$$\hbar(\lambda_0,\lambda_1\mid\tau)\sim\lambda_0^{d_0}\lambda_1^{d_1}\exp\{-[\lambda_0 k_0+\lambda_1(k_1+t_0)]\}. \tag{5.35}$$

which will be used as the basis for obtaining estimates of the probability in the following section.

5.2.2 *The generalized case of a univariate a prior distribution*

This case is characterized by the posterior distribution which has a more complicated form (bearing in mind the numerical aspects). The upper approximations of the resource function $\widetilde{\Lambda}(t;\delta_1,\delta_2)$ and intensity function $\widetilde{\lambda}(t;\delta_1,\delta_2)$ are chosen as the basis for further research. The expression (3.21) for the likelihood function takes on the form

$$\ell(\delta_1,\delta_2 \mid \tau) = c(\tau)\prod_{i=1}^{d}\widetilde{\lambda}(t_i^*;\delta_1,\delta_2)\exp\left[-\sum_{i=1}^{n}\widetilde{\Lambda}(\tau_i;\delta_1,\delta_2)\right]. \tag{5.36}$$

If one substitutes the relation (5.12) and (5.13) into (5.36), it yields

$$\ell(\delta_1,\delta_2 \mid \tau) = c(\tau)\prod_{i=1}^{d}\left\{\delta_1\left[\sum_{j=1}^{n} j\chi_j(t_i^*) + N\sum_{k=1}^{n}\chi_{N+k}(t_i^*) + \delta_2\sum_{k=1}^{n}k\chi_{N+k}(t_i^*)\right]\right\}$$

$$\times\exp\left\{-\delta_1\sum_{j=1}^{n}\left[K_{j-1}\Delta + j(\tau_i - s_{j-1})\right]\chi_j[\tau_i] - \sum_{j=1}^{m}\left\{K_n\delta_1\Delta + \left[N(j-1)\delta_1 + K_{j-2}\delta_2\right]\Delta\right.\right.$$

$$\left.\left.-\left(N\delta_1 + j\delta_2\right)\left(\tau_i - s_{N+j-1}\right)\chi_{N+j}(\tau_i)\right\}\right\}. \tag{5.37}$$

It is impossible to use such an expression of the likelihood function, so we simplify it with the help of the following formulas valid for the functions $\widetilde{\lambda}(t)$ and $\widetilde{\Lambda}(t)$:

$$\widetilde{\lambda}(t) = \sum_{j=1}^{N+M}\lambda_j\chi_j(t), \tag{5.38}$$

$$\widetilde{\Lambda}(t) = \sum_{j=1}^{N+M}\left[\Delta\sum_{k=1}^{j-1}\widetilde{\lambda}_k + \widetilde{\lambda}_j(t - s_{j-1})\right]\chi_j(t) \tag{5.39}$$

Here we use the parameters $\widetilde{\lambda}_j$ $(j = 1, 2, \ldots, N+M)$, the set of which is redundant because all parameters are determined uniquely by δ_1 and δ_2. In view of the expressions (5.38) and (5.11), we may conclude that $\widetilde{\lambda}_j$ depends on δ_1 and δ_2. With the help of (5.38) and (5.39), the likelihood function iswritten as

$$\ell(\delta_1,\delta_2 \mid \tau) = c(\tau)\prod_{i=1}^{d}\sum_{j=1}^{N+M}\widetilde{\lambda}_j\chi_j(t_i^*)$$

$$\times\exp\left\{-\sum_{i=1}^{n}\sum_{j=1}^{N+M}\left[\Delta\sum_{k=1}^{j-1}\widetilde{\lambda}_k + \widetilde{\lambda}_j(t - s_{j-1})\right]\chi_j(\tau_i)\right\}. \tag{5.40}$$

Consider separately each of the multipliers in th expression (5.40),

$$A_1 = \prod_{i=1}^{d}\left[\sum_{j=1}^{N+M}\widetilde{\lambda}_j\chi_j(t_i^*)\right]. \tag{5.41}$$

Denote by $d_j \geqslant 0$ $(j = 1, 2, \ldots, N+M)$ the number of failures observed in the j-th partition interval. Represent the product (5.41) in the form

$$A_1 = \prod_{j=1}^{N+M} \left[\prod_{i_j=1}^{d_j} \sum_{\ell=1}^{N+M} \widetilde{\lambda}_\ell \chi_\ell \left(t_{i_j}^*\right) \right]. \tag{5.42}$$

Since for the expression in the square brackets of the formula (5.42) the index j takes on a completely defined value, one gets

$$A_1 = \prod_{j=1}^{N+M} \left(\prod_{i_j=1}^{d_j} \widetilde{\lambda}_j \right) = \prod_{j=1}^{N+M} \widetilde{\lambda}_j^{d_j}. \tag{5.43}$$

Substituting the expressions (5.11) into (5.43) we obtain

$$A_1 = \delta_1^{D_1} \prod_{j=1}^{n} j^{d_j} \prod_{k=1}^{m} \sum_{i_k=0}^{d_{N+k}} \binom{d_n+k}{i_k} N^{i_k} \delta_1^{i_k} k^{d_{N+k}-i_k} \delta_2^{d_{N+k}-i_k}.$$

The last expression will be represented in the form of a polynomial by means of δ_1 and δ_2. To this end, we unite the similar terms and introduce a new index $I = i_1 + i_2 + \cdots + i_m$. Finally,

$$A_1 = \prod_{j=1}^{n} j^{d_j} \delta_1^{D_1} \sum_{I=0}^{D_2} \alpha_I \delta_1^I \delta_2^{D_2-I}, \tag{5.44}$$

where

$$\alpha_i = N^I \sum_{i_1=0}^{d_{N+1}} \sum_{i_2=0}^{d_{N+2}} \cdots \sum_{i_m=0}^{d_{N+M}} \prod_{k=1}^{m} k^{d_{N+k}-i_k} \binom{d_{N+k}}{i_k}$$

and

$$D_1 = d_1 + \cdots + d_n, \quad D_2 = d_{N+1} + \cdots + d_{N+M}.$$

Define the second multiplier of the likelihood function as

$$A_2 = \exp\left\{ -\sum_{i=1}^{n} \sum_{j=1}^{N+M} \left[\Delta \sum_{k=1}^{j-1} \widetilde{\lambda}_k + \widetilde{\lambda}_j(\tau_i - s_{j-1})\chi_j(\tau_i) \right] \right\}. \tag{5.45}$$

Denote by I_j the set of indices of the sample elements $\tau = (\tau_1, \tau_2, \ldots, \tau_n)$, belonging to the segment μ_j (see Figure 5.3). Thereafter, the expression (5.45) is rewritten in the following manner:

$$-\ln A_2 = \sum_{i \in I_1} \widetilde{\lambda}_1(\tau_i - s_0) + \sum_{i \in I_1} \left[\widetilde{\lambda}_1 \Delta + \widetilde{\lambda}_2(\tau_i - s_1) \right] + \cdots$$

$$+ \sum_{i \in I_{N+M}} \left[\widetilde{\lambda}_1 \Delta + \cdots + \widetilde{\lambda}_{N+M-1} \Delta + \widetilde{\lambda}_{N+M}(\tau_i - s_{N+M-1}) \right]$$

$$= \sum_{j=1}^{N+M} \tilde{\lambda}_j \left[\sum_{i \in I_j} (\tau_i - s_{j-1}) + \sum_{k=j+1}^{N+M} \sum_{i \in I_k} \Delta \right] = \sum_{j-1}^{N+M} \tilde{\lambda}_j k_j.$$

It is easy to see that the obtained statistic

$$k_j = \sum_{i \in I_j} (\tau_i - s_{j-1}) + \sum_{k=j+1}^{N+M} \sum_{i \in I_k} \Delta \tag{5.46}$$

represents by itself a total operating time during the testing, observed in the j-th interval. With the help of (5.46) we represent A_2 in the form

$$A_2 = \exp \left[- \sum_{j=1}^{N+M} \tilde{\lambda}_j k_j \right]. \tag{5.47}$$

The resulting expression for the likelihood multiplier A_2 will be obtained, if we substitute (5.40) into (5.47).

$$A_2 = \exp\left[1(a_1\Delta_1 + a_2\Delta_2)\right]. \tag{5.48}$$

where

$$a_1 = \sum_{j=1}^{N} jk_j + N \sum_{j=N+1}^{N+M} k_j, \quad a_2 = \sum_{j=1}^{N} jk_{N+j}. \tag{5.49}$$

We have found all components of the formula (5.41). Thus,

$$\ell(\delta_1, \delta_2 \mid \tau) = c(\tau) \prod_{j=1}^{N} j^{d_j} \delta_1^{D_1} \sum_{I=0}^{D_2} \alpha_I \delta_1^I \delta_2^{D_2 - I} \mathrm{e}^{-(a_1\delta_1 + a_2\Delta_2)}. \tag{5.50}$$

The coefficient α_I in the function (5.50) depends only on the number of failures $d_{N+1}, d_{N+2}, \ldots, d_{N+M}$, observed in the interval μ_j $(j > N)$. Thus, in view of (5.50), the minimal sufficient statistic is generated by the quantities $D_1, d_{N+1}, d_{N+2}, \ldots, d_{N+M}, a_1, a_2$. The kernel of the likelihood function (5.50) allows us to write the conjugated prior p.d.f. of the form

$$h_p(\delta_1, \delta_2) = B\delta_1^{U_1}\delta_2^{U_2}\mathrm{e}^{-\alpha_1\delta_1 - \alpha_2\delta_2}, \quad (\delta_1, \delta_2) \in D_\delta \tag{5.51}$$

where U_1, U_2, α_1, α_2 are the parameters of a prior distribution, B is the normalized factor, and D_δ has the form (5.17). In view of the Bayes theorem for the posterior p.d.f. of the parameters δ_1, δ_2, we obtain

$$\hbar(\delta_1, \delta_2 \mid \tau) \sim \delta_1^{D_1 + U_1} \delta_2^{U_2} \sum_{I=0}^{D_2} \alpha_I \delta_1^I \delta_2^{D_2 - I}$$
$$\times \exp\left(-\left[(a_1 + \alpha_1)\delta_1 + (a_2 + \alpha_2)\delta_2\right]\right). \tag{5.52}$$

The main difficulties in using the expressions (5.51) and (5.52) in practical situations is the problem of defining the parameters of a prior law.

If one uses as given only the assumption about uniformity of the TTF distribution at the time t_0 in the interval $[R_\ell, R_u]$, a prior p.d.f. can be obtained in the following way. Suppose the parameters δ_1 and δ_2 are independent and a prior p.d.f. is sought in the form

$$h(\delta_1,\delta_2)=h_1(\delta_2)h_2(\delta_2),\quad (\delta_1,\delta_2)\in D_\delta. \tag{5.53}$$

Using the expressions (5.15) and (5.16) and the property of monotonicity of the dependence R_{t_0} on δ_1, we get

$$h_1(\delta_1)=\frac{k_n\Delta}{R_u-R_\ell}\mathrm{e}^{-K_n\Delta\delta_1},\quad \delta_1'\leqslant\delta_1\leqslant\delta_1''. \tag{5.54}$$

The expression for $h_2(\delta_2)$ will be sought in the class of truncated exponential distributions, defined by the density (5.54). The given assumption is justified in view of the same meaning of the parameters δ_1 and δ_2. Since $\delta_2\in[0,\infty)$, for $h_2(\delta_2)$ we obtain

$$h_2(\delta_2)=K_m\Delta\mathrm{e}^{-K_m\Delta\delta_2},\quad 0\leqslant\delta_2<\infty.$$

Denote by $\Delta_1=K_n\Delta$, $\Delta_2=K_m\Delta$. Then the resulting expression for a prior p.d.f. $h(\delta_1,\delta_2)$ takes the form

$$h(\delta_1,\delta_2)=\frac{\Delta_1\Delta_2}{R_u-R_\ell}\mathrm{e}^{-(\Delta_1\delta_1+\Delta_2\delta_2)},\quad (\delta_1,\delta_2)\in D_\delta. \tag{5.55}$$

The obtained p.d.f. appears to be a particular case of a conjugated prior p.d.f. (5.51) with $U_1=U_2=0$, $\alpha_1=\Delta_1$, $\alpha_2=\Delta_2$. The arguments used above may be interpreted as a justification for the method of a choice of the parameters of the conjugate prior p.d.f. if we take into consideration onlythe interval of a prior uncertainty.
With the help of the Bayes theorem we get

$$\hbar(\delta_1,\delta_2\mid\tau)\sim\delta_1^{D_1}\sum_{I=0}^{D_2}\alpha_I\delta_1^I\delta_2^{D_2-I}\times\mathrm{e}^{-[(\alpha_1+\delta_1)\delta_1+(\alpha_2+\delta_2)\delta_2]},\quad (\delta_1,\delta_2)\in D_\delta. \tag{5.56}$$

The expression (5.56) has been obtained with the help of the upper approximation for the resource and intensity functions. Reasoning similarly we may obtain the posterior p.d.f. for the corresponding lower approximations.

5.2.3 *The case of an m-variate prior distribution*

This case was described in §5.1 with the help of approximating the functions of intensity (5.18) and resource (5.19). Each of them depends on $M+1$ parameters $\lambda_1,\lambda_2,\ldots,\lambda_m$, λ_{M+1}, the parameters being the constant values of the intensity in the intervals $[0,t_{10})$,

$[t_{10}, t_{20}), \ldots, [t_{(M-1)0}, t_{M0}), (t_{M0}, \infty)$. Substituting the expressions (5.18) and (5.19) into (3.21), we obtain

$$\ell(\lambda \mid \tau) = c(\tau) \prod_{i=1}^{d} \sum_{j=1}^{M+1} \lambda_j \chi_j(t_i^*)$$
$$\times \exp\left\{ -\sum_{i=1}^{n} \sum_{j=1}^{M+1} \chi_j(\tau_i) \sum_{k=1}^{j-1} \lambda_k \left(t_{k0} - t_{(k-1)0}\right) + \lambda_j \left(\tau_i - t_{(j-1)0}\right) \right\}. \tag{5.57}$$

To simplify the last relation, we introduce statistics $d_1, d_2, \ldots, d_m, d_{M+1}$, being the number of failures observed in the indicated intervals, respectively. It is easy to verify the validity of the expression

$$\prod_{i=1}^{d} \sum_{j=1}^{M+1} \lambda_j \chi_j(t_i^*) = \sum_{j=1}^{M+1} \lambda_j^{d_j}. \tag{5.58}$$

If one denotes by I_j the set of indices of the sample elements belonging to the interval $[t_{(j-1)0}, t_{j0})$, then the second multiplier of the likelihood function can also be simplified:

$$\sum_{i=1}^{n} \sum_{j=1}^{M+1} \left[\chi_j(t) \sum_{k=1}^{j-1} \lambda_k \left(t_{k0} - t_{(k-1)0}\right) + \lambda_j \left(\tau_i - t_{(j-1)0}\right) \right]$$
$$= \sum_{j=1}^{M+1} \lambda_j \left[\sum_{i \in I_j} \left(\tau_i - t_{(j-1)0}\right) + \sum_{k=j+1}^{M+1} \sum_{i \in I_k} \left(t_{k0} - t_{(k-1)0}\right) \right]. \tag{5.59}$$

The obtained statistic

$$k_j \sum_{i \in I_j} \left(\tau_i - t_{(j-1)0}\right) + \sum_{k=j+1}^{M+1} \sum_{i \in I_k} \left(t_{k0} - t_{(k-1)0}\right), \tag{5.60}$$

as already stated, can be interpreted as the total operating time, fixed during the testing in the interval $[t_{(j-1)0}, t_{j0})$. Substituting the expressions (5.58)–(5.60) into the expression (5.57) we obtain the expression for the likelihood function

$$\ell(\lambda \mid \tau) = c(\tau) \prod_{j=1}^{M+1} \lambda_j^{d_j} \exp\left(-\sum_{j=1}^{M+1} \lambda_j k_j \right). \tag{5.61}$$

With the help of this expression, we can represent the kernel of the conjugate prior p.d.f. in the form of

$$h_p(\lambda_1, \ldots, \lambda_{M+1}) \sim \prod_{j=1}^{M+1} \lambda_j^{c_j} \exp\left(-\sum_{j=1}^{M+1} \alpha_j \lambda_j \right), \tag{5.62}$$

where c_j and α_j $(j = 1, 2, \ldots, M+1)$ are the parameters of a priori p.d.f., and the kernel of the posterior p.d.f. in the form

$$\hbar_p(\lambda_1, \ldots, \lambda_{M+1} \mid \tau) \sim \prod_{j=1}^{M+1} \lambda_j^{c_j + d_j} \exp\left[-\sum_{j=1}^{M+1} (\alpha_j + k_j) \lambda_j \right]. \tag{5.63}$$

Here, we restrict ourselves only to obtaining an expression for the posterior probability densities. As is seen from the above arguments, the approach is independent of the method of constructing the parametric approximation. The differences among the approximating functions require us to use various methods of simplification, assigned to determine the sufficient one and write the simplest expression for the likelihood function.

5.3 Bayes estimates of a time to failure probability for the restricted increasing failure rate distributions

In this section we describe the method of obtaining Bayes TTF estimates using a two-linked piecewise-linear approximation of the resource function of the form (5.6). This form is chosen because of its simplicity. The knowledge of the posterior distribution lets us find, in principle, any numerical estimateof the TTF. There are, nevertheless, such cases that make us either apply complicated analytic constructions or use numerical methods. The goal of this section is to obtain finite analytic relations for TTF estimates.

5.3.1 *Bayes TTF estimates for the case* $t \leqslant t_0$

The value of a TTF in the interval $[0,t_0]$, in accordance with the chosen approximation of the resource function (5.6), has the form

$$R(t) = \mathrm{e}^{-\widetilde{\Lambda}(t)} = \mathrm{e}^{-\lambda_0 t}, \quad t \leqslant t_0. \tag{5.64}$$

Since the $R(t)$ is defined by only one parameter λ_0, to define the estimates of r it is necessary to know a marginal posterior density $\hbar_0(\lambda_0 \mid \tau)$. This density is obtained by integrating the joint posterior density $\hbar(\lambda_0,\lambda_1 \mid \tau)$ over the parameter 1:

$$\begin{aligned} \hbar_0(\lambda_0 \mid \tau) &= \int_{\lambda_0}^{\infty} \hbar(\lambda_0,\lambda_1 \mid \tau)\, d\lambda_1 \\ &\sim \lambda_0^{d_0}\mathrm{e}^{-\lambda_0 k_0} \int_{\lambda_0}^{\infty} \lambda_1^{d_1}\mathrm{e}^{-\lambda_1(k_1+t_0)}\, d\lambda_1, \quad \lambda_0' \leqslant \lambda_0 \leqslant \lambda_0'' \end{aligned} \tag{5.65}$$

We shall be using the known integral

$$\int x^n \mathrm{e}^{-\alpha x} dx = -\mathrm{e}^{-\alpha x} \sum_{k=0}^{n} n^{(k)} \frac{x^{n-k}}{\alpha^{k+1}} + C, \tag{5.66}$$

where $n^{(k)} = n!/(n-k)!$. Having performed the integration of (5.65) we obtain

$$\hbar_0(\lambda_0 \mid \tau) \sim \mathrm{e}^{-\lambda_0(k_0+k_1+t_0)} \lambda_0^{d_0} \sum_{i=0}^{d_1} d_1^{(i)} \frac{\lambda_0^{d_1-i}}{(k_1+t_0)^{i+1}}. \tag{5.67}$$

For a quadratic loss function, the desired pointwise estimate $\hat{R}^*(t)$ is written in the form of the posterior mean value

$$\hat{R}^*(t) = \int_{\lambda_0'}^{\lambda_0''} e^{-\lambda_0 t} \hbar_0(\lambda_0 \mid \tau) d\lambda_0. \tag{5.68}$$

The posterior variance $\sigma^2_{\hat{R}^*(t)}$, using the estimate $\hat{R}^*(t)$, is written analogously:

$$\sigma^2_{\hat{R}^*(t)} = \int_{\lambda_0'}^{\lambda_0''} e^{-\lambda_0 t} \hbar_0(\lambda_0 \mid \tau) d\lambda_0 - \left[\hat{R}^*(t)\right]^2. \tag{5.69}$$

The expressions (5.68), (5.69) may be represented in shorter form

$$\hat{R}^*(t) = \frac{H_1(t)}{H_0(t)} \quad \text{and} \quad \sigma^2_{\hat{R}^*(t)} = \frac{H_2(t)}{H_0(t)} - \left[\hat{R}^*(t)\right]^2. \tag{5.70}$$

where

$$H_k(t) = \int_{\lambda_0'}^{\lambda_0''} \exp(-k\lambda_0 t) \left[-\lambda_0(k_0 + k_1 + t_0)\right] \times \lambda_0^{d_0} \sum_{i=0}^{d_1} \frac{d_1^{(i)}}{(k_1 + t_0)^{i+1}} \lambda_0^{d_1 - i} d\lambda_0.$$

Using the integral (5.66) we obtain the resulting expression of the function $H_k(t)$:

$$H_k(t) = \sum_{i=0}^{d_1} \frac{d_1^{(i)}}{(k_1 + t_0)^{i+1}} \sum_{j=0}^{d-i} \frac{(d-i)^{(j)}}{(k_0 + k_1 + t_0 + kt)^{j+1}} \left\{ (\lambda_0')^{d-i-j} \exp\left[-\lambda_0'(k_0 + k_1 + t_0 + kt)\right] \right.$$
$$\left. - (\lambda_0'')^{d-i-j} \exp\left[-\lambda_0''(k_0 + k_1 + t_0 + kt)\right] \right\}. \tag{5.71}$$

Taking into account the form of the expression $H_k(t)$, we introduce the following handy dimensionless statistics:

$$\omega = \frac{k_0 + k_1}{t_0} = \sum_{i=1}^{n} \frac{\tau_i}{t_0} = \sum_{i=1}^{n} \nu_i, \tag{5.72}$$

$$\omega_1 = \frac{k_1}{t_0} = \sum_{i=1}^{n} \left(\frac{\tau_i}{t_0} - 1\right) \chi(\tau_i - t_0) = \sum_{i=1}^{n} (\nu_i - 1)\chi(\nu_i - 1), \tag{5.73}$$

where $\nu_i = \tau_i / t_0$. The use of the statistics ω and ω_1 lets us represent the sample of testing results in the form of relative operating times ν_i. Due to this fact we will use as initial data the vector $\nu = \{\nu^*, \nu'\}$, where $\nu^* = (\nu_1, \ldots, \nu_d)$ is the vector of respective failure moments, and $\nu' = (\nu_1, \ldots, \nu_K)$ is the vector of relative standstills of the testing.

Thereafter, the sufficient Statistic, corresponding to the source sample τ, for the distribution function $\widetilde{F}(t; \lambda_0, \lambda_1)$ is written in the form of the set $\{\omega, \omega_1, d, d_1\}$. The statistic ω represents by itself the total relative operating times during the testing, ω_1 is the total relative operating time after thetime t_0. It is not necessary to divide the vector ν into ν^* and ν' in order to evaluate ω_1 and ω. Information about the partition of the sample into failures and standstills is contained in the statistic d (the total number of failures out of n) and d_1 (the number of failures after the time t_0).

Now the resulting expression for the estimates (5.70) can be written as

$$\hat{R}^*(t) = \frac{I_{1,\nu}(\omega, \omega_1, d, d_1)}{I_{0,\nu}(\omega, \omega_1, d, d_1)}, \tag{5.74}$$

and

$$\sigma^2_{\hat{R}^*(t)} = \frac{I_{2,\nu}(\omega, \omega_1, d, d_1)}{I_{0,\nu}(\omega, \omega_1, d, d_1)} - \left[\hat{R}^*(t)\right]^2. \tag{5.75}$$

The function $I_{k,\nu}(\omega, \omega_1, d, d_1)$ is identically equal to the function $H_k(t)$ except, instead of t, one uses the dimensionless parameter $\nu = t/t_0$. Thus,

$$I_{k,\nu}(\omega, \omega_1, d, d_1) = \sum_{i=0}^{d_1} \frac{d_1^{(i)}}{(\omega_1+1)^{(i+1)}} \sum_{j=0}^{d-i} \frac{(d-i)^{(j)}}{(\omega+k\nu+1)^{j+1}}$$

$$\times \left[R_u^{\omega+k\nu+1} |\ln R_u|^{d-i-j} - R_1^{\omega+k\nu+1} |\ln R_\ell|^{d-i-j}\right]. \tag{5.76}$$

The value of the lower confidence estimate $\underline{R}^*_\gamma(t)$ which characterizes the exactness of the obtained estimate $\hat{R}^*(t)$ may be analogously written:

$$\int_{\underline{R}^*_\gamma(t)\leqslant e^{-\lambda_0 t}\leqslant R_u} \hbar_0(\lambda_0 \mid \tau)d\lambda_0 - \gamma = 0. \tag{5.77}$$

To find $\underline{R}^*_\gamma(t)$, we introduce a new variable x such that $\underline{R}^*_\gamma(t) = \exp(-xt)$. The equation (5.77) is written as

$$\int_{\lambda_0'}^{x} \hbar_0(\lambda_0 \mid \tau)d\lambda_0 - \gamma = 0.$$

Using the relation (5.66), after transformations similar to the procedure of obtaining the function (5.76), we get the resulting expression for $\hat{\underline{R}}^*_\gamma(t)$:

$$\sum_{i=0}^{d_1} \frac{d_1^{(i)}}{(\omega_1+1)^{i+1}} \sum_{j=0}^{d-1} \frac{(d-i)^{(j)}}{(\omega_1+1)^{j+1}} \left[R_u^{\omega+1} |\ln R_u|^{d-i-j}\right.$$

$$\left. -\underline{R}^*_\gamma(t)^{(\omega+1/\nu)} \left|\ln \underline{R}^{*1/\nu}_\gamma(t)\right|^{d-i-j}\right] - \gamma I_{0,\nu}(\omega, \omega_1, d, d_1) = 0. \tag{5.78}$$

If we want to find the TTF estimates for the case $t = t_0$, we should put $\nu = 1$ in the expressions (5.74), (5.75) and (5.78).

Next we investigate the posterior distribution of the estimated TTF index. This investigation is of methodological interest. Consider the case $t = t_0$ ($\nu = 1$). Taking into account the monotonicity of the dependence $R(t_0) = \exp(-\lambda_0 t_0)$, for the posterior density of the index $R(t_0)$ we will have

$$\hbar(r_0 \mid \tau) = \hbar(\lambda_0(r_0) \mid \tau) \left|\lambda_0'(r_0)\right|. \tag{5.79}$$

After substitution of (5.77) into (5.79) and some simplifications we obtain

$$\hbar\,(r_0 \mid \tau) = \frac{1}{\beta} R_0^{\omega} \sum_{i=0}^{d_1} d_1^{(i)} \frac{|\ln R_0|^{d-i}}{(\omega_1+1)^{i+1}}, \tag{5.80}$$

where $\beta = I_{0,1}\,(\omega, \omega_1, d, d_1+1)$.

In Figure 5.7 (a, b), we represent examples of concrete realizations of a posterior density (5.80) with fixed ω and ω_1 and different d and d_1. It can be seen that for the fixed d and increasing d_1 ($d_1 = 0, 1, 2, \ldots, d$) the curve $\hbar_0\,(r_0 \mid \tau)$ biases to the right, which corresponds to the posterior value ofTTF which is larger. This is in full agreement with practice and the engineering interpretation of the considered scheme: while d_1 increases (the other parameters remain fixed), the number of tests, ended by failures, increases too, and the number of failures, occurring before the time t_0, decreases.That is, the considered situation corresponds to the higher reliability level.

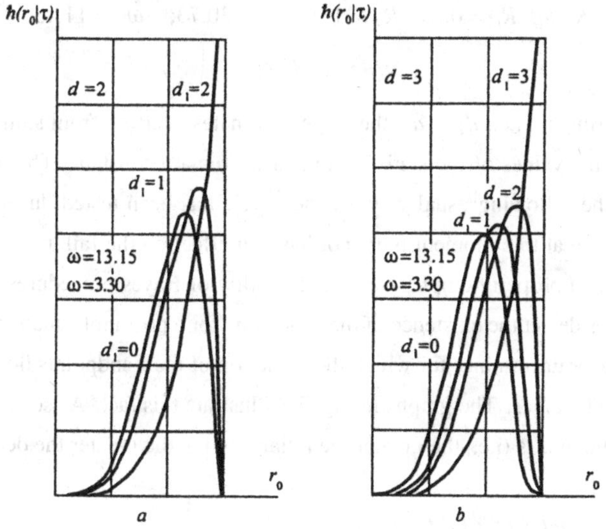

Fig. 5.7 The posterior density of the TTF distribution.

Tables 5.1–5.3 give the calculation results touching upon the values of the estimates $\hat{R}^*(t_0)$, $\sigma_{\hat{R}^*(t_0)}$, $\underline{R}_{\gamma}^*(t)$ carried out with the formulas (5.74)–(5.78) for the fixed sample consisting of 10 elements and different d and d_1. Analyzing these tables we come to the following conclusion. While d_1 increases and d is fixed, $\hat{R}^*(t_0)$ and $\underline{R}_{\gamma}^*(t)$ increase, confirming the obtained earlier qualitative result. Diagonal elements possess the property of asymptotical stability. Therefore, if the number of failures increases (in the case when all failures

Table 5.1 The Bayes point-wise TF estimate.

d_1	d									
	0	1	2	3	4	5	6	7	8	9
0	0.9696	0.9410	0.9152	0.8933	0.8755	0.8616	0.8510	0.8428	0.8364	0.8315
1		0.9617	0.9299	0.9038	0.8830	0.8669	0.8547	0.8455	0.8385	0.8330
2			0.9574	0.9230	0.8963	0.8761	0.8612	0.8511	0.8418	0.8355
3				0.9553	0.9192	0.8919	0.8720	0.8577	0.8472	0.8395
4					0.9544	0.9174	0.8887	0.8699	0.8557	0.8456
5						0.9540	0.9166	0.8887	0.8689	0.8548
6							0.9539	0.9164	0.8884	0.8685
7								0.9539	0.9163	0.8882
8									0.9539	0.9162
9										0.9539

$$\hat{R}^*(t_0)\ R_\ell = 0.8,\quad R_u = 1.0;\quad \omega = 30.73;\quad \omega_1 = 11.13$$

occur after the time t_0, i.e., $d_1 = d$), the Bayes estimates, starting from some value, don't change, unless the values of the statistics ω and ω_1 remain constant. This result may be interpreted in the following usual way. If the article has been tested during the time t_0, then the TTFvalue at this moment must not have an effect on the failures that occur after t_0. The mentioned property emphasizes the flexibility of Bayes procedures. Calculations of TTF estimates detect the existence of the dead zone for a priori information, that is, such intervals of a prior uncertainty for which the deviation of their endpoints does not have an effect on the TTF values. The graphs in Fig. 5.8 illustrate this fact. As seen from Fig. 5.8, the less the value of d is (i.e., the greater the reliability is), the greater the dead zone.

5.3.2 *Bayes estimates of TTF for* $t > t_0$

In accordance with the approximation of (5.6), for $t > t_0$, we have

$$R(t) = R(t;\lambda_0,\lambda_1) = \exp\{-[\lambda_1 t - (\lambda_1 - \lambda_0)t_0]\}. \tag{5.81}$$

In the given case TTF depends on two parameters. Thus, in order to obtain the estimates of the index (5.81) it is necessary to use the posterior density $\hbar(\lambda_0,\lambda_1 \mid \tau)$. Taking into account the expression (5.35), we denote the kernel of the posterior density by

$$C_0(\lambda_0\lambda_1) = \lambda_0^{d_0}\lambda_1^{d_1}\exp\{-[\lambda_0 k_0 + \lambda_1(k_1 + t_0)]\}. \tag{5.82}$$

Table 5.2 The posterior mean squared value.

d_1	d									
	0	1	2	3	4	5	6	7	8	9
0	0.0291	0.0383	0.0422	0.0424	0.0404	0.0373	0.0338	0.0305	0.0274	0.0248
1		0.0344	0.0420	0.0437	0.0421	0.0391	0.0354	0.0319	0.0386	0.0258
2			0.0377	0.0444	0.0446	0.0418	0.0380	0.0341	0.0304	0.0273
3				0.0395	0.0460	0.0452	0.0417	0.0376	0.0333	0.0296
4					0.0404	0.0468	0.0456	0.0417	0.0371	0.0328
5						0.0408	0.0472	0.0459	0.0417	0.0418
6							0.0409	0.0474	0.0460	0.0460
7								0.0410	0.0474	0.0460
8									0.0410	0.0475
9										0.0410

$\sigma_{\hat{R}^*(t_0)}$ $R_\ell = 0.8$, $R_u = 1.0$; $\omega = 30.73$; $\omega_1 = 11.13$

and define the normalizing factor in the form of the following integral:

$$\beta = \iint_d C_0(\lambda_0\lambda_1)\,d\lambda_0\lambda_1 = \left(\frac{1}{t_0}\right)^{d+2} \sum_{i=0}^{d_1} \frac{d_1^{(i)}}{(\omega_1+1)^{i+1}} \sum_{j=0}^{d-i} \frac{(d-i)^{(j)}}{(\omega+1)^{j+1}}$$
$$\times \left(R_u^{\omega+1}|\ln R_u|^{d-i-j} - R_\ell^{\omega+1}|\ln R_\ell|^{d-i-j}\right). \tag{5.83}$$

Let us find the estimate $\hat{R}^*(t)$ for the quadratic loss function in the form of a prior mean value of the function (5.81):

$$\hat{R}^*(t) = \frac{1}{\beta}\exp\left\{-\left[\lambda_0 k_0 + \lambda_1(k_1+t_0)\right]\right\} C_0(\lambda_0,\lambda_1)\,d\lambda_0 d\lambda_1$$
$$= \frac{1}{\beta}\lambda_0^{d_0} e^{-\lambda_0(k_0+t_0)}\,d\lambda_0 \int_{\lambda_0}^{\infty} \lambda_1^{d_1} e^{-\lambda_1(k_1+t_0)}\,d\lambda_1 .$$

Having used the integral (5.66) twice and passed to the dimensionless parameters ω, ω_1, and ν, one finally gets

$$\hat{R}^*(t) = \frac{1}{\beta} \sum_{i=0}^{d_1} \frac{d_1^{(i)}}{(\omega_1+\nu)^{i+1}} \sum_{j=0}^{d-i} \frac{(d-i)^{(j)}}{(\omega+\nu+1)^{j+1}}$$
$$\times \left(R_u^{\omega+\nu+1}|\ln R_u|^{d-i-j} - R_\ell^{\omega+\nu+1}|\ln R_\ell|^{d-i-j}\right).$$

Deviation of the expression for the posterior variance $\sigma^2_{\hat{R}^*(t)}$ is similar to that for $\hat{R}^*(t)$. Introduce the function

$$J_{m,\nu}(\omega,\omega_1,d,d_1) = \sum_{i=0}^{d_1} \frac{d_1^{(i)}}{(\omega_1+\alpha_m)^{i+1}} \sum_{j=0}^{d-i} \frac{(d-i)^{(j)}}{(\omega+m\nu+1)^{j+1}}$$
$$\times \left(R_u^{\omega+m\nu+1}|\ln R_u|^{d-i-j} - R_\ell^{\omega+m\nu+1}|\ln R_\ell|^{d-i-j}\right) \tag{5.84}$$

Table 5.3 The Bayes lower confidence limit.

d_1	d									
	0	1	2	3	4	5	6	7	8	9
0	0.9302	0.8867	0.8544	0.8329	0.8204	0.8134	0.8094	0.8070	0.8055	0.8044
1		0.9137	0.8694	0.8409	0.8244	0.8155	0.8106	0.8077	0.8059	0.8047
2			0.9036	0.8582	0.8327	0.8195	0.8126	0.8089	0.8066	0.8052
3				0.8981	0.8517	0.8282	0.8168	0.8110	0.8079	0.8060
4					0.8945	0.8483	0.8258	0.8153	0.8102	0.8073
5						0.8945	0.8468	0.8246	0.8146	0.8097
6							0.8942	0.8462	0.8241	0.8143
7								0.8941	0.8460	0.8240
8									0.8941	0.8459
9										0.8941

$\underline{R}^*_{0.9}(t_0)$ $R_\ell = 0.8, \quad R_u = 1.0; \quad \omega = 30.73; \quad \omega_1 = 11.13$

where,

$$\alpha_m = \begin{cases} 1, & m = 0, \\ \nu, & m = 1, \\ 2\nu - 1, & m = 2. \end{cases}$$

Then the resulting expressions for the estimates $\hat{R}^*(t)$ and $\sigma^2_{\hat{R}^*(t)}$ are written as

$$\hat{R}^*(t) = \frac{J_{1,\nu}(\omega,\omega_1,d,d_1)}{J_{0,\nu}(\omega,\omega_1,d,d_1)} \quad \text{and} \quad \sigma^2_{\hat{R}^*(t)} \frac{J_{2,\nu}(\omega,\omega_1,d,d_1)}{J_{0,\nu}(\omega,\omega_1,d,d_1)} - \hat{R}^{*2}(t). \tag{5.85}$$

We need to obtain the equation for $\underline{R}^*_\gamma(t)$. Taking into account the relation (2.34) we can write

$$\iint\limits_{\substack{\left[R(t;\lambda_0,\lambda_1)\geqslant \underline{R}^*_\gamma(t)\right] \\ \left[(\lambda_0,\lambda_1)\in D\right]}} \hbar(\lambda_0,\lambda_1 \mid \tau)d\lambda_0 d\lambda_1 - \gamma = 0. \tag{5.86}$$

To simplify the integration domain in (5.86), let $\underline{R}^*_\gamma(t) = \exp(-yt_0)$ and y be an unknown variable. The condition $R(t) \geqslant \underline{R}^*_\gamma(t)$ is rewritten in the form of the inequality

$$\lambda_1 t - (\lambda_1 - \lambda_0)t_0 \leqslant yt_0$$

or, with the help of the dimensionless parameter ν,

$$\lambda_1(\nu - 1) + \lambda_0 \leqslant y. \tag{5.87}$$

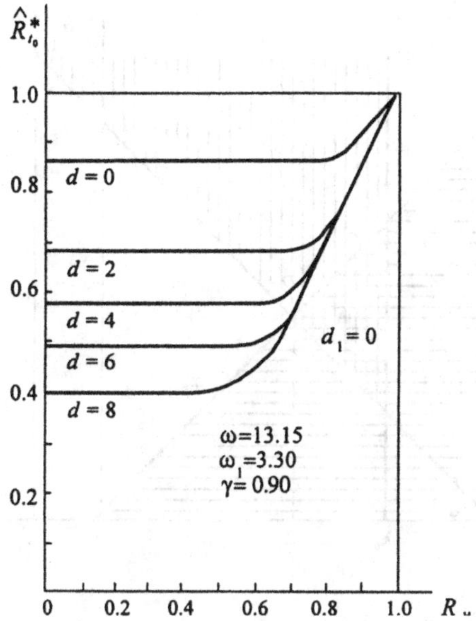

Fig. 5.8 The dependence of the Bayes confidence TTF limit on lower value of the interval of a prior uncertainty.

Domains D and D_γ, defined by (5.87), are shown in Fig. 5.9. The domain D_γ is bounded by the curve α_1, having the equation $y = \lambda_1(\nu-1)+\lambda_0$, and coordinate axes λ_0, λ_1. The domain $D = \{\lambda_0' \leqslant \lambda_0 \leqslant \lambda_0'', \lambda_0 \leqslant \lambda_1\}$ is depicted by the vertical dash lines. The intersection $D \cap D_\gamma$ is written in the form of two inequalities:

$$\lambda_0' \leqslant \lambda_0 \leqslant \lambda_0'', \quad \lambda_0 \leqslant \lambda_1 \leqslant \frac{y-\lambda_0}{\nu-1}.$$

The problem of obtaining y and $\underline{R}^*_\gamma(t) = \exp(-yt_0)$ has the following geometrical interpretation: it is necessary to find a value of the variable y such that the integral from the posterior density $\hbar(\lambda_0, \lambda_1 \mid \tau)$ over the domain $D \cap D_\gamma$ is equal to the confidence probability γ. The resulting equation takes on the form

$$S_1\left(\underline{R}^*_\gamma(t)\right) - S_2\left(\underline{R}^*_\gamma(t)\right) - \gamma J_{0,\nu}(\omega, \omega_1, d, d_1) = 0 \tag{5.88}$$

where

$$S_1(x) = \sum_{i=0}^{d_1} \frac{d_1^{(i)}}{(\omega_1+1)^{i+1}} \sum_{j=0}^{d-i} \frac{(d-i)^{(j)}}{(\omega+1)^{j+1}} \times \left(R_u^{\omega+1} \left|\ln R_u\right|^{d-i-j} - x^{(\omega+1)/\nu} \left|\ln x^{1/\nu}\right|^{d-i-j} \right),$$

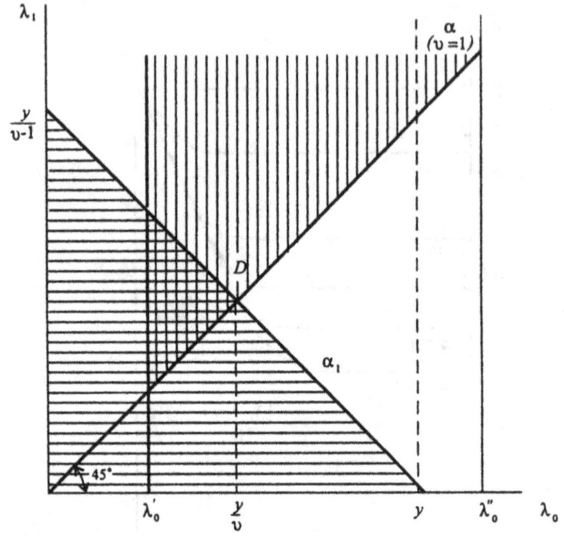

Fig. 5.9 Integration domain for obtaining the Bayes confidence limit of a TTF.

and

$$S_2(x) = \sum_{i=0}^{d_1} \frac{d_1^{(i)}}{(\omega_1+1)^{i+1}} \left(\frac{1}{\nu-1}\right)^{d_1-i} \sum_{k=0}^{d_1-i} \binom{d_1-i}{k} |\ln x|^{d_1-i-k}$$
$$\times \sum_{j==0}^{d_0+k} \frac{(d_0+k)^{(j)}}{a^{j+1}} \left[x^b R_u^a |\ln R_u|^{d_0-k-j} - x^{(\omega+1)/\nu} \left|\ln x^{1/\nu}\right|^{d_0-k-j}\right],$$

where

$$\alpha = \frac{\nu(\omega-\omega_1)-(\omega-1)}{\nu-1}, \quad b = \frac{\omega_1+1}{\nu-1}, \text{ and } d_0 = d-d_1.$$

The equation (5.88) is transcendental and quite complicated. However, the numerical integration may be performed without any difficulties since this equation has only one root in the interval $[R_\ell, R_u]$.

The calculation results, obtained with the help of expressions (5.85) and (5.87), are presented in Tables 5.4-5.6. The table data emphasize the inconsistency of the chosen method. Actually, for a fixed d_1 the estimates $\hat{R}^*(t)$ and $\underline{R}^*_\gamma(t)$ are decreasing while d is increasing. In contrast to Tables 5.1–5.3, Tables 5.4–5.6 don't contain equal diagonal elements. It appears to be natural, since for $R(t_0)$ the failures, occurred after t_0, are insignificant. At the same time, this fact plays the leading role for $R(t)$ when $t > t_0$.

The length of the interval $[R_\ell, R_u]$ effects the TTF estimates similarly to the one in the previous case. It should be noted that decrease of the difference $R_u - R_\ell$ induces the estimates

Table 5.4 The Bayes point-wise TTF estimate $\hat{R}^*(t)$ as $t > t_0$.

d_1	d									
	0	1	2	3	4	5	6	7	8	9
0	0.9318	0.9053	0.8875	0.8756	0.8675	0.8618	0.8577	0.8546	0.8522	0.8501
1		0.9029	0.8805	0.8662	0.8569	0.8506	0.8461	0.8427	0.8403	0.8382
2			0.8750	0.8553	0.8432	0.8354	0.8302	0.8265	0.8237	0.8216
3				0.8475	0.8293	0.8184	0.8116	0.8070	0.8037	0.8013
4					0.8207	0.8033	0.7931	0.7867	0.7824	0.7794
5						0.7945	0.8468	0.7680	0.7619	0.7578
6							0.7778	0.7530	0.7435	0.7376
7								0.7446	0.7290	0.7198
8									0.7208	0.7057
9										0.6978c

$$R_\ell = 0.9; \quad R_u = 1.0; \quad \omega = 30.73; \quad \omega_1 = 11.13; \quad \nu = \frac{t}{t_0} = 1.4$$

$\hat{R}^*(t)$ and $\underline{R}^*_\gamma(t)$ to approach each other while the parameter ν increases. This property is illustrated in Figure 5.10.

As can be seen from Fig. 5.10, the TTF estimates decrease while ν increases. This emphasizes the naturalness of the dependence of TTF estimates on the dimensionless parameter ν.

5.3.3 *Investigation of the certainty of the derived estimates*

The exact error estimate of the proposed method in the class of failure rate distributions has not been found yet. Therefore, we have used a statistical model to justify the obtained results. We model successively samples of sizes 20, 40, 60, 80 of the random variable having the Weibull distribution with c.d.f.

$$F(t) = F(t;\sigma,\alpha) - 1 - \exp\left[\left(\frac{t}{\sigma}\right)^\alpha\right],$$

belonging to the class of failure rate distributions. Censoring from the right is carried out for $\alpha = 1, 2, 3$ and different intervals of a prior uncertainty $[R_\ell, R_u]$. In Table 5.7 we represent a fragment of the results of modeling, namely, the point-wise TTF estimates $\hat{R}^*(t_0)$, obtained with the help of (4.38) for $\nu = 1$, $t = t_0 = 100$ s, $\sigma = 350$ s, $k_1 = 0.75$, $k_2 = 2.0$, and $\delta = 0.8$. Comparing these estimates with the exact value of TTF, we may draw the following conclusions:

Table 5.5 The posterior mean squared value $\sigma_{\hat{R}^*(t)}$ for $t > t_0$.

d_1	d									
	0	1	2	3	4	5	6	7	8	9
0	0.0427	0.0439	0.0416	0.0388	0.0363	0.0343	0.0329	0.0318	0.297	0.0288
1		0.0489	0.0480	0.0455	0.0431	0.0412	0.0398	0.0388	0.0375	0.0368
2			0.0543	0.0528	0.0506	0.0487	0.0472	0.0462	0.0453	0.0448
3				0.0589	0.0574	0.0555	0.0540	0.0529	0.0520	0.0515
4					0.0628	0.0613	0.0596	0.0583	0.0574	0.0567
5						0.0659	0.0644	0.0628	0.0616	0.0608
6							0.0684	0.0669	0.0653	0.0642
7								0.0704	0.0688	0.0673
8									0.0720	0.0704
9										0.0732

$$R_\ell = 0.9; \quad R_u = 1.0; \quad \omega = 30.73; \quad \omega_1 = 11.13; \quad \nu = \frac{t}{t_0} = 1.4$$

1) With increase of a sample volume, the estimate $\hat{R}^*(t_0)$ tends to the exact value of $R(t_0)$;
2) Construction of the interval of a prior uncertainty $[R_\ell, R_u]$ induces a more precise (with respect to $R(t_0)$) value of the estimate.

For $t \neq t_0$ ($\nu \neq 1$) the Bayes estimate $\hat{R}^*(t)$ behaves in the following way: the approach of the pointwise estimate approximation to the exact value $R(t)$ in the interval $[0.9t_0, 1.1t_0]$ is analogous to the one represented in Table 5.7, that is, it is satisfactory; outside of this interval, it is not satisfactory. This fact is illustrated in Fig. 5.11. Consequently, we identify the following important practical recommendation: for a priori information for the TTF $R(t)$ estimating the intervals of a prior uncertainty for the times near to t should be chosen.

5.4 Bayes estimates of a TTF probability for the restricted increasing failure rate distributions

In this section, we shall discuss a method of approximation of the cumulative distribution function $F(t)$, based on the expression (5.6), and apply it to the TTF probability estimation in the case of so called restricted failure rate distributions, defined by the limit value of the growth rate for the intensity function. The use of such a method enables us to estimate the limit error with the help of the chosen approximation. We will study the case of censored testing results and a prior information that reduces to a uniform prior distribution of the

Table 5.6 The Bayes lower confidence limit $R^*_{0.9}(t_0)$ for $t > t_0$.

d_1	d									
	0	1	2	3	4	5	6	7	8	9
0	0.8722	0.8507	0.8446	0.8433	0.8424	0.8315	0.8287	0.8243	0.8238	0.8230
1		0.8400	0.8308	0.8289	0.8261	0.8209	0.8191	0.8170	0.8152	0.8144
2			0.8112	0.8102	0.8094	0.8081	0.8075	0.8068	0.8051	0.8047
3				0.7829	0.7812	0.7801	0.7792	0.7783	0.7772	0.7766
4					0.7549	0.7538	0.7524	0.7513	0.7503	0.7496
5						0.7274	0.7266	0.7258	0.7249	0.7239
6							0.7008	0.6998	0.6990	0.6987
7								0.6753	0.6740	0.6731
8									0.6507	0.6492
9										0.6271

$$R_\ell = 0.9; \quad R_u = 1.0; \quad \omega = 30.73; \quad \omega_1 = 11.13; \quad \nu = \frac{t}{t_0} = 1.4$$

required TTF in the interval $\left[R_\ell, R_u\right] \subset [0,1]$.

5.4.1 *Parametric approximation on the class of restricted failure rate distributions*

We will use a two parametric approximation of the resource function (5.6) in application to certain subclasses of increasing failure rate distributions.

Definition of a class of restricted increasing failure rate distributions A class of probability distributions $S_0(\delta) \subset S_0$ is said to be a *restricted failure rate*class or δ-failure rate class, if for any distributionfunction $F(x) \in S_0(\delta)$ the relation

$$0 \leqslant \lambda'(x) \leqslant \delta \tag{5.89}$$

holds, where $\lambda(x) = F'(x)/(1-F(x))$ is the failure rate function.

It is clear that for $\delta \geqslant 0$ the class $S_0(\delta)$ is nonempty and $S_0(\infty) = S_0$. For $\delta = 0$, the class $S_0(\delta)$ degenerates into a parametric family of exponential distributions.

A probability distribution function

$$F_{LS}(x) = F_{LS}(x;\alpha,c) = 1 - \exp\left[-\left(\alpha x + \frac{c}{2}x^2\right)\right]$$

for $c \geqslant 0$ will be called, by analogy, the linear failure rate. The class of all linear failure rate distributions, determined by the condition $c \leqslant \Delta$, will be denoted by $S_{LS}(\delta)$. It is clear that $S_{LS}(\delta) \subset S_0(\delta)$, where, $\delta \geqslant 0$ the class $S_{LS}(\delta)$ is nonempty. We will approximate

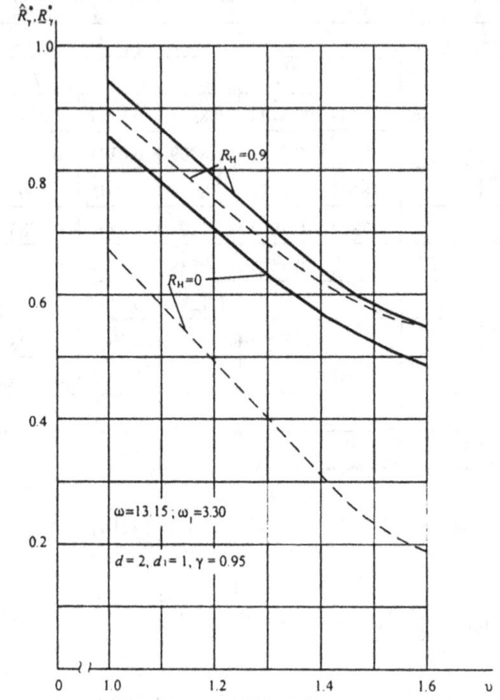

Fig. 5.10 Dependence of the Bayes TTF estimates on dimensionless parameter.

an unknown time to failure distribution function $F(x) \in S_0(\delta)$ with the help of a function $\widetilde{F}(x) = \widetilde{F}(x;\alpha,\theta) = 1 - \exp\left[\widetilde{\Lambda}(x;\alpha,\theta)\right]$. Here

$$\widetilde{\Lambda}(x;\alpha,\theta) = \chi(t-x)\alpha x + \chi(x-t)\left[\theta x - (\theta-\alpha)t\right], \tag{5.90}$$

t is the time for which the TTF is defined, α, θ are parameters. The following lemma clarifies the relationship between $\widetilde{F}(x)$ and a class of linear failure rate distributions.

Lemma 5.1. *Let parameters α and θ belong to the set*

$$\Omega(\delta) = \{(\alpha,\theta): \quad \alpha \geqslant 0, \quad \alpha \leqslant \theta\alpha + \delta t\}.$$

Then for the approximating function $\widetilde{F}(x)$ the following relation holds:

$$F_{LS}(x;\alpha,0) \leqslant \widetilde{F}(x;\alpha,\theta) \leqslant F_{LS}(x;\alpha,\delta).$$

Proof. The failure rate function $\lambda(x) = \widetilde{\Lambda}'(x;\alpha,\theta)$ can be written with the help of (5.90) in the form $\lambda(x) = \chi(t-x)\alpha + \chi(x-t)\theta$. Under the lemma conditions $(\alpha,\theta) \in \Omega(\delta)$ the relation

$$\lambda_1 \leqslant \widetilde{\lambda}(x;\alpha,\theta) \leqslant \lambda_2(x)$$

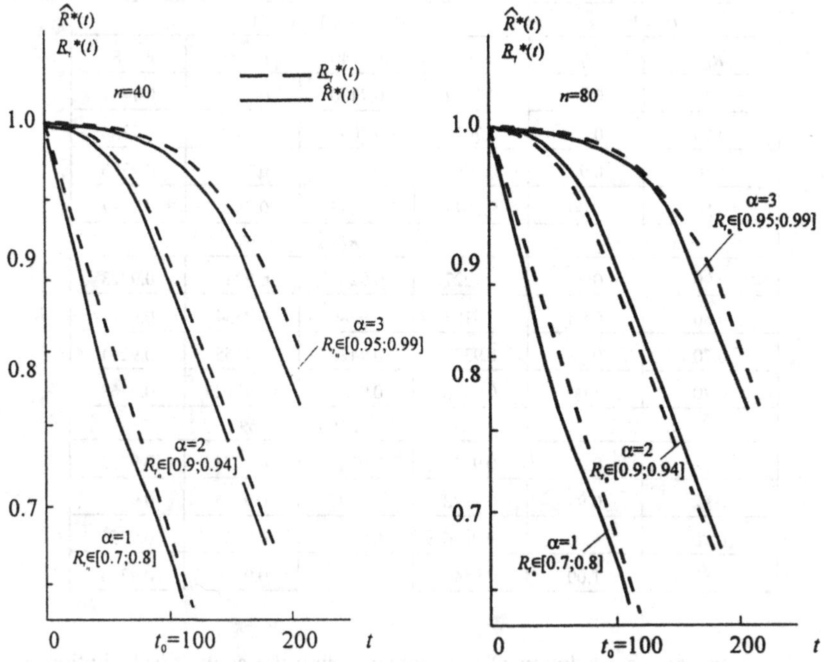

Fig. 5.11 Comparison of the Bayes TTF estimate with its exact values for the Weibull distribution.

holds; moreover, $\lambda_1 = \alpha$ and $\lambda_2(x) = \alpha + \delta(x)$ appear to be, respectively, the intensity functions of the distributions $F_{LS}(x;\alpha,0)$ and $F_{LS}(x;\alpha,\delta)$. The proof of the lemma follows from the above double inequality after the transformation of the failure rate function into a distribution function. □

5.4.2 *Approximate estimates TTF of Bayes for the class* $S_0(\delta)$

To formulate the problem, let us assume the following:

(1) $F(x) \in S_0(\delta)$, with the value δ given;

(2) The estimating TTF $R(t) = 1 - F(t)$ during the given time interval has a uniform prior distribution in the segment $[R_\ell, R_u] \subset [0,1]$;

(3) The testing results have the form of a censored sample $\tau = \{\mathbf{t}^*, \mathbf{t}\}$, obtained after the NC-plan realization. The problem is to obtain the posterior density $\hbar_r(r \mid \tau)$ of the required TTF and estimate $\hat{R}^*(t)$ for a quadratic loss function.

Table 5.7 Comparison of the Bayes posterior pointwise estimate (t_0) with a real TTF value $R(t_0)$ for the Weibull distribution.

$\alpha = 1$		$R(t_0) = 0.7515$			
R_H	R_B	$n = 20$	$n = 40$	$n = 60$	$n = 80$
0.70	0.80	0.7432	0.7420	0.7548	0.7449
0.60	0.85	0.7074	0.7098	0.7618	0.7384
0.50	0.90	0.6945	0.7044	0.7654	0.7386
0.50	1.00	0.6947	0.7045	0.7655	0.7387
$\alpha = 2$		$R(t_0) = 0.9216$			
0.90	0.94	0.9227	0.9237	0.9247	0.9223
0.80	0.96	0.9183	0.9280	0.9334	0.9219
0.70	0.98	0.9337	0.9429	0.9465	0.9264
0.70	1.00	0.9526	0.9515	0.9512	0.9268
$\alpha = 3$		$R(t_0) = 0.9769$			
0.95	0.99	0.9726	0.9751	0.9774	0.9752
0.92	0.99	0.9628	0.9697	0.9746	0.9718
0.90	1.00	0.9636	0.9771	0.9838	0.9756
0.80	1.00	0.9546	0.9756	0.9836	0.9754

We seek the approximate solution of the problem using the analytic substitution of the function $\widetilde{F}(x) \in S_0(\delta)$, given by the expression (5.90), instead of the unknown distribution function $F(x) \in S_0(\delta)$. We additionally require that the relation $F(t) = \widetilde{F}(t)$ (i.e., the values of the true unknown distribution function and the values of its approximating function coincide at time t for which the TTF $R(t)$ is defined). In view of this assumption, the parameter a is uniquely determined by the unknown value of $R(t)$:

$$\alpha = \alpha(R(t)) = -\ln R(t)/t. \tag{5.91}$$

Thus, we will determine the posterior density of the TTF and the corresponding pointwise estimate for the parametric class of distribution functions $\widetilde{F}(x;\alpha,\theta)$, where $(\alpha,\theta) \in \Omega(\delta;R_\ell,R_u) \subseteq \Omega(\delta)$, where $\Omega(\delta;R_\ell,R_u) = \{(\alpha,\theta)\colon \alpha' \leqslant \alpha \leqslant \alpha'',\ \alpha \leqslant \theta \leqslant \alpha + \delta t\}$, $\alpha' = -\ln R_u/t$, $\alpha'' = -\ln R_\ell/t$. A prior density $h(\alpha,\theta)$ is sought in the form

$$h(\alpha,\theta) = h_1(\alpha)h_2(\theta \mid \alpha). \tag{5.92}$$

Taking into account the assumption (2) and the monotonic dependence (5.91), we obtain

$$h_1(\alpha) = \frac{t}{R_u - R_1} e^{-\alpha t}, \quad \alpha \in [\alpha', \alpha''] \in [0, \infty). \tag{5.93}$$

Requiring additionally that the conditional density $h_2(\theta, \alpha)$ belongs to the class of truncated exponential densities given by the relation (5.93), we find

$$h_2(\theta \mid \alpha) = \frac{t\,\mathrm{e}^{-(\theta-\alpha)t}}{1-\mathrm{e}^{-\delta t^2}}, \quad \theta \in [\alpha, \alpha + \delta t]. \tag{5.94}$$

$h_2(\theta \mid \alpha)$ degenerates into the delta-function when $t = 0$. We write the joint prior density $h(\theta, \alpha)$ having substituted (5.93) and (5.94) into (5.92):

$$h(\theta, \alpha) = \frac{t^2 \exp(-\theta t)}{(R_u - R_\ell)\,(1 - \exp(-\delta t^2))}, \quad (\alpha, \theta) \in \Omega(\delta, R_\ell, R_u). \tag{5.95}$$

The likelihood function $\ell(\alpha, \theta \mid \tau)$ for $\widetilde{F}(x; \alpha, \theta)$ can be found analogously to (5.26) and has the following form:

$$\ell(\alpha, \theta \mid \tau) = K(\tau)\alpha^{d_0}\theta^{d_1} \exp\left[-(\alpha K_0 + \theta K_1)\right], \tag{5.96}$$

where

$$K_0 = \sum_{i=1}^{n} \tau_i \chi\,(t - \tau_i) + n_1 t, \quad K_1 = \sum_{i=1}^{n} \tau_i \chi(\tau_i - t) - n_1 t,$$

and

$$n_1 = \sum_{i=1}^{n} \chi(\tau_i - t), \quad d_0 = \sum_{i=1}^{n} \chi(t - \tau_i^*), \quad d_1 = \sum_{i=1}^{n} \chi(\tau_i^* - t),$$

where $K(\tau)$ is a function which depends only on the data τ.
The posterior density $\hbar_r(r \mid \tau)$ is uniquely determined by the prior density $h(\alpha, \theta)$ and the likelihood function $\ell(\alpha, \theta \mid \tau)$.

Theorem 5.1. *Suppose a prior density $h(\alpha, \theta)$ has the form* (5.95). *Then the following relation holds true for the posterior density $\hbar_r(r \mid \tau)$ of the TTF probability $R(t) = 1 - \widetilde{F}(t; \alpha, \theta) \in [R_\ell, R_u]$:*

$$\hbar_r(r \mid \tau) \sim r^{\omega}(-\ln r)^{d_0} \sum_{k=0}^{d_1} \frac{d_1^{(k)}}{(\omega+1)^{k+1}} \left[(-\ln r)^{d_1 - k} - \mathrm{e}^{-\delta t^2(\omega_1 + 1)}(\delta t^2 - \ln r)^{d_1 - k}\right]$$

for $\delta > 0$ and

$$\hbar_r(r \mid \tau) \sim r^{\omega}(-\ln r)^{d_0 + d_1}$$

for $\delta = 0$, where $\omega_1 = K_1/t$, $\omega = (K_0 + K_1)/t$.

Proof. Taking into account the expression (5.91), we obtain

$$R(t) = \exp(-\alpha t).$$

Therefore, in order to obtain $\hbar_r(r \mid \tau)$, we have to find $\hbar_1(\alpha \mid \tau)$.

First, let $\delta > 0$. In accordance with the Bayes theorem $\hbar(\alpha,\theta \mid \tau) \sim h(\alpha,\theta)\ell(\alpha,\theta \mid \tau)$, whence, using the expressions (5.95) and (5.96), we obtain

$$\hbar(\alpha,\theta \mid \tau) \sim \alpha^{d_0}\theta^{d_1}\exp\{-[\alpha K_0 + \theta(K_1+t)]\}, \quad (\alpha,\theta) \in \Omega(\delta; R_\ell, R_u). \tag{5.97}$$

Integration of (5.97) with respect to q over the interval $[\alpha, \alpha+\delta t]$ yields

$$\hbar(\alpha \mid \tau) \sim \alpha^{d_0} e^{-\alpha K_0} e^{-\alpha(K_1+t)} \sum_{k=0}^{d_1} \frac{d_1^{(k)}}{(K_1+t)^{k+t}} \left[\alpha^{d_1-k} e^{-\delta(K_1+t)} (\alpha+\delta t)^{d_1-k}\right],$$
$$\alpha \leqslant \alpha \leqslant \alpha''. \tag{5.98}$$

Since $\alpha = \alpha(r) = -\ln r/t$, for $h_R(r \mid \tau)$ we have

$$\hbar_R(r \mid \tau) = |\alpha'(r)|\hbar_1(\alpha(r) \mid \tau) \sim \frac{1}{t^{d+2}} r^{\omega}(-\ln r)^{d_0}$$
$$\times \sum_{k=0}^{d_1} \frac{d_1^{(k)}}{(\omega_1+1)^{k+1}} \left[(-\ln r)^{d_1-k} - e^{-\delta t^2(\omega_1+1)}(\delta t^2 - \ln r)^{d_1-k}\right], \tag{5.99}$$

which proves the first part of the theorem.

For $\delta = 0$ a prior density $\hbar_2(\theta \mid \alpha)$ degenerates into a delta-function, and for $\hbar(\alpha,\theta \mid \tau)$ the expression

$$\hbar(\alpha,\theta \mid \tau) \sim \alpha^{d_0}\theta^{d_1}\exp\{-[\alpha(K_0+t) + \theta K_1]\}\,\Delta_0(\theta-\alpha)$$

holds, where $\Delta_\theta(x)$ denotes the delta-function of the variable θ. Using the filtering property of the delta-function, we obtain

$$\hbar(\alpha \mid \tau) = \int_{-\infty}^{\infty} \hbar(\alpha,\theta \mid \tau)d\theta \sim \alpha^{d_0+d_1} e^{-\alpha(K_0+K_1+t)}.$$

Now, by analogy with (5.99), we can write

$$\hbar_r(r \mid \tau) \sim \frac{1}{t^{d+1}} r^{\omega}(-\ln r)^{d_0+d_1},$$

which proves the second part of the theorem. □

Using Theorem 5.1, it is easy to find the posterior pointwise TTF estimate for $\delta > 0$ and the quadratic loss function:

$$\hat{R}^*(t) = \int_0^1 r\hbar_r(r \mid \tau)dr = \frac{I_1(R_\ell,R_u)}{I_0(R_\ell,R_u)}, \tag{5.100}$$

where

$$I_m(R_\ell,R_u) = \sum_{k=0}^{d_1} \frac{d_1^{(k)}}{(\omega_1+1)^{k+1}} \left[\sum_{\ell=0}^{d-k} \frac{(d-k)^{(\ell)}}{(\omega+m+1)^{\ell+1}} \left(R_u^{\omega+m}|\ln R_u|^{d-k-1}\right.\right.$$
$$-\left(R_u^{\omega+m}|\ln R_u|^{d-k-1} - e^{-\delta t^2(\omega_1+1)} \sum_{j=1}^{d_1-k} \delta t^2 \sum_{\ell=0}^{d-k-j} \frac{(d-k-j)^{(\ell)}}{(\omega+m+1)^{\ell+1}}\right.$$

$$\times\left(R_u^{\omega+m}|\ln R_u|^{d-k-j-\ell}-R_\ell^{\omega+m}|\ln R_\ell|^{d-k-j-\ell}\right)\Big],\quad d=d_0+d_1.$$

For $R_\ell=0$ and $R_u=1$, the function I_m takes on the following simple form:

$$\begin{aligned}I_m(0,1)=\sum_{k=0}^{d_1}\frac{1}{(\omega_1+1)^{k+1}}&\left[\frac{(d-k)!}{(d_1-k)!}\cdot\frac{1}{(\omega+m+1)^{d-k+1}}\right.\\ -e^{-\delta t^2(\omega_1+1)}&\left.\sum_{j=0}^{d_1-k}\frac{(d-k-j)!}{j!(d_i-k-j)!}\cdot\frac{\delta t^2}{(\omega+m+1)^{d-k-j+1}}\right].\end{aligned}\tag{5.101}$$

By analogy with (5.100), the expression for the posterior variance is written as

$$D[R(t)\mid\tau]=\frac{I_2(R_\ell,R_u)}{I_0(R_\ell,R_u)}-\left[\frac{I_1(R_\ell,R_u)}{I_0(R_\ell,R_u)}\right]^2.$$

Later we shall restrict ourselves to the case $R_\ell=0$, $R_u=1$ corresponding to the absence of a priori information.

5.4.3 *Error approximation*

Information about the error of the approximation used for the distribution function can be obtained with the help of the above lemma. Due to this lemma, the function $\widetilde{F}(x;\alpha,\theta)$ for $(\alpha,\theta)\in\Omega(\delta)$ is situated between the two failure rate distributions. In the following theorem we present the methodfor obtaining the TTF, constructed on linear failure rate distributions.

Theorem 5.2. *The posterior distribution density $\hbar_{LS}(r\mid\tau)$ of the TTF $R_{LS}(t)=1-F_{LS}(t;\alpha,\beta)$ for given β and uniform prior distribution $R_{S(t)}$ satisfies in $[0,1]$ the relation*

$$\hbar_{LS}(r\mid\tau)\sim r^\omega\sum_{k=0}^{d}(\beta t^2)^k\omega_K^*|\ln r|^{d-k},\quad r\in[0,1],$$

where,

$$\omega_0^*=1,\quad \omega_1^*=\sum_{i=1}^{d}\nu_i^*,\quad \omega_2^*=\sum_{1\leqslant i\leqslant}\sum_{j\leqslant d}\nu_i^*\nu_j^*,\ldots,\quad \omega_d^*=\prod_{i=1}^{d}\nu_i^*,$$

$\nu_i^*=\frac{t_i^*}{t}-\frac{1}{2}$, $t^*=(t_1^*,t_2^*,\ldots,t_d^*)$ *is the set of all failure times in τ.*

Proof. In accordance with the expression for $F_{LS}(t;\alpha,\beta)$, we have

$$R(t)=\exp\left[-\left(\frac{\beta}{2}t^2+\alpha t\right)\right].\tag{5.102}$$

Introduce a new parameterization for $F_{LS}(t;\alpha,\beta)$, using the parameter $r=R(t)$. According to (5.102),

$$\alpha=-\frac{\ln r}{t}-\frac{\beta}{2}t.$$

Thereafter, we obtain the following relation for the density function of the linear failure rate distribution:

$$f_{LS}(x) = (\beta x+\alpha)e^{-\frac{\beta}{2}x^2-\alpha x} = \left[\beta\left(x-\frac{t}{2}\right)-\frac{\ln r}{r}\right] r^{\frac{x}{t}} e^{-\frac{\beta}{2}x(x+t)}.$$

Using the common expression of the likelihood function (3.20) for the samples derived after the realization of NC-plan, we can write

$$\ell_{LS}(r \mid \tau) = K(\tau)\prod_{i=1}^{d}\left[\beta t^2\left(\frac{t_i^*}{t}-\frac{1}{2}\right)-\ln r\right] r^{\omega}, \tag{5.103}$$

where $\omega = (\tau_1+\tau_2+\cdots+\tau_n)/t_q$, $K(\tau)$ is a function independent of r. Transforming the product into a sum, we get from (5.103)

$$\ell_{LS}(r \mid \tau) = K(\tau)\sum_{k=0}^{d}(\beta t^2)^k \omega_k^* (-\ln r)^{d-k}.$$

Since the random parameter r is distributed uniformly in the interval $[0,1]$, in accordance with Bayes theorem $\hbar_{LS}(r \mid \tau) \sim \ell_{LS}(r \mid \tau)$, as desired. □

Theorem 5.2 lets us find the corresponding osterior pointwise estimate of TTF:

$$\hat{R}_{LS}^*(t) = \hat{R}_{LS}^*(t;\beta) = \int_0^1 r\hbar_{LS}(r \mid \tau)\,dr = \frac{J_1(\beta)}{J_0(\beta)},$$

where

$$J_m(\beta) = \sum_{k=0}^{d}(\beta t^2)^k \omega_k^* \frac{(d-k)!}{(\omega+m+1)^{d-k+1}}.$$

The relations among the estimates $\hat{R}_{LS}^*(t;\beta)$ for different β will be established in the following theorem. First we introduce a statistic

$$\varepsilon = \sum_{i=1}^{n}\left(\frac{\tau_i}{t}\right)^2.$$

Theorem 5.3. *Let $\varepsilon \geqslant \omega$. Then for any nonnegative β_1 and β_2 such that $\beta_1 \leqslant \beta_2$, the relation*

$$\hat{R}_{LS}^*(t;\beta_1) \leqslant \hat{R}_{LS}^*(t;\beta_2)$$

holds if one uses as a sample of the testing results the same sample τ, and the probability $R_{LS}(t)$ is uniformly distributed a priori in $[0,1]$.

Proof. Parameterize the distribution function $F_{LS}(x;\alpha,\beta)$ using as parameters $r = R(t)$ and $y = \lambda(t)/\lambda(0)$, where $\lambda(x) = \alpha+\beta x$. It is easy to verify that for $\beta \geqslant 0$, $y \geqslant 1$ and, in addition, the condition $\beta_1 \leqslant \beta_2$ implies $y_1 \leqslant y_2$. Therefore, for the theorem proof it suffices to prove that $\hat{R}^*(t;y)$ is a nondecreasing function of y when $y \geqslant 1$.

Write the expression for the distribution function $F_{LS}(x;\alpha,\beta)$ depending on the parameters r and y:

$$F_{LS}(x;r,y) = 1 - r^{\frac{1}{y+1}\left[(y-1)\frac{x^2}{t^2}+2\frac{x}{t}\right]},$$

whence it follows the expression for the density function

$$F_{LS}(x;r,y) = \frac{2}{t}\cdot\frac{(-\ln r)}{y+1}\left[(y-1)\frac{x}{t}+1\right] r^{\frac{1}{y+1}\left[(y-1)\frac{x^2}{t^2}+2\frac{x}{t}\right]}.$$

With the help of the obtained expression for the distribution function and density function of TTF, and the general expression (3.20), we can write the likelihood function, assuming that y is given:

$$\ell_{LS}(r \mid \tau) = K(\tau,y)(-\ln r)^d r^{b(y)}.$$

where $K(\tau,y)$ is a function independent of r, $b(y) = \frac{(y-1)\varepsilon+2\omega}{y+1}$. Since the random parameter is subjected to a uniform prior distribution in $[0,1]$ and, in view of Bayes theorem, we have

$$\hbar_{LS}(r \mid \tau) \sim \ell_{LS}(r \mid \tau),$$

whence

$$\hat{R}^*_{LS}(t;y) = \frac{\displaystyle\int_0^1 \ln^d r \cdot r^{b(y)+1} dr}{\displaystyle\int_0^1 \ln^d r \cdot r^{b(y)} dr} = \left[1 - \frac{1}{b(y)+2}\right]^{d+1}.$$

Investigating the derivative of the function $\hat{R}^*_{LS}(t;y)$ with respect to t, we can write

$$\phi(y) = \left[1 - \frac{1}{b(y)+2}\right]^d \frac{d+1}{(b(y)+2)^2}\cdot\frac{2(\varepsilon-\omega)}{(y+1)^2},$$

we observe that for $\varepsilon \geqslant \omega$, $\phi(y) \geqslant 0$, i.e., the function $\hat{R}^*_{LS}(t;y)$ is nondecreasing with respect to y. □

Observe that the condition $\varepsilon \geqslant \omega$ is always fulfilled when the highly reliable devices for which most of the tests are terminated after the time t is recorded.

Taking into account Theorem 5.2, Theorem 5.3, and the Lemma, we can draw the following conclusion: the approximate estimate $\hat{R}^*_{LS}(t)$ obtained for the class $S_0(\delta)$ for $\varepsilon \geqslant \omega$ lies in the interval $\mu\left(\delta = \left[\hat{R}^*_{LS}(t;0),\, \hat{R}^*_{LS}(t;\delta)\right]\right)$. Moreover, the length of the interval is determined by the value of the limiting failure rate δ and the test results. In Fig. 5.12 we present the graphs of the functions $\hat{R}^*(t)$ and $\mu(\delta)$ as functions of the dimensionless parameter δt^2 under the assumption $R(t) \in [0,1]$ for different values of sufficient statistics. Beginning with some value δ, the estimate $\hat{R}^*_{LS}(t)$ and the upper limit $\hat{R}^*_{LS}(t;\delta)$ remain practically unchanged, having achieved their limit values $\hat{R}^*_{\infty}(t)$ and $\hat{R}^*_{LS}(t;\infty)$. The estimate $\hat{R}^*(t)$ is

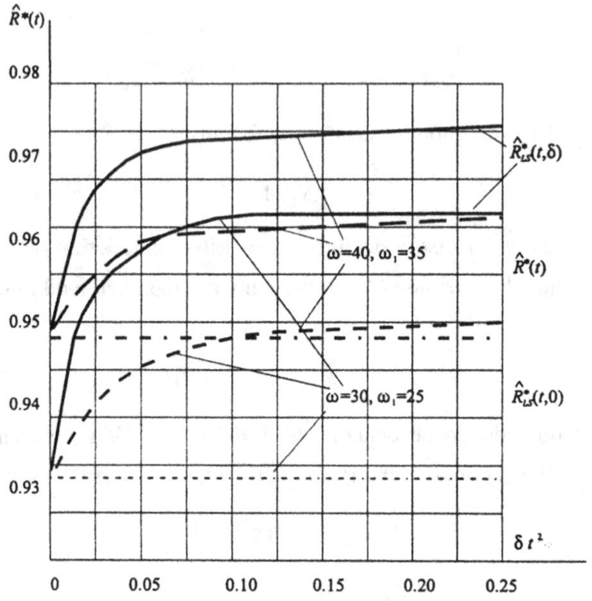

Fig. 5.12 The pointwise TTF estimates and endpoints of the interval $\mu(\delta)$.

determined by the expressions (5.100) and (5.101) which coincide, as $\delta \to \infty$, with the pointwise estimate of the TTF (5.74) for $\nu = 1$. For $\hat{R}^*_{LS}(t;\infty)$ we have

$$\hat{R}^*_{LS}(t;\infty) = \frac{\omega+1}{\omega+2}$$

corresponding to the pointwise estimate of TTF for the exponential distribution of the time to failure under the condition of no failures. The length of the interval $\mu(\delta)$ may be used as a qualitative characteristic for the approximation of an unknown distribution function. We can construct confidence intervals for TTF with the help of the procedure for the posterior density represented in § 5.3 by Theorem 5.1.

Chapter 6

Estimates of the TTF Probability under the Conditions of a Partial Prior Uncertainty

6.1 The setting of a problem and its general solution

In the problem of estimating the reliability of many technical devices, we often meet a situation which is characterized by incomplete or partial prior uncertainty when the given a priori information doesn't allow us to determine uniquely the prior distribution.

The following example may be considered as typical for such a situation. We construct a system containing model elements produced by an industrial complex. We have catalogs with the values of failure rates for each model device. In accordance with the methods of Reliability Theory devoted to complicated multi element systems [256], one defines the TTF value of the model element during the given time interval. The obtained value is a priori for the TTF estimate with respect to a whole complex of the conducted measures and doesn't allow us to form a prior distribution. We need to find a method of estimating TTF based on a pointwise a priori value and testing reliability results. Such a method is initiated in [222, 225].

The theoretical solution of the problem in case of absence of a prior data is known [210, 257]; here the authors use different modifications of a minimax principle. In the work [210] a problem of searching for the optimal solution on the set of all Bayes solutions, corresponding to a definite class of prior distributions, is formulated. In this chapter we shall give a solution of the problem for the class of prior distributions conjugated with the kernel of a likelihood function. A priori information is given in the form of a set of restrictions of the equality and inequality type applied to some functionalisms from unknown prior density. These restrictions make practical sense similar to the problem that we considered above.

6.1.1 *The mathematical setting of the problem*

Let a distribution function of a random time-to-failure be given by a parametric family $F(t) = F(t;\theta)$, where θ is a vector of parameters, $\theta = (\theta_1, \theta_2, \ldots \theta_m)$. Since the problem is formulated in the Bayes form, the parameter is assumed to be random. The system testing is carried out in accordance with some plan P which gives a censored sample τ. The testing plan P and distribution function F generate a class of prior distributions H_{PF}, conjugated with the likelihood kernel. The following restrictions a replaced on the unknown prior density $h(\theta)$ from this class, that is,

$$\begin{aligned} S_j[h(\theta)] &\leqslant 0, \quad j = 1, 2, \ldots, p, \\ S_j[h(\theta)] &= 0, \quad j = p+1, \ldots, p+q, \end{aligned} \tag{6.1}$$

where $S_j[h(\theta)]$ is some functional, determined by the form of given a priori information. For example, if only a prior value R_0 of TTF is known during the time t_0, then the set of conditions (6.1) are reduced to the equality

$$\int_{\Theta} [1 - F(t_0;\theta)]h(\theta)d\theta - R_0 = 0, \tag{6.2}$$

characterizing the coincidence of the theoretical prior mean value of TTF with R_0. In practice, the expressions having the form (6.2) are used most often.

In the general case, the restrictions (6.1) construct the class of prior distributions generating a subclass $H_{PF}^{pq} \subset H_{PF}$. The subject of consideration is some functional $R[(F(t)]$, characterizing the system reliability. In particular, it may be a TTF during some time interval. Then $R = R(t) = 1 - F(t)$. If a mean operating time is used as a reliability index, the functional has the form

$$T = T(\theta) = \int_0^{\infty} [1 - F(t;\theta)]dt.$$

It is assumed that a loss function $L(\hat{R}, R(F(t))$, is given allowing us to write a function of the posterior risk $G(\hat{R}, h)$. The problem is to find the estimate $\hat{R}$, minimizing the risk function in the class of prior distributions H_{PF}^{pq}.

6.1.2 *Determination of a class of prior distributions* H_{PF}

In accordance with the problem setting, the sample τ is censored, i.e., it is represented by the union of two vectors: $\tau = \{\mathbf{t}^*, t\}$, where $t^* = (t_1^*, \ldots, t_d^*)$ is a vector of failure times, and $t = (t_1, \ldots, t_K)$ is a vector of censoring elements. In accordance with the expression (3.21), a likelihood function for an arbitrary parametric family $F(t;\theta)$ may be written as

$$\ell(\theta \mid \tau) = K(\tau) \prod_{i=1}^{d} \lambda(t_i^*;\theta) \exp\left[-\sum_{j=1}^{n} \Lambda(T_j;\theta) \right],$$

where $K(\tau)$ is a sample function independent of the parameter θ:

$$\lambda(t;\theta) = F'(t;\theta)/[1-F(t;\theta)], \quad \Lambda(t;\theta) = \ln[1-F(t;\theta)].$$

We have to find, with the help of the expression for $\ell(\theta \mid \tau)$, a minimal sufficient statistic $\alpha = \alpha(P,F)$ which is defined by the testing plan P and the form of the distribution function F. In the general case a sufficient statistic appears to be a vector $\alpha = (\alpha_1,\dots,\alpha_s) \in \Omega_\alpha$ which allows us to write the likelihood function in the form

$$\ell(\theta \mid \tau) = c_0(\tau)\ell_0(\theta,\alpha), \tag{6.3}$$

where $\ell_0(\theta,\alpha)$ is the likelihood kernel, and the function $c_0(\tau)$ is independent of α and θ, and, generally speaking, doesn't coincide with $K(\tau)$. In accordance with the theory of conjugate prior distributions [202], the kernel of a prior density $h(\theta)$ coincides with the likelihood kernel, i.e.,

$$h(\theta;\alpha') \sim \ell_0(\theta;\alpha'), \tag{6.4}$$

where $\alpha' = (\alpha_1',\dots,\alpha_s')$ is a vector of parameters of a prior density. Also, α' has the same dimension as the one for α, and $\alpha' \in \Omega_\alpha$. Thus, the class of prior distributions H_{PF} is completely determined by the form of the function $\ell_0(\theta;\alpha)$ and the set Ω_α. It is possible to broaden this class if one uses a set Ω_α' such that $\Omega_\alpha \subseteq \Omega_\alpha'$ [202]. We can do this, for example, by using real parameters in the vector α' instead of the corresponding integer components of the vector α. This method will be used later in 6.2 and 6.3. In the common case we assume that $\alpha' \in \Omega_\alpha' \supseteq \Omega_\alpha$.

6.1.3 *Construction of the class H_{PF}*

Since the prior density represented depends on the parameter α', the restrictions (6.1) are transformed into functional inequalities and equalities of the form

$$\psi_j(\alpha') \leqslant 0, \quad j = 1,2,\dots,p, \tag{6.5}$$

and

$$\psi_j(\alpha') = 0, \quad j = p+1,\dots,p+q, \tag{6.6}$$

where $\psi_j(\alpha') = S_j[h(\theta;\alpha')]$, $j = 1,\dots,p+q$. The restrictions (6.5) and (6.6) generate the set $D = D_p \cap D_Q$ in the parametric space of the vector α', where D_Q is the set of values of the parameter α' satisfying the equalities (6.6), and D_p is the set of values of the parameter which satisfy all inequalities (6.5). It is assumed that conditions (6.6) are independent, i.e., there are no additional conditions which may be found from these conditions by transformations. The analysis of (6.5) and (6.6) shows that, first of all, D is nonempty. Because the functions $\psi_j(\alpha)$ are nonlinear in a general case, the analysis of the domain D will be very complicated. It should be noted that only for $s < q$ the set of equations (6.6) is unsolvable, and the set D is empty. In the general case for $s \geqslant q$ the set D is nonempty, where, for $s = q$ the set D is countable.

Introduce a class of prior distributions H_{PF}^{pq} represented by the contraction of the class H_{PF}.The class H_{PF}^{pq} is generated by all prior distributions from H_{PF} which satisfy the expressions (6.5) and (6.6), or, is the same as, (6.1). Since the class H_{PF}^{pq} is also defined by the relation (6.4), the parameter α'must belong to the set $\Omega_H = \Omega'_\alpha \cap D \subseteq \Omega'_\alpha$. The resulting formula for the class H_{PF}^{pq} is written as

$$h(\theta;\alpha') \sim \ell_0(\theta;\alpha'), \quad \alpha' \in \Omega_H = \Omega'_\alpha \cap D \Rightarrow h(\theta;\alpha') \in H_{PF}^{pq}. \tag{6.7}$$

6.1.4 *Choice of a prior density from the class H_{PF}^{pq}*

If the set D is nonempty and contains more than one point, each of which corresponds to a concretely defined prior distribution density, then we are faced with a problem of choice of the unique prior density $h_*(\theta) = h(\theta;\alpha'_*)$. To this end, we will use a posterior risk criterion, i.e., $h_*(\theta)$ will be chosen as a prior density that guarantees the maximum of the function of the posterior risk. In other words, the worst prior distribution giving the most pessimistic (in the sense of the posterior risk) estimates of the reliability index is chosen.

Choose some loss function $L\left(\hat{R},R\right)$ expressing the losses occurred after the replacement of the reliability index $R[T(t;\theta)]$ by the estimate $\hat{R}$. With the help of the function $L\left(\hat{R},R\right)$, the function of the mean posterior risk is written as

$$G\left(\hat{R},h\right) = \int_\Theta L\left(\hat{R},R[F(t)]\right)\bar{h}(\theta \mid \tau)d\theta, \tag{6.8}$$

where $\bar{h}(\theta \mid \tau)$ is the posterior distribution density of the parameter $\theta \in \theta$. To find $\bar{h}(\theta \mid \tau)$ we apply the Bayes theorem. It yields

$$\bar{h}(\theta \mid \tau) = \bar{h}\left(\theta,\alpha''\right) \sim h\left(\theta,\alpha'\right)\ell_0(\theta,\alpha),$$

where $\alpha''$is the parameter of the posterior density. Applying relation (6.4) we obtain

$$\bar{h}\left(\theta,\alpha''\right) \sim \ell_0\left(\theta,\alpha'\right)\ell_0(\theta,\alpha), \tag{6.9}$$

For the vector parameters we will use a binary operation $\alpha'' = \alpha' * \alpha$ which determines the following transformation of two equal functions with different parameters: $p(x;\alpha'') = p(x;\alpha')p(x;\alpha)$. Using this operation, we can rewrite the expression (6.9) in the form

$$\bar{h}(\theta \mid \tau) = \bar{h}(\theta;\alpha'') \sim \ell_0(\theta;\alpha' * \alpha). \tag{6.10}$$

If instead of a prior density $h_*(\theta)$ one uses a distribution density, ensuring the maximum of a mean posterior risk, the problem of obtaining the Bayes posterior estimate $\hat{R}^*$ of the reliability index can be reduced to the following minimax problem:

$$G(\hat{R}^*, h_*) = \min_{\hat{R}} \max_{h \in H_{PF}^{pq}} G(\hat{R}, h). \tag{6.11}$$

Taking into account that $h_*(\theta) = h(\theta; \alpha'_*) \sim \ell_0(\theta; \alpha'_*)$, the problem (6.11) can be reduced to a problem of finding the parameter α'_*. Let us denote $R(\theta) = R[F(t;\theta)]$. Using the equations (6.8)–(6.10) we can write the mean posterior risk function as follows

$$G(\hat{R}, h(\theta; \alpha')) = G_\alpha(\hat{R}, \alpha') = \frac{1}{\beta} \int_\Theta L(\hat{R}, R(\theta)) \ell_0(\theta; \alpha * \alpha') d\theta, \tag{6.12}$$

where β is the normalizing factor of the posterior density. In view of (6.10) we have

$$\beta = \int_\Theta \ell_0(\theta; \alpha * \alpha') \, d\theta.$$

Taking into account the obtained expression (6.12), we can reduce the problem (6.11) to the following minimax problem:

$$G_\alpha(\hat{R}^*; \alpha'_*) = \min_{\hat{R}} \max_{\alpha' \in \Omega_H} G(\hat{R}, \alpha'). \tag{6.13}$$

For many practical problems, it is very difficult to represent the set $\Omega_H = \Omega'_\alpha \cap D$ explicitly. Therefore, it is more convenient to define a by solving the following conditional minimax problem:

$$G_\alpha(\hat{R}^*, \alpha'_*) = \min_{\hat{R}} \max_{\alpha' \in \Omega'_\alpha} G(\hat{R}, \alpha'),$$

$$\psi(\alpha') \leqslant 0, \quad j = 1, \ldots, p, \quad \psi(\alpha') = 0, \quad j = p+1, \ldots, p+q. \tag{6.14}$$

6.1.5 *Solution of the minimax problem*

When solving problem (6.14) we meet many mathematical difficulties arising from the nonlinearity of the functions used. In addition, in some cases we can not write the function of mean posterior risk in an explicit form, and therefore we have to use numerical methods of integration. The problem is simplified essentially if one uses a quadratic loss function. The following theorem is valid for this case.

Theorem 6.1. *Suppose that the loss function* $L(\hat{R}, R) = (R - \hat{R})^2$. *Then the problem* (6.14) *is equivalent to the problem of finding maximum of the posterior variance.*

$$U(\alpha') = \int_\Theta R^2(\theta) \hbar(\theta; \alpha * \alpha') d\theta - \left[\int_\Theta R(\theta) \hbar(\theta; \alpha * \alpha') d\theta \right]^2 \tag{6.15}$$

on the set Ω'_α under the restrictions

$$\psi_j(\alpha') \leqslant 0, \quad j = 1, 2, \ldots, p,$$

and

$$\psi_j(\alpha') = 0, \quad j = p+1, \ldots, p+q.$$

Proof. In accordance with the Walde theorem [257], the following equality of minimax and maximum takes place:

$$\min_{\hat{R}} \max_{\alpha' \in \Omega_H} G_\alpha\left(\hat{R}, \alpha'\right) = \max_{\alpha' \in \Omega_H} \min_{\hat{R}} G_\alpha\left(\hat{R}, \alpha'\right). \tag{6.16}$$

Consider the problem of minimization of the function $G_\alpha\left(\hat{R}, \alpha'\right)$ for each $\alpha' \in \Omega_H$ for a fixed value of the sufficient statistic α:

$$G_\alpha\left(\hat{R}^*, \alpha'\right) = \min_{\hat{R}} \int_\Theta \ell(\hat{R}, R(\theta))\hbar(\theta; \alpha * \alpha')d\theta.$$

The solution of the problem for the quadratic loss function $L(\hat{R}, R) = \left(R - \hat{R}\right)^2$ is represented by the posterior mean value

$$\hat{R}^* = \int_\Theta R(\theta)\hbar(\theta; \alpha * \alpha')d\theta, \tag{6.17}$$

which gives the following posterior risk function:

$$G_\alpha\left(\hat{R}^*, \alpha'\right) = \min_{\hat{R}} \int_\Theta \left[R(\theta) - \hat{R}^*\right] \hbar(\theta; \alpha * \alpha')d\theta. \tag{6.18}$$

The estimate (6.17) is conditionally optimal, i.e., it enables us to find the posterior mean value of a TTF for a given α'. Substituting the expression (6.18) into (6.14) and taking into account the expressions (6.16) and (6.17), we obtain the following formulation of the problem:

$$G_\alpha\left(\hat{R}^*, \alpha'\right) = \max_{\alpha' \in \Omega'_\alpha} \left\{ \int_\Theta R^2(\theta)\,\hbar(\theta; \alpha * \alpha')d\theta - \left[\int_\Theta R(\theta)\,\hbar(\theta; \alpha * \alpha')d\theta\right]^2 \right\}$$

$$\psi_j(\alpha') \leqslant 0, \quad j = 1, \ldots, p, \quad \psi_j(\alpha') = 0, \quad j = p+1, \ldots, p+q,$$

which proves Theorem 6.1. In order to obtain the Bayes lower confidence limit $\underline{R}^*_\gamma$ with given α'_*, we need to solve, in accordance with (2.34), the equation

$$\int_{R(\theta \geqslant R^*_\gamma)} \hbar(\theta; \alpha * \alpha')d\theta - \gamma = 0. \tag{6.19}$$

□

Formulation of the problem (6.14) together with the equation (6.19) gives us the method of obtaining TTF estimates. These estimates are called conditionally minimaximal in view of the special form of the problem arising from the estimation method.

6.2 A partial prior information for the Bernoulli trials

6.2.1 *Formulation of the problem*

Consider the following testing plan P_B. n devices are being tested having a single-use purpose. Each device during the test period has a capacity for performing with a constant probability p and fails with a probability $1-p$. The unknown quantity p will be considered as a parameter in the interval of admissible values $[0,1]$. Assume that during the testing $d \geqslant 0$ devices fail. The likelihood function for the subject scheme has the form

$$\ell(p;n,d) = \binom{n}{d} p^{n-d}(1-p)^d. \qquad (6.20)$$

In this case the following beta-distribution plays the role of a prior distribution conjugated with the likelihood kernel (6.20), that is,

$$h(p) = h(p;\alpha,\beta) = \frac{p^{\alpha-1}(1-p)^{\beta-1}}{\beta(\alpha,\beta)}, \quad \alpha \geqslant 0,\ \beta \geqslant 0, \qquad (6.21)$$

where $\beta(\alpha,\beta)$ is a beta-function. Note that in the subject case the expansion of the class of a conjugate prior distribution takes place because the sufficient likelihood statistics are integer constants, and parameters α and β are real numbers. Let us denote the beta-distribution with the parameters α and β by $Be(\alpha,\beta)$.

Consider the problem of obtaining the TTF $R = p$ which, in the given case, will be out-of-time characteristic, under the conditions of a partial prior uncertainty, expressed in the form of a single restriction. Let us assume that at first a prior TTF value R_0 is known. This condition has the following mathematical interpretation:

$$\int_0^1 ph(p;\alpha,\beta)dp = R_0.$$

After integration

$$\frac{\alpha}{\alpha+\beta} = R_0. \qquad (6.22)$$

The posterior distribution, corresponding to the likelihood (6.20) and a prior density (6.21), is $Be(\alpha+n-d,\beta+d)$.

In order to find optimal values α_* and β_* of the parameters of a prior density $h_*(p) = h(p;\alpha_*,\beta_*)$, we will use the quadratic loss function $L(\hat{p},p) = (p-\hat{p})^2$. In view of Theorem 6.1, the problem is reduced to the minimization of the function of the posterior variance

$$U(\alpha,\beta) = \int_0^1 \frac{x^{\alpha+n-d-1}(1-x)^{\beta+d-1}}{B(\alpha+n-d,\beta+d)}dx - \left[\int_0^1 \frac{x^{\alpha+n-d-1}(1-x)^{\beta+d-1}}{B(\alpha+n-d,\beta+d)}dx\right]^2$$

under the restriction (6.22). Carrying out the calculations, we obtain

$$U(\alpha_*,\beta_*) = \max_{\substack{\alpha\geqslant 0\\ \beta\geqslant 0}} U(\alpha,\beta) = \max_{\substack{\alpha\geqslant 0\\ \beta\geqslant 0}} \frac{(\alpha+n-d)(\beta+d)}{(\alpha+\beta+n)^2(\alpha+\beta+1)}, \quad \frac{\alpha}{\alpha+\beta} - R_0 = 0. \qquad (6.23)$$

6.2.2 *Peculiarities of the problem solution*

Let us clarify some characteristics of the problem (6.23) useful for applications. At first we will investigate the case when there is no information about experiment outcomes, i.e., in the problem (6.23) $n = d = 0$. This, and other cases in which we are interested, will be formulated and provided when it is necessary.

Theorem 6.2. *Suppose that the posterior variance is represented by the formula*

$$U(\alpha,\beta) = \frac{\alpha\beta}{(\alpha+\beta)(\alpha+\beta+1)}, \quad \alpha \geqslant 0,\ \beta \geqslant 0.$$

Then the point (α_*,β_*), corresponding to maximum of the function $U(\alpha,\beta)$ under the restriction $\alpha/(\alpha+\beta) = R_0$ is $(0,0)$ for any R_0. Moreover, the maximum value of U will be $R_0(1-R_0)$.

Proof. Introduce the variable $z = \alpha+\beta$. With the help of this variable and the equality $\alpha/z = R_0$, the function $U(\alpha,\beta)$ may be written as

$$F(z) \equiv U(\alpha,\beta) = \frac{R_0(1-R_0)}{z+1}.$$

Since $\alpha \geqslant 0$, $\beta \geqslant 0$, one has $z \geqslant 0$. The function $F(z)$ in the domain of its nonnegative values has a supremum at the point $z = 0$ equal to $F(0) = R_0(1-R_0)$. Taking into account our assumption $\alpha = R_0 z$ for $z = 0$, we obtain $\alpha = \beta = 0$ as was desired. □

Due to the proved property, the optimal values of the parameters α_* and β_* in absence of experimental data are independent of the a priori value of TTF R_0, and the desired TTF estimate equals the, prior one R_0, and has the variance $R_0(1-R_0)$.

Consider now the more general case $n \geqslant 0$. The solution of the problem (6.23) for this case is represented by the following statement.

Theorem 6.3. *Suppose the function of the posterior variance of the index R_0 is written as*

$$U(\alpha,\beta) = \frac{(\alpha+n-d)(\beta+d)}{(\alpha+\beta+n)^2(\alpha+\beta+n+1)}$$

for $\alpha \geqslant 0$, $\beta \geqslant 0$, $n > 0$, $d \geqslant 0$. Then the function U is monotonically decreasing along any straight line of the form $\alpha/(\alpha+\beta) = R_0$, if the following inequality holds

$$\left(\frac{1-R_0}{R_0} - g\right)\left(d - \frac{n}{2}\right) \geqslant 0, \tag{6.24}$$

where

$$g = \frac{d}{n-d} \cdot \frac{(d+1)(n-2d)+2(n-d)^2}{(n-d+1)(n-2d)-2d^2}. \tag{6.25}$$

Proof. Introduce the variables $x + \alpha + m$, where $m = n - d$, and $y = \beta + d$. The function $U(\alpha, \beta)$ changes into

$$\widetilde{U}(x,y) = \frac{xy}{(x+y)^2(x+y+1)}, \quad x \geqslant m,\ y \geqslant d.$$

In view of Theorem 6.2, the function $\widetilde{U}(x,y)$ for $x \geqslant 0$, $y \geqslant 0$ is monotonically decreasing along any straight line of the form $y = px$ for $p > 0$, and attains its maximum at the point $x = y = 0$. At the same time, the absolute maximum can't be attained at the point $x = y = 0$, i.e., the point $(0,0)$ is an isolated singular point. It is easy to prove that $U(x,y) < 0.25$, for all $x > 0$, $y > 0$. Investigate the function $y = \phi(x)$ obtained in the result of cross-cutting of the function $z = \widetilde{U}(x,y)$ by the plane $z = h$ (for $h < 0.25$). The implicit form of the function $y = \phi(x)$ is $F(x,y) = xy - h(x+y)^2(x+y+1) = 0$. The point $x = y = 0$ is a node for the given function, since $\Delta = F''^2_{xy}(0,0) - F''_{xx}(0,0)F''_{yy}(0,0) = 1 - 4h > 0$. It is easy to check also that the function $y = \phi(x)$ is symmetric with respect to the straight line $y = x$. In view of the mentioned properties, the function $F(x,y) = 0$ has the form shown in Fig. 6.1. □

In order to find the form of the function represented by the implicit equation $U(\alpha, \beta) = h$, we have to transfer the origin into the point $x = m = n - d$, $y = d$. As seen from Fig. 6.1, the function $U(\alpha, \beta)$ will not be monotonic along any straight line of the form

$$\frac{\alpha}{\alpha + \beta R} = R_0 \iff \beta = \frac{1 - R_0}{R_0}\alpha.$$

The monotonicity domain is ended by the tangent to the equal-level line $U(\alpha, \beta) = h$ at the point $\alpha = \beta = 0$, or is the same, to the equal-level line $\widetilde{U}(x,y) = h$ at the point $x = m$, $y = d$.

We proceed to find the slope g of this tangent. By definition,

$$g = -\frac{F'_x(m,d)}{F'_y(m,d)} = \frac{d}{m} \cdot \frac{(d+1)(m-d) + 2m^2}{(m+1)(m-d) - 2d^2}. \tag{6.26}$$

As seen from Fig. 6.1, for $m \geqslant d$ ($n \geqslant d/2$) the function $U(\alpha, \beta)$ will be monotonically decreasing along any straight line whose slope doesn't exceed g. For $m < d$ ($n < d/2$), vice versa, the function $U(\alpha, \beta)$ is monotonically decreasing along any straight line with the slope which is greater or equal to g. In other words, the monotonicity condition for the function $U(\alpha, \beta)$ along the straight line $\alpha/(\alpha + \beta) = R_0$ takes on the following form

$$\frac{1 - R_0}{R_0} \leqslant g, \quad \text{if } d \leqslant \frac{n}{2},$$

and

$$\frac{1 - R_0}{R_0} > g, \quad \text{if } d > \frac{n}{2},$$

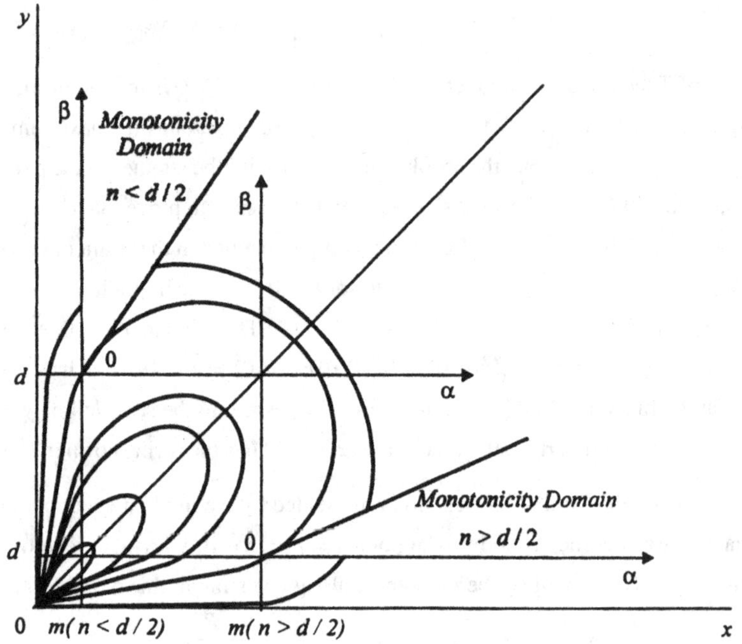

Fig. 6.1 Curves with equal levels for the function $U(x,y)$ and $U(\alpha,\beta)$.

which may be written with the help of (6.24).

In view of this theorem we can easily obtain the following two corollaries:

Corollary 6.1. *The solution of problem* (6.23) *under the condition* (6.24) *is independent of* R_0, *and is written as* $\alpha_* = \beta_* = 0$. *The posterior Bayes estimate for this case coincides with the maximum likelihood estimate:*

$$\hat{R}^* = 1 - \frac{d}{n} \quad and \quad \sigma^2_{\hat{R}^*} = \frac{\left(1 - \frac{d}{n}\right)\frac{d}{n}}{n+1}.$$

Thereby the Bayes conditionally minimax estimate may ignore a priori information, if the last one contradicts the results of testing.

Corollary 6.2. *For completely successful tests* ($d = 0$), *the condition of monotonicity* (6.2) *is never fulfilled.*

The following statement establishes the relationship between the Bayes and maximum likelihood estimates.

Theorem 6.4. *Suppose the condition* (6.24) *is not fulfilled and the solution of the problem* (6.23) *differs from the trivial one. Then the Bayes pointwise TTF estimate* $\hat{R}^*$ *for the quadratic loss function exceeds the maximum likelihood estimate, if* $R_0 \leqslant 1 - d/n$.

Proof. The Bayes estimate $\hat{R}^*$ for the quadratic loss function coincides with the posterior mean value, that is,

$$\hat{R}^* = \hat{R}^*(\alpha,\beta) = \frac{\alpha+n-d}{\alpha+\beta+n}.$$

Investigate the behavior of the function $\hat{R}^*(\alpha,\beta)$ along the straight line $\alpha/(\alpha+\beta) = R_0$. To this end, we express $\hat{R}^*(\alpha,\beta)$ as a function of a single variable α:

$$\left.\hat{R}^* = \frac{\alpha+n-d}{\alpha+\beta+n}\;\frac{\alpha}{\alpha+\beta} = n_0\right\} \Longrightarrow \hat{R}^*(\alpha,\beta) = \phi(\alpha) = \frac{\alpha+n-d}{\alpha/R_0+n}.$$

The derivative of the function $\phi(\alpha)$ will be

$$\phi'(\alpha) = \frac{d+(1-R_0)n}{R_0\left(\frac{\alpha}{R_0}+n\right)}.$$

As seen from the last expression $\phi'(\alpha) > 0$, if $R_0 > 1-d/n$, and $\phi'(\alpha) \leqslant 0$, if $R_0 \leqslant 1-d/n$. Therefore, since $\alpha_* > 0$, under the condition $R_0 > 1-d/n$, we have

$$\hat{R}^*(\alpha_*,\beta_*) = \phi(\alpha_*) > \phi(0) = 1-\frac{d}{n}.$$

Otherwise, i.e., when $R_0 \leqslant 1-d/n$, we have

$$\hat{R}^*(\alpha_*,\beta_*) = \phi(\alpha_*) \leqslant \phi(0) = 1-\frac{d}{n}.$$

and the theorem is now proved. □

If the condition (6.24) is not fulfilled, the problem of obtaining optimal values of the parameters α_* and β_* can be reduced to the solution of a cubic equation. Introduce a new variable $z = \alpha+\beta+n$. After this the problem (6.23) represents by itself the problem of finding a maximum for the following function of variable z:

$$T(z) = \frac{[R_0(z-n)+n-d]\,[(z-n)(1-R_0)+d]}{z^2(1+z)}.$$

Applying Calculus methods to the last problem we arrive at the equation

$$z^3 + Az^2 + Bz + C = 0, \tag{6.27}$$

where

$$A=-\frac{2s(2R_0-1)}{R_0(1-R_0)},\quad B=-\frac{s(3s+2R_0-1)}{R_0(1-R_0)},$$
$$C=-\frac{2s^2}{R_0(1-R_0)},\quad \text{and}\quad s=n(1-R_0)-d. \tag{6.28}$$

The equation (6.27) has a single root z_* in the domain $z>n$. Thereafter we obtain the resulting expression for the parameters α_* and β_*, that is,

$$\alpha_*=(z_*-n)R_0\quad\text{and}\quad \beta_*=(z_*-n)(1-R_0). \tag{6.29}$$

6.2.3 *A scheme for evaluating TTF estimates*

A prior pointwise estimate of TTF R_0, the total number of tests n and the number of failures d are the input data for calculation. The following scheme will be applied for finding pointwise estimates $\hat{R}^*$ and $\sigma_{\hat{R}^*}$:

a) By the formula (6.25) we find the slope g of the tangent and verify the condition (6.24).

b) If the condition (6.24) is fulfilled, then we evaluate the desired estimates

$$\hat{R}^*=1-\frac{d}{n}\quad\text{and}\quad \sigma_{\hat{R}^*}=\frac{(n-d)d}{n^2(n+1)},$$

and the algorithm terminates. Otherwise we pass to the next step.

c) With the help of (6.28) we Bud the values of the coefficients A, B, C and solve equation (6.27) in the domain $z>n$. Having solved the problem, we obtain the single root z_*.

d) Using (6.29) we obtain the optimal values of α_*, β_*.

e) Calculations are terminated with

$$\hat{R}^*=\frac{\alpha_*+n-d}{\alpha_*+\beta_*+n},\quad \sigma_{\hat{R}^*}=\frac{(\alpha_*+n-d)(\beta_*+d)}{(\alpha_*+\beta_*+n)^2(\alpha_*+\beta_*+n+1)}. \tag{6.30}$$

6.2.4 *Numerical analysis for TTF estimates*

Consider the case of non-failure testing ($d=0$) frequently exploited in practice. In Table 6.1 we represent the graphs of dependence of the parameters α_*, β_* on the number of tests n and a prior value of TTF R_0.

As seen from Table 6.1, the estimates of α_*, β_* for the constant value of R_0 change proportionally, and in addition, α_* and β_* increase together with the increase of n and R_0. In Figures 6.2 and 6.3 we represent the dependencies of the estimates $\hat{R}^*$ and $\sigma_{\hat{R}^*}$ on the

Table 6.1 Optimal values of the parameters of a prior distribution (the first number is α_*, the second is β_*).

N	n_N				
	20	40	60	80	100
Homogeneous data					
0	0.9732	0.9740	0.9753	0.9787	0.9755
2	0.9740	0.9751	0.9788	0.9753	0.9761
4	0.9737	0.9744	0.9760	0.9780	0.9772
Nonhomogeneous data					
0	0.9732	0.9740	0.9753	0.9787	0.9755
2	0.9731	0.9740	0.9779	0.9744	0.9773
4	0.9729	0.9749	0.9735	0.9731	0.9761

number of tests and a prior value of TTF R_0. They demonstrate the behavior of approximations of prior estimates. We can see that as $n \to \infty$ the estimate $\hat{R}^*$ tends to the maximum likelihood estimate, and for $d = 0$ tends to 1. However, as it is seen from Figure 6.2, the convergence rate depends substantially on a prior value of TTF. The same conclusion may be drawn for the posterior mean-squared value.

6.2.5 *A different way to calculate a lower confidence limit of TTF*

In accordance with the definition, the estimate $\underline{R}_\gamma^*$ is defined by the equation

$$\int_{\underline{R}_\gamma^*}^1 \hbar(p;\alpha_*,\beta_*,n,d)\,dp - \gamma = 0, \tag{6.31}$$

where $\hbar(p)$ is the posterior density of the beta-distribution, given by the expression

$$\hbar(p) = \frac{p^{\alpha_*+n-d-1}(1-p)^{\beta_*+d-1}}{B(\alpha_*+n-d,\,\beta_*+d)}, \quad 0 \leqslant p \leqslant 1.$$

The first method for obtaining the estimate $\underline{R}_\gamma^*$ is based on the numerical solution of the equation (6.31) for the function $\hbar(p)$. Unfortunately this method has a disadvantage. For large values of TTF ($R \geqslant 0.99$) and $d = 0$, the posterior density is concentrated in a very small neighborhood of the point $p = 1$. Because of this we can meet serious calculation obstacles: the error of numerical integration may be large.

The second method is based on the known results about a completely defined binomial scheme. The use of such a method is possible because of the following fact: after determination of the parameters α_* and β_*, the considered scheme will be completely determined. Due to this reason, satisfies the relation [120]:

$$\underline{R}_\gamma^* = \left[1 + \frac{\beta_*+d}{\alpha+n-d} F_{1-\gamma;2(\beta_*+d);2(\alpha_*+n-d)}\right]^{-1}. \tag{6.32}$$

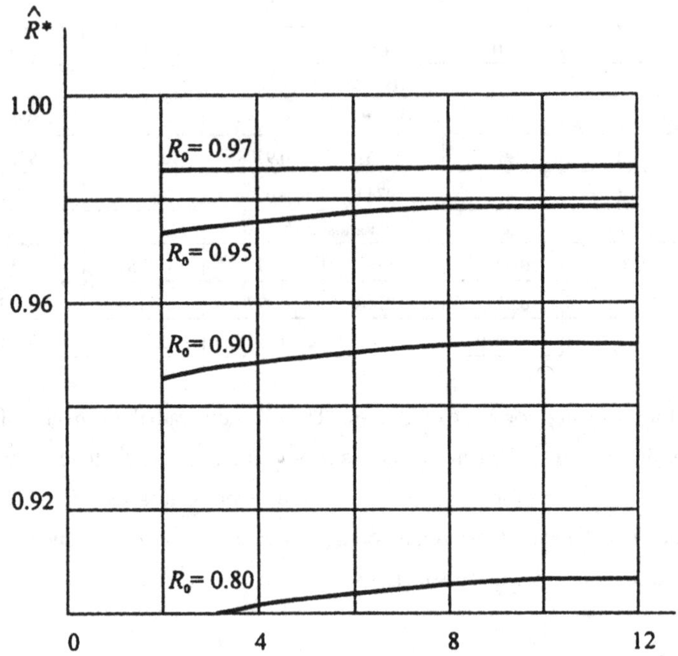

Fig. 6.2 The posterior pointwise TTF estimate.

where $F_{\delta;\nu_1,\nu_2}$ is the 100 δ-percent point of the F-distribution with ν_1, ν_2 degrees of freedom which is found from the tables [160]. The difficulties arising from practical use of the expression (6.32) are characterized by the following: even the fullest tables [160] contain the values of percentiles of the F-distribution beginning with the value of the degree of freedom $\nu_1 = 0.1$. At the same time, if we carry out the practical calculations for highly reliable devices, we need to have the percentile values for $\nu_1 < 0.1$ (see, for example, the data from Table 6.1). In Table 6.2 we represent the calculated values of the estimate for different n and R_0. It is easy to see that $\underline{R}_\gamma^*$ increases more rapidly in comparison with $\hat{R}^*$ as R_0 and n increase.

We present a third method to obtain approximate estimates of $\underline{R}_\gamma^*$. It is based on the analytical change of the posterior density $\hbar\,[p]$ by the density $\underset{\underset{\sim}{\hbar}(p)}{\rightarrow}$, corresponding to the prior

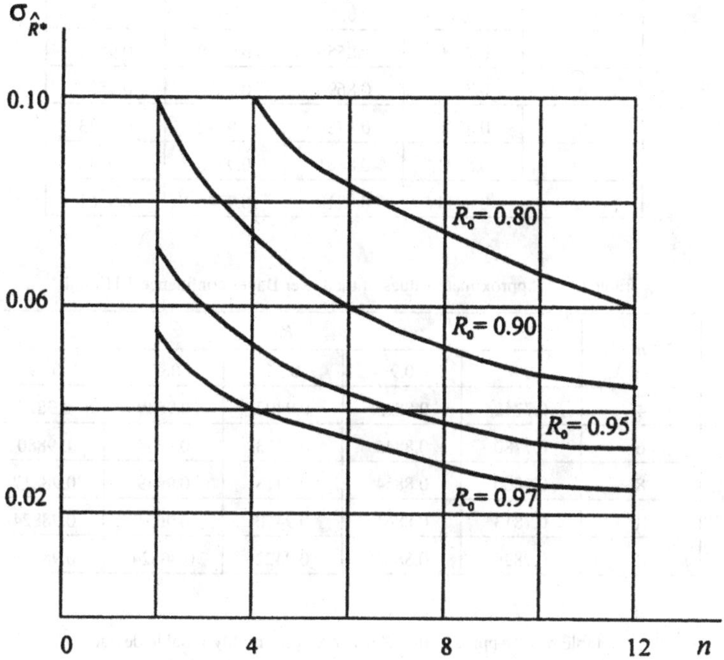

Fig. 6.3 The posterior mean squared value of a TTF.

scheme. The corresponding conditions for $\hbar$ and $\underset{\underset{\sim}{\hbar}(p)}{\rightarrow}$ is written in the form of equality of their first times

$$\int_0^1 p\hbar(p)\,dp = \int_0^1 p\,\underset{\sim}{\hbar}(p)\,dp.$$

Taking into account the above assumptions, we obtain

$$\underset{\sim}{\hbar}(p) = \frac{p^{c-1}}{B(c,1)}, \quad 0 \leqslant p \leqslant 1, \tag{6.33}$$

where $c = \hat{R}^*/(1-\hat{R}^*)$. Then (6.30) may be rewritten as

$$\int_{\underline{R}^*_\gamma}^1 \underset{\sim}{\hbar}(p)(p;c,1)\,dp - \gamma = 0,$$

and thereby we can obtain the analytical solution

$$\underline{R}^*_\gamma = (1-\gamma)^{1/c}. \tag{6.34}$$

Table 6.2 The values of the lower Bayes confidence limit of the TTF.

n	R_0			
	0.8	0.9	0.95	0.97
4	0.7500	0.8556	0.9188	0.9432
6	0.7855	0.8690	0.9237	0.9523
8	0.8018	0.8789	0.9282	0.9533
10	0.8131	0.8861	0.9315	0.9548
12	0.8211	0.8910	0.9340	0.9561

Table 6.3 Approximate values of the lower Bayes confidence TTF limit.

n	R_0				
	0.8	0.9	0.95	0.97	0.99
4	0.7742	0.8825	0.9402	0.9639	0.9878
6	0.7780	0.8845	0.9413	0.9644	0.9880
8	0.7800	0.8854	0.9418	0.9649	0.98817
10	0.7813	0.8861	0.9420	0.9651	0.98824
12	0.7820	0.8865	0.9422	0.96524	0.98829

Table 6.4 Approximate values of $R^*_{0.9}$ for highly-reliable devices.

n	R_0			
	0.9990	0.9992	0.9994	0.9996
6	0.9988048	0.9990438	0.9992888	0.9995217
10	0.9988259	0.9990574	0.9992929	0.9995286

Table 6.5 Approximate values of $\bar{Q}_{0.9}$ for highly-reliable devices.

n	R_0			
	0.9990	0.9992	0.9994	0.9996
6	$1.1952 \cdot 10^{-3}$	$9.562 \cdot 10^{-4}$	$7.172 \cdot 10^{-4}$	$4.783 \cdot 10^{-4}$
10	$1.1784 \cdot 10^{-3}$	$9.426 \cdot 10^{-4}$	$7.071 \cdot 10^{-4}$	$4.714 \cdot 10^{-4}$

In Table 6.3 we represent the values of $\underline{R}^*_{0.9}$, obtained with the third method, for different R_0 and n for tests with no failures. Comparison of the data from Tables 6.2 and 6.3 characterize the exactness of approximate methods.

In Table 6.4 we give the values of $\underline{R}^*_{0.9}$ for $d = 0$.

Representation of the final result in the form of the lower confidence limit $\bar{Q}_\gamma$ of the probability of failure is more observable. In Table 6.5 we represent the values of $\bar{Q}_{0.9}$ corresponding to the data from Table 6.4.

The results, represented in Table 6.5, are more suitable for applied analysis for the following reasons. What matters is that for large values of TTF (greater than 0.999) the values of the estimates we obtain are slightly distinguishable from the point of view of traditional numerical methods (the values differ beginning only with the fifth digit). At the same time, if one uses for the purpose of comparative applied analysis, a probability of failure, then the differences among the estimates will be more essential (beginning with the first valuable digit). In accordance with this, it should be more preferable to define the confidence requirement in the form of a probability of failure Q_{req} which must be ensured with the confidence level γ. As a corollary of this, the procedure of control of the achieved confidence level must be established in accordance with the condition $\bar{Q}_\gamma \leqslant Q_{\text{req}}$.

6.2.6 *Comparison with known results*

Next we consider the following example, touching upon the estimate of TTF by the results of natural tests, and give its solution using different methods.

Example 6.1. From a priori information we know a prior pointwise estimate of TTF $R_0 = 0.9576$ and its error characteristic $\sigma_{R_0} = 0.0333$ during the experiment 12 tests with no failures of the device have been carried out. We need to estimate the TTF with the confidence level $\gamma = 0.9$.

Solution. Since R_0 and σ_{R_0} are given, the considered scheme is completely defined. Determine the parameters of a prior distribution α and β by the following known formula:

$$\alpha = R_0\rho, \quad \beta = (1-R_0)\rho \ \text{ and } \ \rho = \frac{1}{\sigma_{R_0}^2}(1-R_0)R_0 - 1.$$

For the initial example data we have $\alpha = 19.97$, $\beta = 0.499$. Putting $\alpha_* = \alpha$, $\beta_* = \beta$ in (6.31), for $n = 12$, $d = 0$, we obtain $\hat{R}^* = 0.9846$, $\sigma_{\hat{R}^*} = 0.0213$. With the help of tables [160] we find the corresponding percentage point of the F-distribution: $F_{0.1,0.998,64} = 2.79$. Thereafter by the formula (6.32) we find the lower confidence limit $\underline{R}^*_{0.9} = 0.9583$. Note, by the way, that for ensuring the confidence level $R_{\text{req}} = 0.9583$ without using a priori information, it would be necessary to carry out 54 tests with no failures.

Consider another example where the scheme of estimating TTF doesn't have a complete prior definiteness.

Example 6.2. The data of this example are almost the same as those in Example 6.1, except that the condition σ_{R_0} is unknown.

Solution. Thus, we have a scheme with a partial prior definiteness, scrupulously investigated in the preceding section. Return to Section 6.2.3. Since $d = 0$, we have $g = 0$ and therefore the condition (6.24) is not fulfilled. Consequently, to find the optimal values of the parameters α_* and β_*, we need to solve the cubic equation (6.27). Using formulas (6.28) we get the value of the equation coefficient $A = -22.94$, $B = -30.60$, $C = -12.75$. Solving the cubic equation we obtain $z_* = 24.22$. With the help of (6.29) we calculate the optimal values of the parameters: $\alpha_* = 11.92$, $\beta_* = 0.52$. Evaluation of the TTF estimates is carried out with the help of expressions (6.30) and (6.32). Finally, $\hat{R}^* = 0.9788$, $\sigma_{\hat{R}^*} = 0.0286$, $\underline{R}^*_{0.9} = 0.9425$. □

Let us compare the solutions of Example 6.1 and Example 6.2. At first, the TTF estimate obtained in the first case has an error less than the one for the second case. Such a conclusion is unavoidable, since the first calculation scheme is completely a priori determined. Therefore, estimating the reliability in the more general case of a partial prior definiteness, we lose in the exactness of obtained estimates. This can be considered as the price we have to pay for the solution of the problem in the more general case. Later, the estimate $\underline{R}^*_\gamma$ in the second case appeared to be less, and consequently, to ensure the same reliability level under the conditions of a partial prior definiteness, we need to carry out more tests than have been done earlier. This may be also interpreted in other words: lack of a priori information is compensated by additional data.

In conclusion, we note that the winnings in the number of tests, in comparison with the traditional Bayes approach, remain more valuable in the case of realization of the scheme with a partial prior definiteness. Thus, in the conditions of Example 6.2 for ensuring the reliability level $R_{\text{req}} = 0.9425$ in the case of absence of a priori information, we need to carry out 39 tests without any observed failures, against 12, under the assumption that the value of R_0 is known. The gain is three times as much as it was earlier. The greater the required values are, the more precise our end result.

6.3 Partial prior information for the constant failure rate

We will assume that the random time to failure obeys the exponential distribution with the function

$$F(t) = F(t;\lambda) = 1 - e^{-\lambda t}, \quad t \geqslant 0, \ \kappa \geqslant 0. \tag{6.35}$$

The tests are carried out in accordance with the plan giving the censored sample $\tau = \{t^*, t\}$, where $t^* = (t_1^*, \ldots, t_d^*)$ is a sample of failure moments, and $t = (t_1, \ldots, t_K)$ is a sample of censoring times.

6.3.1 *A problem of estimating TTF, $R(t)$, for an arbitrary time*

Suppose that as a priori information is used a prior value of TTF, R_0, for a given t_0. We have to find the estimate of $R(t)$ for the time t different (in a general case) from t_0. The solution of the problem will be obtained in accordance with the approach given in § 6.1. Taking into account the general relation (6.3), we write down the likelihood function for the parametric family (6.35):

$$\ell(\lambda \mid \tau) = K(\tau)\lambda^d e^{-K\lambda}, \quad d \geqslant 0, \; K > 0, \tag{6.36}$$

where $K = \tau_1 + \cdots + \tau_n$ is a total test operating time. In view of (6.36), we conclude that the following density of a gamma-distribution with some unknown parameters s and ε is a conjugated prior density for the parameter λ:

$$h(\lambda) = h(\lambda; s, \varepsilon) = \frac{\varepsilon^{s+1}}{\Gamma(s+1)} \lambda^s e^{-\lambda\varepsilon}, \quad \varepsilon \leqslant 0, \quad s \geqslant 0, \tag{6.37}$$

or, in a brief form, we will note that λ fits the distribution $\Gamma(s, \varepsilon)$. The parameter s, in contrast to d, is real, i.e., we meet the expansion of the range of the sufficient statistic (d, k). In accordance with the Bayes theorem $(d, k) * (s, \varepsilon) = (d + s, \, K + \varepsilon)$, thereby the posterior distribution for λ will be $\Gamma(d + s, \, K + \varepsilon)$, i.e.,

$$\hbar(\lambda \mid \tau) = \hbar(d, s, K, \varepsilon) = \frac{(k+\varepsilon)^{d+s+1}}{\Gamma(d+s+1)} \lambda^{d+s} e^{-\lambda(k+\varepsilon)}. \tag{6.38}$$

The parameters s and ε are unknown. Define their optimal values s_* and ε_*, using the minimax principle given in § 6.1. Choose a quadratic loss function and apply Theorem 6.1. The problem of calculating s_* and ε_* is reduced to the maximization of the posterior variance of the function $R(t) = 1 - F(t)$ under the restriction on the prior mean value of this function:

$$U_R(s, \varepsilon) = \int_0^\infty R^2(t; \lambda)\hbar(\pi; d, s, K, \varepsilon) d\lambda - \left[\int_0^\infty R(t; \lambda)\hbar(\lambda, d, K, \varepsilon) d\lambda \right]^2 \Longrightarrow \max, \tag{6.39}$$

$$\int_0^\infty R(t_0; \lambda) h(\lambda; s, \varepsilon) d\lambda = R_0.$$

Having carried out some calculations, one can rewrite the problem (6.39) in the final form

$$U(s_*, \varepsilon_*) = \max_{s, \varepsilon} \left[\left(\frac{K+\varepsilon}{K+\varepsilon+2t} \right)^{d+s+1} - \left(\frac{K+\varepsilon}{K+\varepsilon+t} \right)^{2(d+s+1)} \right], \tag{6.40}$$

As in the preceding paragraph, we come to the problem of the conditional maximum which can only be solved using numerical methods.

6.3.2 *A problem of estimating the failure rate*

Let us change the problem in the following way. First, suppose that we have to estimate the parameter λ, and thereafter, with the help of the obtained estimate, find the estimate of TTF $R(t)$. As before, we will use a quadratic loss function and Theorem 6.1. As a priori information, we will choose a prior value of the failure rate λ_0, i.e., the restriction of the problem will now be written as

$$\int_0^\infty \lambda h(\lambda; s, \varepsilon)\, d\lambda = \lambda_0,$$

or, after substitution of 6.37, and further integration, we have

$$\frac{s+1}{\varepsilon} = \lambda_0. \tag{6.41}$$

Let us write the function of the posterior variance of the parameter λ as a function of the unknown parameters d and ε:

$$U_\lambda(s,\varepsilon) = \int_0^\infty \lambda^2 \hbar(\lambda; d, s, k, \varepsilon) d\lambda - \left[\int_0^\infty \lambda \hbar(\lambda; d, s, k, \varepsilon) d\lambda\right]^2 = \frac{d+s+1}{(k+\varepsilon)^2}. \tag{6.42}$$

Taking into account the expressions (6.42) and (6.41), in accordance with Theorem 6.1, we represent the problem of finding optimal values of the parameters ε_* and s_* in the following form

$$U_\lambda(s_*, \varepsilon_*) = \max_{\substack{s\geqslant 0\\ \varepsilon\geqslant 0}} U_\lambda(s,\varepsilon) = \max_{\substack{s\geqslant 0\\ \varepsilon\geqslant 0}} \frac{d+s+1}{(k+\varepsilon)^2}, \quad \frac{s+1}{\varepsilon} = \lambda_0. \tag{6.43}$$

The problem (6.43) may be solved analytically.

6.3.3 *Solution of problem* (6.43)

Taking into account the restrictions of the problem, we have $\varepsilon = (s+1)/\lambda_0$. Define a function

$$\phi(s) \equiv U_\lambda\left(s, \frac{s+1}{\lambda_0}\right) = \lambda_0^2 \frac{d+s+1}{(\lambda_0 k + s + 1)^2}, \quad s \geqslant 0$$

whose greatest value corresponds to the solution of the problem (6.43). Its derivative is given by

$$\phi'(s) = \lambda_0^2 \frac{(\lambda_0 k - 2d - 1) - s}{(\lambda_0 k + s + 1)^3} \tag{6.44}$$

for $s \geqslant 0$. It is easy to see from (6.44) that the condition

$$\lambda_0 k - 2d - 1 \leqslant 0 \iff \lambda_0 \leqslant \frac{2d+1}{k} \tag{6.45}$$

implies the nonpositiveness of the derivative $\phi'(s)$ for $s \geqslant 0$, where the function $\phi(s)$ is monotonic as $s \geqslant 0$ and reaches its greatest value at the point $s_* = 0$. Otherwise, the function $\phi(s)$ has a single maximum at the point $s_* = \lambda_0 k - 2d - 1$. Thereby, the general solution of the problem (6.43) takes on the form

$$\begin{cases} 0, \dfrac{1}{\lambda_0}, & \text{if } \lambda_0 \leqslant \dfrac{2d+1}{k}, \\ \left(\lambda_0 k - 2d - 1,\ k - \dfrac{d}{\lambda_0}\right), & \text{if } \lambda_0 > \dfrac{2d+1}{k}. \end{cases} \tag{6.46}$$

With the help of the obtained values s_* and ε_*, we find the posterior estimates of the failure rate in the form

$$\hat{\lambda}^* = \frac{d+s+1}{k+\varepsilon_*} \quad \text{and} \quad \sigma^2_{\hat{\lambda}^*} = \frac{d+s+1}{(k+\varepsilon_*)^2}. \tag{6.47}$$

In order to find the upper confidence limit, we apply the results of the work [120] for a completely determined scheme with a constant failure rate. Then

$$\bar{\lambda}_\gamma = \frac{\chi^2_{1-\gamma;2(d+s_*+1)}}{2(k+\varepsilon_*)}, \tag{6.48}$$

where $\chi^2_{\alpha;v}$ is the 100α percent point of the χ^2_v distribution.

6.3.4 *Estimation of the TTF with the help of the failure rate estimates*

When the parameters s_* and ε_*, defined by the expression (6.46), are unknown, the posterior density of the parameter λ (6.38) is determined. It enables us to find, without any difficulties, corresponding TTF estimates $R(t) = 1 - F(t;\lambda) = \exp(-\lambda t)$. In particular,

$$\begin{aligned} \hat{R}^*(t) &= \int_0^\infty e^{\lambda t} \hbar(\lambda; d, s_*, k, \varepsilon_*) d\lambda \\ &= \frac{(k+\varepsilon_*)^{d+s_*+1}}{\Gamma(d+s_*+1)} \int_0^\infty \lambda^{d+s_*\varepsilon^{-\lambda(k+\varepsilon_*+t)}} d\lambda \\ &= \frac{(k+\varepsilon_*)^{d+s_*+1}}{\Gamma(d+s_*+1)} \int_0^\infty \frac{z^{d+s_*\varepsilon} e^{-z} dz}{(k+\varepsilon_*+t)^{d+s_*}} \\ &= \left(\frac{k+\varepsilon_*}{k+\varepsilon_*+t}\right)^{d+s_*+1}. \end{aligned}$$

For the posterior variance $\sigma^2_{\hat{R}^*(t)}$ we apply a similar scheme. Introduce dimensionless parameters

$$u_* = (\varepsilon_* + k)/t \quad \text{and} \quad v_* = s_* + d. \tag{6.49}$$

Thereafter TTF estimates may be rewritten with the help of the following simple formulas:

$$\hat{R}^*(t) = \left(\frac{u_*}{u_*+1}\right)^{v_*+1}, \tag{6.50}$$

Table 6.6 Bayes estimation of TTF with testing without failures $\hat{R}^*(t_0)/\underline{R}^*_{0.9}(t_0)$.

ω	R_0			
	0.9992	0.9994	0.9996	0.9998
2	0.99920153	0.99940095	0.99960045	0.99980003
	0.99816168	0.99862060	0.99907984	0.99953951
6	0.99920413	0.99940235	0.99960105	0.99980023
	0.99816746	0.99862388	0.99908134	0.99953991
10	0.9992066	0.9994038	0.99960165	0.99980033
	0.9981733	0.9986272	0.99808284	0.99954031

and

$$\sigma^2_{\hat{R}^*(t)} = \left(\frac{u_*}{u_*+2}\right)^{v_*+1} - \left(\frac{u_*}{u_*+1}\right)^{2(v_*+1)}$$

For the estimate $\underline{R}^*_\gamma$ the relation $P\{R(t) \geqslant \underline{R}^*_\gamma(t)\} = P\{\bar{\lambda}_\gamma \leqslant \lambda\}$, holds, whence

$$\underline{R}^*_\gamma(t) = \exp\left[-\frac{\chi^2_{1-\gamma;2(d+s_*+1)}}{2u_*}\right]. \tag{6.51}$$

The estimate $\underline{R}^*_\gamma(t)$ also may be found with the help of the equation (6.19) which for the given case takes on the form

$$\int_{e^{-\lambda t} \geqslant \underline{R}^*_\gamma(t)} \hbar(\lambda; d, s_*, k, \varepsilon_*) d\lambda - \gamma = 0,$$

and may be rewritten as

$$\left(\underline{R}^*_\gamma(t)\right)^{u_*}\left[1 + \sum_{k=1}^{d} \frac{1}{k!} u \left|\ln \underline{R}^*_\gamma(t)\right|^k\right] = 1 - \gamma. \tag{6.52}$$

This equation is recommended for the estimation of a TTF as a compound part of some numerical algorithm when it is inexpedient to use the table values of the percent points of the *chi*^{2} distribution. In the case $d = 0$, (6.52) has a simple analytical solution:

$$\underline{R}^*_\gamma(t) = (1-\gamma)^{1/u^*}. \tag{6.53}$$

6.3.5 *Numerical analysis for TTF estimates*

In Tables 6.6 and 6.7 we represent the results of calculations of TTF estimates by the formulas (6.50) and (6.52), depending on a prior value $R_0 = R(t_0)$ and reduced testing statistic $\omega = k/t$. Calculations of TTF, carried out for the time $t = t_0$, allow us to observe the evolution of the posterior estimate $\hat{R}^*$in accordance with the character of empirical data. Comparing Tables 6.6 and 6.7 we conclude that for $d = 1$, TTF estimates are less

Table 6.7 Bayes estimation of TTF with one failure $\hat{R}^*(t_0)/\underline{R}^*_{0.9}$.

ω	R_0			
	0.9990	0.9994	0.9996	0.9998
2	0.99840370	0.99880226	0.99920106	0.99960001
	0.99689645	0.99767105	0.99844630	0.99922240
6	0.998409	0.9988051	0.99920226	0.99960050
	0.9969065	0.9976767	0.99844881	0.9992231
10	0.99841387	0.99880786	0.99920346	0.99960071
	0.99691900	0.99768205	0.99845125	0.99922370

than corresponding estimates in a testing without failures. The increasing of ω and R_0 induces the increasing of TTF estimates.

In Tables 6.8 and 6.9, we present the results of the reliability calculations which depend on the probability of failures. As in § 6.2, we again deal with a visually and practical form of representation to obtain reliability estimates.

6.4 Bayes estimates of the time to failures probability for the restricted increasing failure rate distributions

In Chapters 3 and 5 we have used as a priori information the intervals of prior uncertainty of the estimated parameter. It is assumed also that the estimated index or parameter lies in the indicated interval with the probability equal to 1. Superfluous categoricity of the assertion about the domain of possible values of the parameter is the main drawback of this method. In this section, we will investigate a modification of the method of representation of a priori information in the form of the interval of a prior uncertainty. The essence of such a modification is interpreted as follows: the indicated interval of a priori uncertainty contains the estimated parameter with some probability $\mu < 1$, i.e., it doesn't appear to be completely ensured. Such a form is more preferable because it is less categorical. If one uses conjugated prior distributions, then the reliability estimates belong to the class of Bayes conditional minimax estimates.

6.4.1 *Setting of the problem*

Let a TTF of the investigated device obey the probability distribution with a function $F(t;\theta)$, where $\theta \in \Omega$ is some vector parameter. The parameter θ is distributed in accordance with a probability density $h(\theta)$ which is unknown. As a priori information is

Table 6.8 Bayes estimation of TTF with failure free testing $Q^*(t_0)/Q^*_{0.9}(t_0)$.

ω	R_0			
	0.9992	0.9994	0.9996	0.9998
2	$7.985\cdot 10^{-4}$ $1.838\cdot 10^{-3}$	$5.990\cdot 10^{-4}$ $1.379\cdot 10^{-3}$	$3.995\cdot 10^{-4}$ $9.202\cdot 10^{-4}$	$2.001\cdot 10^{-4}$ $4.605\cdot 10^{-4}$
6	$7.959\cdot 10^{-4}$ $1.833\cdot 10^{-3}$	$5.976\cdot 10^{-4}$ $1.376\cdot 10^{-3}$	$3.989\cdot 10^{-4}$ $9.187\cdot 10^{-4}$	$1.988\cdot 10^{-4}$ $4.601\cdot 10^{-4}$
10	$7.934\cdot 10^{-4}$ $1.827\cdot 10^{-3}$	$5.962\cdot 10^{-4}$ $1.373\cdot 10^{-3}$	$3.983\cdot 10^{-4}$ $9.172\cdot 10^{-4}$	$1.997\cdot 10^{-4}$ $4.597\cdot 10^{-4}$

Table 6.9 Bayes estimation of TTF with failure-free testing $Q^*(t_0)/Q^*_{0.9}(t_0)$.

ω	R_0			
	0.9992	0.9994	0.9996	0.9998
2	$7.985\cdot 10^{-4}$ $1.838\cdot 10^{-3}$	$5.990\cdot 10^{-4}$ $1.379\cdot 10^{-3}$	$3.995\cdot 10^{-4}$ $9.202\cdot 10^{-4}$	$2.001\cdot 10^{-4}$ $4.605\cdot 10^{-4}$
6	$7.959\cdot 10^{-4}$ $1.833\cdot 10^{-3}$	$5.976\cdot 10^{-4}$ $1.376\cdot 10^{-3}$	$3.989\cdot 10^{-4}$ $9.187\cdot 10^{-4}$	$1.988\cdot 10^{-4}$ $4.601\cdot 10^{-4}$
10	$7.934\cdot 10^{-4}$ $1.827\cdot 10^{-3}$	$5.962\cdot 10^{-4}$ $1.373\cdot 10^{-3}$	$3.983\cdot 10^{-4}$ $9.172\cdot 10^{-4}$	$1.997\cdot 10^{-4}$ $4.597\cdot 10^{-4}$

used, a pair (Θ,μ), where $\Theta\in\Omega$, and $\mu\in[0,1]$, satisfy the relation

$$\int_{\Theta} h(\theta)d\theta \geqslant \mu. \tag{6.54}$$

Definition 6.1. The set $\Theta\subset\Omega$ will be called a Bayes prior confidence set, if it satisfies the relation (6.54). In the case of a one-dimensional parameter, the interval $\Theta=[\theta',\theta'']$ is called a prior confidence interval.

We will assume that tests are carried out by the NC-plan and we have obtained the sample $\tau=\{\mathbf{t}^*,\mathbf{t}\}$, where $\mathbf{t}^*=(t_1^*,\ldots,t_d^*)$ is the vector of failure times, and $\mathbf{t}=(t_1,\ldots,t_k)$ is the vector of standstills of tests which are not connected with a failure. The problem is to Bud the posterior estimate of TTF $R(t)=1-F(t)$ for the quadratic loss function.

6.4.2 *General solution of the problem*

Taking into account the restriction (6.54) imposed on a prior density, we can draw the following conclusion: the considered problem coincides with the problem of estimating TTF under the conditions of a partial prior definiteness. As was the case in a general solution (see § 6.1), we will use a conjugate a priori distribution, whose kernel coincides with the likelihood kernel

$$h(\theta) = h(\theta;\alpha') \sim \ell_0(\theta;\alpha'), \tag{6.55}$$

where α' is a vector of parameters of a prior density, and $\ell_0(\theta;\alpha')$ is the likelihood kernel written with the help of the general formula (3.20).

Later on we will use the general (for the class of Bayes estimates under the conditions of a partial prior definiteness) principle of a choice of the parameter α' which leads, in the final form, to the solution of the minimax problem (6.14). Substituting the expression (6.55) into (6.54), we arrive at the following partial formulation of the problem (6.14) for obtaining the Bayes estimate R^* and the vector of parameters of a prior density α'_*:

$$\begin{gathered} G\left(\hat{R}^*,\alpha'_*\right) = \min_{\hat{R}}\max_{\alpha'} \int_{\Omega} L\left(\hat{R},R(\theta)\right)\ell_0(\theta,\alpha*\alpha')d\theta, \\ \int_{\Theta}\ell_0(\theta;\alpha')d\theta \geqslant \mu\int_{\Omega}\ell_0(\theta;\alpha')d\theta. \end{gathered} \tag{6.56}$$

Given below are two cases frequently encountered in practice: the first one has an exponential distribution $F(t;\theta)$, the second has a binomial.

6.4.3 *Estimate of the TTF for the exponential distribution of the time-to-failure*

Let $F(t;\lambda) = 1-\exp(-\lambda t)$, $\lambda > 0$; we need to estimate the TTF

$$R(t) = P\{\xi > t\} = \mathrm{e}^{-\lambda t} \tag{6.57}$$

under the condition that given prior μ-confidence interval $[R_\ell, R_u]$ such that

$$P\{R_\ell \leqslant R(t_0) \leqslant R_u\} \geqslant \mu, \tag{6.58}$$

where, generally speaking, $t_0 \neq t$. The results of testing are represented by the parameter τ, introduced in § 6.1.

Let us find first a prior distribution for λ. In view of the monotonicity of the dependence (6.57), a prior confidence interval for λ has the form $[\lambda',\lambda'']$, where $\lambda' = -\ln R_u/t_0$, $\lambda'' = -\ln R_\ell/t_0$. By the definition of a prior confidence interval, for a prior density $h(\lambda)$ of the parameter λ we have

$$\int_{\lambda'}^{\lambda''} h(\lambda)d\lambda \geqslant \mu. \tag{6.59}$$

For the exponential distribution, a prior density $h(\lambda)$, conjugate to the likelihood kernel, is represented by the formula (6.37). The final formulation of the problem of finding optimal values of the parameters of a prior density s_* and ε_* and, in view of (6.56), is written similarly to (6.43)

$$\begin{gathered} U(s_*,\varepsilon_*) = \max_{s,\varepsilon} U(s,\varepsilon) = \max_{s,\varepsilon} \frac{d+s+1}{(k+\varepsilon)^2}, \\ \int_{\lambda'}^{\lambda''} \lambda^s e^{-\lambda\varepsilon} d\lambda \geqslant \mu \frac{\Gamma(s+1)}{e^{s+1}}, \end{gathered} \tag{6.60}$$

where $k = \tau_1 + \cdots + \tau_n$, and $U(s,\varepsilon)$ is the posterior variance of the parameter.

The problem (6.60) belongs to the class of problems of Nonlinear Programming, and can be solved only numerically with computer tools. For the approximate solution of the problem (6.60), we consider the so-called case of tests without failures which can be associated with a highly-reliable technical device. This case is introduced by the condition $s_* = 0$, since the parameter s has the sense of the prior number of failures that occurred during the total operating time ε. Suppose also that $R(t_0) \in [R_\ell, 1]$. Thereby it follows $\lambda' = 0$, $\lambda'' = -\ln R_\ell / t_0$. The problem (6.60) takes on the form

$$U_0(\varepsilon_*) = U(0,\varepsilon_*) = \max_{\varepsilon>0} \frac{d+1}{(k+\varepsilon)^2}, \quad \int_0^{\lambda''} e^{-\lambda\varepsilon} d\lambda \geqslant \frac{\mu}{\varepsilon}. \tag{6.61}$$

Since the parameter ε is continuous, the solution of the problem (6.61) belongs to the boundary of the domain of admissible solutions, i.e., it is defined by the condition

$$R_\ell^{\varepsilon_*/t_0} = 1 - \mu,$$

or

$$\varepsilon_* = \frac{\ln(1-\mu)}{\ln R_\ell} t_0. \tag{6.62}$$

After we apply the formula similar to (6.50), we have

$$\hat{R}^*(t) = \left(\frac{u_*}{u_*+1}\right)^{d+1}, \quad u_* = \frac{\varepsilon_*}{t} + \frac{k}{t}, \tag{6.63}$$

and

$$\sigma^2_{\hat{R}^*(t)} = \left(\frac{u_*}{u_*+2}\right)^{d+1} - \left(\frac{u_*}{u_*+1}\right)^{2(d+1)}. \tag{6.64}$$

For the lower Bayes confidence limit, we recommend the use of the formula (6.51) with $s_* = 1$. In Table 6.10 we present the estimates TTF, obtained by the formulas (6.62)–(6.64), and (6.51) for different values of characteristics of a priori information R_ℓ and μ and experimental data, expressed by the statistics $\omega = k/t_0$ and $d = 0$. For each computing variant we determine three estimates $\hat{R}^*$, $\sigma_{\hat{R}^*}$ and $\underline{R}^*_{0.9}$, situated successively one after another. As can be seen from the table, the TTF estimates improve as the prior confidence level increases: the pointwise estimate and confidence limit increase while the posterior mean-squared value decreases.

Table 6.10 Bayes estimation of TTF with one failure $\bar{Q}^*(t_0)/\bar{Q}^*_{0.9}(t_0)$.

ω	R_0			
	0.9990	0.9994	0.9996	0.9998
2	$1.596\cdot10^{-4}$	$1.198\cdot10^{-3}$	$7.989\cdot10^{-4}$	$3.999\cdot10^{-4}$
	$3.103\cdot10^{-3}$	$1.329\cdot10^{-3}$	$1.554\cdot10^{-3}$	$7.776\cdot10^{-4}$
6	$1.591\cdot10^{-3}$	$1.195\cdot10^{-3}$	$7.977\cdot10^{-4}$	$3.995\cdot10^{-4}$
	$3.094\cdot10^{-3}$	$2.323\cdot10^{-3}$	$1.551\cdot10^{-3}$	$7.770\cdot10^{-4}$
10	$1.596\cdot10^{-3}$	$1.192\cdot10^{-3}$	$7.965\cdot10^{-4}$	$3.993\cdot10^{-4}$
	$3.081\cdot10^{-3}$	$2.318\cdot10^{-3}$	$1.548\cdot10^{-3}$	$7.763\cdot10^{-4}$

6.4.4 *The TTF estimate for the binomial distribution*

Consider a case of independent tests, when the results are fixed in the form "success or failure" and represented in the final form by the total number of tests n and by the number of failures d. The likelihood function for the considered scheme has the form (6.20), and the beta-distribution with the density (6.21) plays the role of a conjugate prior distribution. The common minimax problem of finding unknown parameters of the a priori distribution α_* and β_* and TTF estimate, $R = p$, in the given case will be formulated as

$$G(\hat{p}^*;\alpha_*,\beta_*) = \min_{\hat{p}} \max_{\substack{\alpha\geqslant 0\\ \beta\geqslant 0}} \int_0^1 L(\hat{p},p)p^{n-d+\alpha-1}(1-p)^{d+\beta-1}dp,$$
$$\int_{R_\ell}^{R_u} p^{\alpha-1}(1-p)^{\beta-1}dp \geqslant \mu B(\alpha,\beta). \tag{6.65}$$

The problem corresponds to the case of defining a prior confidence interval $[R_\ell, R_u]$ with a probability μ. Solving the problem, we again meet the necessity of using numerical methods. In the case of the quadratic loss function $L(\hat{p},p) = (\hat{p}-p)^2$, as shown in § 6.1, the minimax of the function of the posterior risk is reduced to the maximum of a prior variance $U(\alpha,\beta)$ of the parameter p. In the final form, the problem (6.65) is reduced to the problem of Nonlinear Programming:

$$U(\alpha_*,\beta_*) = \max_{\substack{\alpha\geqslant 0\\ \beta\geqslant 0}} U(\alpha,\beta) = \max \frac{(\alpha+n-d)(\beta+d)}{(\alpha+\beta+n)^2(\alpha+\beta+n+1)},$$
$$\int_{R_\ell}^{R_u} p^{\alpha-1}(1-p)^{\beta-1}dp \geqslant \mu B(\alpha,\beta). \tag{6.66}$$

This problem doesn't have an analytical solution, and requires applying one of the methods of Numerical Optimization. We will assume that $R_u = 1$ and $\beta_* = 1$. This case is associated with the practical situation when the reliability of a tested device is large, and a priori information has been obtained in the form of the μ-confidence Bayes interval with the help

Table 6.11 A posteriori TTF for exponential distribution.

ω	$\mu = 0.90$			$\mu = 0.95$		
	$R_{\rm H} = 0.90$	$R_{\rm H} = 0.95$	$R_{\rm H} = 0.99$	$R_{\rm H} = 0.90$	$R_{\rm H} = 0.95$	$R_{\rm H} = 0.99$
5	0.9641	0.9803	0.9957	0.9709	0.9845	0.99671
	0.0346	0.0192	0.0042	0.0282	0.0153	0.00334
	0.9178	0.9549	0.9902	0.9334	0.9643	0.99242
10	0.9696	0.9841	0.9958	0.9746	0.9856	0.99676
	0.0295	0.0176	0.0041	0.0247	0.0142	0.00326
	0.9303	0.9589	0.9906	0.9418	0.9669	0.99255
15	0.9736	0.9836	0.9959	0.9775	0.9865	0.99680
	0.0257	0.0162	0.0041	0.0220	0.0132	0.00316
	0.9394	0.9623	0.9906	0.9484	0.9691	0.99267
20	0.9767	0.9848	0.9960	0.9798	0.9874	0.99696
	0.0227	0.0149	0.0040	0.0198	0.0124	0.00314
	0.9465	0.9651	0.9908	0.9536	0.9711	0.99279
50	0.9863	0.9896	0.9964	0.9874	0.9909	0.99714
	0.0135	0.0103	0.0035	0.0124	0.0091	0.00287
	0.9685	0.9760	0.9918	0.9711	0.9790	0.99341

of tests without failures. The problem is simplified, and takes on the form

$$U(\alpha_*,0) = \max_{\alpha>0} \frac{(\alpha+n-d)(d+1)}{(\alpha+n+1)^2(\alpha+n+2)}, \qquad R_\ell^\alpha \leqslant 1-\mu.$$

It is easy to see that the solution to the problem lies on the boundary of the domain of admissible solutions, i.e.,

$$\alpha_* = \frac{\ln(1-\mu)}{\ln R_\ell}. \tag{6.67}$$

Now, for the estimate of TTF we should only apply the formulas (6.30) and (6.32) which take on the form

$$\hat{R}^* = \hat{p}^* = \frac{\alpha_* + n - d}{\alpha_* + n + 1}, \tag{6.68}$$

$$\sigma_{\hat{R}^*} = \frac{(\alpha_* + n - d)(d+1)}{(\alpha_* + n + 1)^2(\alpha_* + n + 2)}, \tag{6.69}$$

and

$$\underline{R}_\gamma^* = \left[1 + \frac{d+1}{\alpha_* + n - d} F_{1-\gamma;2(d+1);2(\alpha_*+n-d)}\right]^{-1}. \tag{6.70}$$

It should be noted that in the calculation algorithm for obtaining TTF estimates, based on the formulas (6.68)–(6.70), the parameter α_* plays the role of the number of successful tests

Table 6.12 Bayes lower confidence bound of TTF for binomial testing.

μ	R_H				
	0.80	0.90	0.95	0.97	0.99
0.90	0.9289	0.9413	0.9498	0.9536	0.9622
0.95	0.9527	0.9626	0.9696	0.9733	0.9787
0.99	0.9871	0.9907	0.9907	0.9937	0.9952

which are equivalent to using a priori information. Table 6.11 illustrates the dependence of the estimate $\underline{R}^*_{0.9}$ on R_ℓ and a prior confidence probability μ.

Chapter 7

Empirical Bayes Estimates of Reliability

7.1 Setting of the problem and the state of the theory of empirical Bayes estimation

In many problems frequently encountered in practice, a scientific designer possesses information on the reliability of technical devices appearing to be prototypes or analogs of the contemplated system. These analogs may be put into operation during a long period of time so that the information about characteristics of their reliability is certain. As prototypes with respect to contemplating technical device, the devices having analogous functional assignment and structure but differing from the original device by some new elements or parameters may be used (in this case, the device of interest appears to be a modification of a previous one); devices of the same type but made with the help of another technology or produced by another firm; the device which is being operated under the conditions slightly different from those applied to the original device.

The following approach is preferable and perspective for elaboration of technical devices. Designer organizations contemplating model units accumulate statistical information about object properties represented in the form of testing results and exploitation characteristics of each model device. To design a new variant of the analogous technical device, engineers apply all their past experience in the field. This information is reflected reasonably in the methods of estimating the reliability, based on all preceding information about reliability characteristics of devices which already have been put into operation. This situation compels us to develop a method of reliability estimating under the conditions of data accumulation. This corresponds to the tendency of a modern technology development in the conditions of an automatized project and production systems that use various databases. One method of estimating the reliability under the conditions of data accumulation can be based on empirical Bayes approach which uses a priori information, for example, in the form of reliability estimates of all preceding types of the device, and doesn't require determination of a prior distribution in a unique way.

In this Chapter we carry out a brief analysis of all existing estimation methods within the framework of the empirical Bayes approach, and present practical recommendations touching upon the calculations of TTF estimates frequently used in practical situations. We propose also a new method of obtaining empirical Bayes estimates under the conditions of data accumulation.

For the sake of simplicity of exposition of the foundations of the theory of empirical Bayes estimates, we consider the case of obtaining the Bayes estimate for the scalar, parameter θ and the connected reliability function, $R(\theta)$. Using an empirical Bayes approach, we have to postulate the existence of a prior distribution of the parameter θ which is assumed to be unknown. The main idea of such approach lies in the use of a general scheme of Bayes estimation (see Chapter 2) of the approximation of either a Bayes decision rule or a prior distribution. Approximation in both of these cases is the basis for the previous observations. The Bayes empirical approach was initiated by Robbins [211] and developed in the works of many. Authors (we shall only mention three such works in this field: [168, 194, and 229]).

7.1.1 *Setting of the problem of empirical Bayes estimates*

Let $\tau^{(j)} = \left(\tau_1^{(j)}, \ldots, \tau_{n_j}^{(j)}\right)$ be the testing results (represented, for example, in the form of total operating times) which have been fixed in the j-th series of tests. Systems which have been tested in the 1-st, 2-nd,…, $(N-1)$-th series are analogs to the device examined in the N-th series. Following a formalized description of the empirical Bayes approach [16, 208], we will assume that there exists a stable statistical mechanism leading to a prior distribution of $h(\theta)$, unknown in general. The problem is to find a Bayes estimate of the parameter θ of reliability function $R(\theta)$ with the help of the results obtained in the N-th series, taking into consideration the testing results of the previous series. Following the earlier mentioned method of estimate representation, we will consider the following estimates: For the parameter θ consider the pointwise estimate $\hat{\theta}_e^*$, the posterior mean value $\sigma_{\hat{\theta}_e^*}$, the Bayes confidence interval $[\underline{\theta}, \bar{\theta}]_\gamma$;
For a TTF consider the pointwise estimate$\hat{R}_e^*$, the posterior mean value $\sigma_{\hat{R}_e^*}$, and the lower confidence limit $\underline{R}_{\gamma e}^*$.

7.1.2 *Classification of methods*

In Figure 7.1 we present an integrated classification of empirical Bayes methods. In the first place, all methods are divided into two kinds: *parametric* ones which touch upon the case with unknown parametric family of a probability distribution $F(t;\theta)$ of the trouble-free time ξ, and *nonparametric* methods which are based on the assumption that $F(t;\theta)$ belongs to some nonparametric class S which is more or less broad.

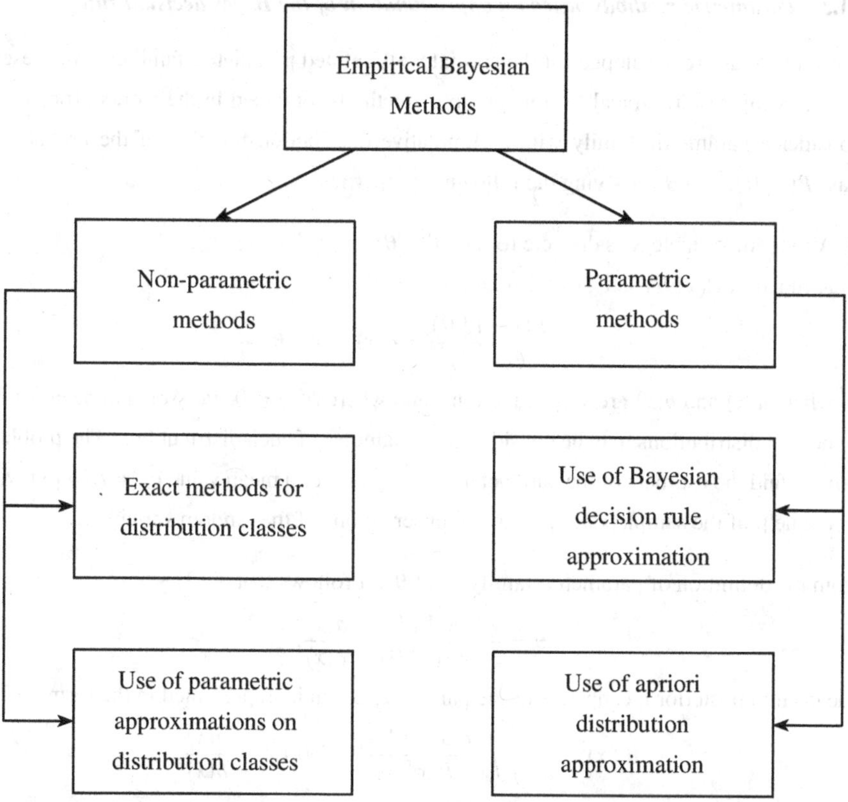

Fig. 7.1 Classification of Bayes empirical methods.

In the group of parametric methods we distinguish two classes. The methods belonging to the first class use an empirical approximation of the Bayes decision rule without approximation of a prior distribution. The methods belonging to the second class are nearer to the general scheme of Bayes estimates. They are based on empirical approximation of a prior distribution and successive use of the standard Bayes procedure. These methods form the base for practical procedures of empirical Bayes estimates.

In the group of nonparametric methods we also distinguish two classes. The first one, named by the class of exact methods, uses tools analogous to Ferguson constructions, considered in Chapter 4. We shall revisit these methods in the third section of Chapter 7.

7.1.3 *Parametric methods based on approximation of the Bayes decision rule*

These methods are developed for the special well-defined parametric families. We present the following result, typical for this group of methods, obtained in the works [168, 170]. Consider a parametric family with a cumulative distribution function of the probability mass $P(x \mid \theta)$, $\theta \in \theta$ satisfying the following properties:

1) A random variable X is discrete for any $\theta \in \theta$;
2) A function $P(x \mid \theta)$ satisfies the relation
$$\frac{P(x+1 \mid \theta)}{P(x \mid \theta)} = a(x) + b(x)\theta.$$
where $a(x)$ and $b(x)$ are some functions, and where $b(x) \neq 0$. Poisson and negative binomial distributions may be considered as examples of such distributions. The problem is to find the estimate of the parameter θ in the form of a mean value $\hat{\theta}_N = E(\theta \mid x)$ with the help of the sample $x_1, x_2, \ldots, x_N$ of observations of the random variable X.

From the definition of parametric family $P(x \mid \theta)$, it follows that
$$\theta = \frac{P(x+1 \mid \theta)}{b(x)P(x \mid \theta)} - \frac{a(x)}{b(x)}.$$
The desired posterior mean value of the parameter θ can be represented in the form
$$E(\theta \mid x) = \frac{1}{b(x)} \int_{\Theta} \frac{P(x+1 \mid \theta)}{P(x \mid \theta)} dH(\theta \mid x) - \frac{a(x)}{b(x)},$$
where $H(\theta)$ and $H(\theta \mid x) = P(x \mid \theta)H(\theta)/P(x)$ are, respectively, the prior and posterior distribution functions of the parameter θ. The parametric family is of a type that the expression for $E(\theta \mid x)$may be simplified as
$$E(\theta \mid x) = \frac{P(x+1)}{P(x)b(x)} - \frac{a(x)}{b(x)}.$$
In this expression $a(x)$ and $b(x)$ are unknown, while $P(x)$ and $P(x+1)$ are known. For obtaining the estimate $\hat{\theta}_N = E_N(\theta \mid x)$, we will use the corresponding estimates of the

functions $\hat{P}_N(x)$ and $\hat{P}_N(x+1)$ obtained with the help of the observed sample $x_1, x_2, \ldots, x_N$, where for estimates $\hat{P}_N(x)$, $\hat{P}_N(x+1)$ may be used usually as nonparametric estimates. The given method has a shortcoming, the strict restriction on the type of parametric family $P(x \mid \theta)$.

7.1.4 *Parametric methods, based on approximation of a prior distribution*

In this class, representing the largest group of methods, one may distinguish two subclasses: The first one uses a parametric empirical approximation of a prior distribution, the second class is based, following the same purposes, on some parametric family of prior distributions and estimated parameters of this family. Presentation of the methods belonging to the first class will be carried out in accordance with the results of the works [17, 48, 162, 229]. The methods considered don't have, unlike the proceeding case, any restrictions on the parametric family $F(t;\theta)$.

As a starting point, the traditional Bayes formula for estimating the parameter θ with respect to arbitrary sample τ is chosen, that is,

$$E(\theta \mid \tau) = \frac{\int_{\Theta} \theta f_{\tau}(\tau \mid \theta) dH(\theta)}{\int_{\Theta} f_{\tau}(\tau \mid \theta) dH(\theta)}, \tag{7.1}$$

where $f_{\tau}(\tau \mid \theta)$ is the density of the distribution of observations. It is assumed that each observation $\tau^{(j)}$ $(j = 1, 2, \ldots, N)$ is a vector of the same dimension n; Note that this is a simplification of the more general case when each vector $\tau^{(j)}$ has a dimension n_j. There is a statistic $\hat{\theta} = \hat{\theta}(\tau)$ which is sufficient for each realization of the parameter θ from the set $\theta_1, \ldots, \theta_N$. In this case, in accordance with the factorization theorem [208],

$$E(\theta \mid \tau) = E(\theta \mid \hat{\theta}(\tau)) = E(\theta \mid \hat{\theta}).$$

Then expression (7.1) may be rewritten as

$$E(\theta \mid \hat{\theta}) = \frac{\int_{\Theta} \theta f(\hat{\theta} \mid \theta) dH(\theta)}{\int_{\Theta} f(\hat{\theta} \mid \theta) dH(\theta)}, \tag{7.2}$$

where, it is assumed that the distribution density of the statistic $f(\hat{\theta} \mid \theta)$ is known. The method proposed in [16] lies in approximating a prior distribution function with the help of step-functions having the increment $1/N$ in each of the estimates $\hat{\theta}_1, \ldots, \hat{\theta}_N$. The indicated approximation for $dH(\theta)$ has the form

$$d\hat{H}(\theta) = \frac{1}{N} \sum_{i=1}^{N} \delta(\hat{\theta}_i; \theta), \tag{7.3}$$

where

$$\delta(\hat{\theta}_i;\theta)=\begin{cases}\ell & \text{if } \theta=\theta_i,\\ 0 & \text{if } \theta\neq\theta_i.\end{cases}$$

Substituting (7.3) into (7.2) yields the resulting expression for the estimate of the parameter θ over the sample $\tau^{(N)}$:

$$\hat{\theta}^*=E_N(\theta\mid\hat{\theta})=\frac{\sum_{j=1}^{N}\hat{\theta}_j f(\hat{\theta}_N\mid\hat{\theta}_j)}{\sum_{j=1}^{N} f(\hat{\theta}_N\mid\hat{\theta}_j)}. \tag{7.4}$$

The estimate $\hat{\theta}^*$ obtained with the help of (7.4) is called the first approximation estimate in [16]. It can be defined more exactly if one uses the following simple idea. Instead of each estimate $\hat{\theta}_j$ in the formula (7.4), we will use an empirical Bayes estimate $\hat{\theta}_j^{(1)}=\hat{\theta}_j^*$ of the first approximation obtained from the formula (7.4) over the set of data $\tau^{(1)},\tau^{(2)},\ldots,\tau^{(j)}$. Thereby we have the following procedure for obtaining the empirical Bayes estimate $\hat{\theta}^2$ of the second approximation. At first for each $j=1,2,\ldots,N$ we find the first-approximation estimate:

$$\hat{\theta}_j^{(1)}=\hat{\theta}_j^*=\frac{\sum_{i=1}^{j}\hat{\theta}_j f(\hat{\theta}_j\mid\hat{\theta}_i)}{\sum_{i=1}^{j} f(\hat{\theta}_j\mid\hat{\theta}_i)},\qquad j=1,2,\ldots,N. \tag{7.5}$$

Then we evaluate the second approximation estimate $\hat{\theta}^{(2)}$:

$$\hat{\theta}^{(2)}=\frac{\sum_{j=1}^{N}\hat{\theta}_j^{(1)} f(\hat{\theta}_N^{(1)}\mid\hat{\theta}_j^{(1)})}{\sum_{j=1}^{N} f(\hat{\theta}_N^{(1)}\mid\hat{\theta}_j^{(1)})}. \tag{7.6}$$

As stated in the work [162], the second approximation estimate appears to be more exact. In [16], Bennett proposes to use for obtaining a more exact value of the estimate the third, fourth, etc., approximations. However, the exact measure of the estimate is not improved as much as desired. Procedures for obtaining empirical Bayes estimates for different parametric families are the subject of consideration in the work by Lemon [137]. These works give great attention to the questions of empirical Bayes estimates of the parametric Weibull family see [16, 17, 48, 107, and 163]. The discrete character of approximation of a prior distribution is a serious shortcoming of the proposed method. This obstacle doesn't allow us, in particular, to construct confidence intervals for the parameter θ and the reliability functions connected with it. To this end, we apply the proposition given by Bennett and

Martz [18], which consists of using a continuous nonparametric approximation introduced by Parzen [191] for approximating a prior probability density $h(\theta)$ having the following form

$$h(\theta) = \hat{h}_N(\theta) = \frac{1}{Nk(N)} \sum_{j=1}^{N} w\left(\frac{\theta - \theta_j}{k(N)}\right), \tag{7.7}$$

where $w(\cdot)$is a function, satisfying the conditions of boundness and regularity, and $k(N)$ is independent of θ, such that

$$\lim_{N\to\infty} k(N) = 0 \quad \text{and} \quad \lim_{N\to\infty} Nk(N) = \infty.$$

Bennett and Martz use, in particular, approximation (7.7) for which

$$w(y) = \left(\frac{\sin y}{y}\right)^2, \; y = \frac{\theta - \theta_j}{2k(N)} \quad \text{and} \quad k(N) = N^{-1/s}.$$

For this case, the Bayes parametric estimate of the parameter θ takes on the following form:

$$\hat{\theta}^* = \frac{1}{\beta}\int_{\Theta} \theta f(\theta \mid \hat{\theta}_N)\hat{h}(\theta)d\theta, \tag{7.8}$$

where β is a normalizing constant. Now we can find the Bayes lower confidence limit of TTF from the equation

$$\int_{R(\theta)\geqslant \underline{R}_\gamma} f(\theta \mid \hat{\theta}_N)\hat{h}(\theta)d\theta = \gamma \int_{\Theta} f(\theta \mid \hat{\theta}_N)\hat{h}(\theta)d\theta. \tag{7.9}$$

The subclass of parametric methods used for approximation of a prior distribution of some parametric families gives us the methods, constructed in accordance with the following natural scheme [229]. For a given parametric family $F(t;\theta)$, a likelihood function is constructed and a prior distribution is identified, conjugated with the likelihood kernel. The parameters of a prior distribution are assumed to be unknown, and are estimated using the estimates $\hat{\theta}_1, \hat{\theta}_2, \ldots, \hat{\theta}_N$. In the work [212], Robbins shows that with the growth of N an empirical Bayes estimate begins to "forget" the type of prior distribution. This procedure may be improved with the help of the specific properties associated with the estimating scheme. The work by Higgins and Tsokos [107] gives us an example of such a modification. They prove the following: if one carries out the estimation of a prior gamma-distribution in a Poisson scheme using the variation coefficient, it is possible to increase the effectiveness of the Bayes TTF estimate.

7.1.5 *Nonparametric empirical Bayes methods*

Most of the known results arise from the Ferguson theory that we explained in §4.1. The first extension of this theory to the case of empirical Bayes estimates was done by Korwar and Hollander [128]. In the work [245], Susarla and Van Ryzin generalize these results to the case of censored samples. Phadia [194] considers the particular case which is important for practice. Here all censoring moments are distributed by the same probability law. All obtained results are based on approximation of a prior measure α with the help of the preceding censored test outcomes $(\delta_1,\tau_1),(\delta_2,\tau_2),\ldots,(\delta_{N-1},\tau_{N-1})$, where $\tau_i=\min\{\xi_i,\zeta_i\}$, ξ_i are failure times, ζ_i are censoring times, $\delta_j=1$, if the failure is observed and $\delta_j=0$, if the failure has been censored. The estimate of the TTF, $R(t)$, is constructed by the results of the N-th observation (δ_N,τ_N) with regard to the mentioned approximation of the measure α of a prior Dirichlet process. Let us find the estimate $\hat{R}^*(t)$ obtained in the work [194] for the case when all censoring times have the same distribution while failure times have different ones. Assuming that the parameter of significance of the a priori information $\beta=\alpha([0,\infty))$ is known,

$$\hat{R}^*(t)=\frac{1}{\beta+1}\{I[t<\tau_N]+\hat{\alpha}([t;\infty))+I[\delta_N=0,\ t\geqslant\tau_N]\}\frac{\hat{\alpha}([t;\infty))}{\hat{\alpha}([\tau_N,\infty))},$$

where

$$\hat{\alpha}([t,\infty))=\frac{N^+(t)}{N-1}\prod_{i=1}^{N-1}\left(\frac{N^+(\tau_i)+c+1}{N^+(\tau_i)+c}\right)^{I[\delta_i=0,t\geqslant\tau_i]}.$$

$N^+(t)$is the number of observations from the set $\tau_1,\tau_2,\ldots,\tau_{N-1}$, exceeding t; $I[A]$ the indicator of the event A: if the event A has occurred $I=1$, otherwise $I=0$, c is a positive constant, controlling the smoothness of the estimate (in practical calculations one often puts $c=1$).

It should be noted that all considered methods have the following shortcoming: they don't allow us to estimate the exact identification of $\hat{R}^*(t)$ and to find its interval estimate.

7.2 Empirical Bayes estimation of the survival probability for the most extended parametric distributions

In this section we shall consider the more general procedure of parametric Bayes TTF estimates and its particular realizations for the cases of binomial, exponential and Weibull probability distributions, as well as for the case of a linearly increasing failure rate function.

7.2.1 *General procedure for obtaining estimates*

Suppose that the random time to failure obeys the distribution with c.d.f. $F(t;\theta)$, and we are given the information of the results of N tests $\tau^{(1)},\tau^{(2)},\ldots,\tau^{(N)}$ having sizes $n_1,n_2,\ldots,n_N$, respectively. Each vector $\tau^{(j)}$ represents the union of two vectors: $t^{*(j)}$ the failure times,

$t^{(j)}$ the censoring times having sizes d_j and k_j, respectively, such that $n_j = d_j + k_j$. We need to find an empirical Bayes estimate of the TTF, $R(t;\theta) = 1 - F(t;\theta)$, for the sample $\tau^{(N)}$ using the results of the preceding tests.

The presence of a parametric family allows us to write with the help of expression (3.20) or (3.21) the likelihood function $\ell(\theta \mid \tau)$ for an arbitrary sample τ, and having generated the sufficient statistic α, in the form $\ell(\theta \mid \tau) = K(\tau)\ell_0(\theta;\alpha)$.

The desired TTF estimate of $R(\theta)$ may be found if for results of the N-th series of tests a prior density of the parameter θ is known. In view of Bayes theorem we get

$$\hbar(\theta \mid \tau^{(N)}) = \hbar(\theta \mid \alpha^{(N)}) \sim h(\theta)\ell_0(\theta;\alpha^{(N)}). \tag{7.10}$$

A prior density $h(\theta)$ is unknown, and we will approximate it. To this end, we assume that there are estimates $\hat{\theta}^{(1)}, \hat{\theta}^{(2)}, \ldots, \hat{\theta}^{(N)}$, each of which has been obtained with the help of its "own" sample $\tau^{(j)}$ ($j = 1, 2, \ldots, N$). For obtaining the estimate $\hat{\theta}^{(j)}$ we may use any statistical method suitable for these purposes, it is desirable certainly that the obtained estimate is as effective as possible. In particular, we may use a maximum likelihood method, then components of the estimate $\hat{\theta}^{(j)}$ should be found by solving the set of equations

$$\frac{\partial \ell(\theta;\alpha^{(j)})}{\partial \theta_i} = 0 \Longrightarrow \hat{\theta}_i^{(j)} = \theta_i, \quad i = 1, 2, \ldots, m, \tag{7.11}$$

where m is the dimension of the vector θ. For the same purposes we also may use the methods which determine the estimate $\hat{\theta}_i^{(j)}$ as the posterior mean value for the sample $\tau^{(j)}$:

$$\hat{\theta}_i^{(j)} = \frac{1}{\beta_j} \int_{\Theta} \theta_i \ell_0(\theta;\alpha^{(j)}) h_j(\theta) d\theta, \quad i = 1, 2, \ldots, m, \tag{7.12}$$

where β_j is a normalizing factor, and $h_j(\theta)$ is a prior probability density of the parameter θ which possibly exists when we investigate the reliability for the j-th series. If there is no a priori information in the j-th series, one should use as $h_j(\theta)$ the uninformative Jeffrey's density [114].

For approximation of $h(\theta)$ we will use in the relation (7.10) a nonparametric discrete estimate of the density for which

$$d\hat{H}(\theta) = \frac{1}{n} \sum_{j=1}^{N} n_j \delta(\hat{\theta}^{(j)}, \theta), \tag{7.13}$$

where

$$\delta(x,y) = \begin{Bmatrix} 1 & \text{if } x = y \\ 0 & \text{if } x \neq y, \end{Bmatrix} \quad \text{and} \quad n = \sum_{j=1}^{N} n_j.$$

The obtained estimate generalizes the estimate (7.3), used in the work [16], for the case of the samples $\tau^{(j)}$ having different sizes. The corresponding estimate of the empirical function of a prior distribution $\hat{H}(\theta)$ has the form of the step-function with the increment n_j/n at each point $\hat{\theta}^{(j)}$.

Now, suppose that we need to find the estimate $\hat{R}_e^* = \hat{R}_e^*(t_0)$ in the form of the posterior mean value (if we use a quadratic loss function). This estimate, based on approximation of a prior distribution, is defined by the integral

$$\hat{R}_e^*(t_0) = \frac{\int_\Theta R(t_0;\theta)\ell_0\big(\theta;\alpha^{(N)}\big)d\hat{H}(\theta)}{\int_\Theta \ell_0\big(\theta;\alpha^{(N)}\big)d\hat{H}(\theta)}, \tag{7.14}$$

where $\alpha^{(N)}$ is a sufficient statistic, corresponding to the sample $\tau^{(N)}$. Let us substitute approximation (7.13) into (7.14) and simplify the obtained formula. This yields:

$$\hat{R}_e^*(t_0) = \frac{\sum_{j=1}^{N} n_j R\big(t_0;\hat{\theta}^{(j)}\big)\ell_0\big(\hat{\theta}^{(j)};\alpha^{(N)}\big)}{\sum_{j=1}^{N} n_j \ell_0\big(\hat{\theta}^{(j)};\alpha^{(N)}\big)}. \tag{7.15}$$

The empirical estimate of the posterior variance can be found analogously without any difficulties:

$$\sigma^2_{\hat{R}_e^*(t_0)} = \frac{\sum_{j=1}^{N} n_j R^2\big(t_0;\hat{\theta}^{(j)}\big)\ell_0\big(\hat{\theta}^{(j)};\alpha^{(N)}\big)}{\sum_{j=1}^{N} n_j \ell_0\big(\hat{\theta}^{(j)};\alpha^{(N)}\big)} - \hat{R}_e^*(t_0). \tag{7.16}$$

Note that we don't meet such a form of a parametric empirical Bayes procedure in all of the works cited above. We believe that the empirical Bayes procedure given above appears to be the most general among all the procedures that use a discrete approximation of a prior distribution. Unfortunately we cannot find interval estimate $\underline{R}_\gamma^*$ of TTF with the help of this procedure. For this purpose we recommend using some approximate methods, based on the knowledge of the pointwise estimate $\hat{R}_e^*(t)$ and mean-squared value $\sigma^2_{\hat{R}_e^*(t_0)}$.

In conclusion, we note that the general procedure given above lets us find empirical Bayes estimates of the second and successive approximations. To do this, we need to first find empirical Bayes estimates of the parameters $\hat{\theta}^{(j)}$ of the first approximation

$$\hat{\theta}_{i(1)}^{(j)} = \frac{\sum_{k=1}^{j} n_k \hat{\theta}_i^{(k)} \ell_0\big(\hat{\theta}^{(k)};\alpha^{(j)}\big)}{\sum_{k=1}^{j} n_k \ell_0\big(\hat{\theta}^{(k)};\alpha^{(j)}\big)}, \tag{7.17}$$

and thereafter replace in (7.15) and (7.16) the estimates $\hat{\theta}^{(j)}$ by the first approximation estimates.

7.2.2 *Binomial scheme*

First we consider the simplest binomial case, when the data $\tau^{(j)}$ $(j=1,\ldots,N)$ represent by themselves the set of 0 and 1, and the sufficient statistic $\alpha^{(j)} = (n_j, d_j)$ contains the total number of tests n_j and number of failures d_j. A TTF, in the given case, coincides with the value of a single parameter p, and the likelihood function has the form

$$\ell(p;n,d) = \binom{n}{d} p^{n-d}(1-p)^d.$$

In accordance with the common expressions (7.15) and (7.16), the empirical Bayes estimate may be written as

$$\hat{R}_e^* = \frac{\sum\limits_{j=1}^{N} n_j \hat{p}_j^{n_N-d_N+1}(1-\hat{p}_j)^{d_N}}{\sum\limits_{j=1}^{N} n_j \hat{p}_j^{n_N-d_N}(1-\hat{p}_j)^{d_N}}, \tag{7.18}$$

and

$$\sigma^2_{\hat{R}_e^*} = \frac{\sum\limits_{j=1}^{N} n_j \hat{p}_j^{n_N-d_N+2}(1-\hat{p}_j)^{d_N}}{\sum\limits_{j=1}^{N} n_j \hat{p}_j^{n_N-d_N}(1-\hat{p}_j)^{d_N}} - \hat{R}_e^*. \tag{7.19}$$

Instead of $\hat{p}_j$ we may use the maximum likelihood estimates $\hat{p}_j = 1 - d_j/n_j$. However, in the case $d_j = 0$ we have $\hat{p}_j = 1$ which makes the estimate (7.18) inaccurate. It is advisable to use the Bayes estimate $\hat{p}_j^*$ obtained for the uniform prior distribution. In this case,

$$\hat{p}_j^* = \frac{\sum\limits_{i=0}^{d_j} (-1)^i \frac{d_j}{(d_j-i)!\,i!\,(n_j+i+2)}}{\sum\limits_{i=0}^{d_j} (-1)^i \frac{d_j}{(d_j-i)!\,i!\,(n_j+i+1)}},$$

and for $d_j = 0$ we have $\hat{p}_j^* = 1 - 1/(n_j+2)$ which mostly corresponds to the real situation.

7.2.3 *Exponential distribution*

For the parametric family

$$F(t;\lambda) = 1 - \exp(-\lambda t),$$

the likelihood function of the sample $\tau^{(j)}$ has the form

$$\ell(\lambda \mid \tau^{(j)}) \sim \ell_0(\lambda; d_j, K_j) = \lambda^{d_j} e^{-\lambda K_j},$$

where $K_j = \tau_1^{(j)} + \tau_2^{(j)} + \cdots + \tau_{n_j}^{(j)}$, and d_j is the number of failures in the j-th sample. Due to this fact, the empirical Bayes estimate of the failure rate λ is computed by the formulas

$$\hat{\lambda}_e^* = \frac{\sum_{j=1}^{N} n_j \hat{\lambda}_j^{d_{N+1}} \mathrm{e}^{-\hat{\lambda}_j K_N}}{\sum_{j=1}^{N} n_j \hat{\lambda}_j^{d_N} \mathrm{e}^{-\hat{\lambda}_j K_N}}, \tag{7.20}$$

and

$$\sigma_{\hat{\lambda}_e^*}^2 = \frac{\sum_{j=1}^{N} n_j \hat{\lambda}_j^{d_{N+2}} \mathrm{e}^{-\hat{\lambda}_j K_N}}{\sum_{j=1}^{N} n_j \hat{\lambda}_j^{d_N} \mathrm{e}^{-\hat{\lambda}_j K_N}} - \hat{\lambda}_e^{*2}. \tag{7.21}$$

The problem is in what way should we construct the estimate $\hat{\lambda}_j$ with the help of the sample $\tau^{(j)}$. For many empirical Bayes procedures one proposes to use maximum likelihood estimates. Solving the likelihood equation inconformity for the given case, we obtain the estimate of the form $\hat{\lambda}_j = d_j/k_j$.

For highly reliable devices it is possible to meet a situation when there are no failures during the testing. This automatically gives us zero estimate $\hat{\lambda}_j$. If one fixes in all N series only successful outcomes (all samples $\tau^{(j)}$ consist of only stopping times without failure), then the formulas (7.20) and(7.21) don't hold. It is more advisable to choose as $\hat{\lambda}_j$. the Bayes estimate constructed with the help of the sample $\tau^{(j)}$ which corresponds to the case of trivial prior information. Such an estimate may be found if we put a uniform prior distribution for λ in the interval $[0,\infty)$. In this case the estimate $\hat{\lambda}_j^* = (d_j+1)/K_j$ and formulas (7.20) and (7.21) hold for any outcomes in each of the N series of test.

7.2.4 *Distribution with a linearly-increasing failure rate*

The Bayes TTF estimate for this case was obtained in §3.4. Let us apply the results of this section. In accordance with (3.54), the kernel of the likelihood function for the sample $\tau^{(j)}$ has the form

$$\ell_0(r,z,w_j,K_j) = a_j(z) r^{b_j(z)} |\ln r|^{d_j}, \tag{7.22}$$

where

$$\begin{aligned} a_j(z) &= \frac{1}{(z+1)^{d_j}} \prod_{i=1}^{d_j} \left[(z-1)\frac{t_i^{(j)*}}{t_0} + 1 \right], \\ b_j(z) &= \frac{1}{z+1}[(z-1)K_j + 2\omega_j], \\ \omega_j &= \frac{1}{t_0}\sum_{i=1}^{n_j} \tau_i^{(j)} \ \text{ and } \ K_j = \frac{1}{t_0^2}\sum_{i=1}^{n_j} \tau_i^{(j)2}, \end{aligned} \tag{7.23}$$

t_0 is the time during which we define the device TTF.

Consider first the case when the degradation parameter z is assumed to be given. We will find empirical Bayes TTF estimates using the likelihood kernel $r^{b_j(z)}|\ln r|^{d_j}$. The resulting expressions for these estimates have the form

$$\hat{R}_e^* = \frac{\sum\limits_{j=1}^{N} n_j \hat{R}_j^{b_{N(z)+1}} |\ln \hat{R}_j|^{d_N}}{\sum\limits_{j=1}^{N} n_j \hat{R}_j^{b_{N(z)}} |\ln \hat{R}_j|^{d_N}}, \tag{7.24}$$

and

$$\sigma^2_{\hat{R}_e^*} = \frac{\sum\limits_{j=1}^{N} n_j \hat{R}_j^{b_{N(z)+2}} |\ln \hat{R}_j|^{d_N}}{\sum\limits_{j=1}^{N} n_j \hat{R}_j^{b_{N(z)}} |\ln \hat{R}_j|^{d_N}} - \hat{R}_e^{*2}, \tag{7.25}$$

where

$$b_N(z) = \frac{1}{z+1}\left[(z-1)\frac{1}{t_0}\sum_{i=1}^{n_N} \tau_i^{(N)} + \frac{2}{t_0^2}\sum_{i=1}^{n_N} \tau_i^{(N)2}\right].$$

For $\hat{R}_j$ we recommend using the Bayes TTF estimates with a linearly increasing failure rate for the uniform prior distribution in $[0,1]$. In view of this and with the help of the function $I_{(z,R_\ell,R_u,m,d)}$ we obtain

$$\hat{R}_j = \frac{I_L(z,0,1,1,d_j)}{I_L(z,0,1,0,d_j)} = \left[1 - \frac{1}{b_j(z)+1}\right]^{d_j+1} \tag{7.26}$$

where b_j is computed by the formula (7.23).

Consider the more common case when the value of the failure rate degradation coefficient z in the interval $[0,t_0]$ is unknown. We will assume that only the limit value z_m is known such that the degradation coefficient is always less than this value. To obtain the empirical Bayes estimate we have to use the likelihood kernel (7.22). The resulting expressions have the form

$$\hat{R}_e^*(t_0) = \frac{\sum\limits_{j=1}^{N} n_j a_N(\hat{z}_j) \hat{R}_j^{b_{N(\hat{z}_j)+1}} |\ln \hat{R}_j|^{d_N}}{\sum\limits_{j=1}^{N} n_j a_N(\hat{z}_j) \hat{R}_j^{b_{N(\hat{z}_j)}} |\ln \hat{R}_j|^{d_N}}, \tag{7.27}$$

and

$$\sigma^2_{\hat{R}_e^*(t_0)} = \frac{\sum\limits_{j=1}^{N} n_j a_N(\hat{z}_j) \hat{R}_j^{b_{N(\hat{z}_j)+1}} |\ln \hat{R}_j|^{d_N}}{\sum\limits_{j=1}^{N} n_j a_N(\hat{z}_j) \hat{R}_j^{b_{N(\hat{z}_j)}} |\ln \hat{R}_j|^{d_N}} - \hat{R}_e^{*2}(t_0). \tag{7.28}$$

We again recommend using as estimates $\hat{R}_j$ and $\hat{z}_j$ ($j = 1, 2, \ldots, N$), the Bayes estimates corresponding to the case of trivial a priori information, that is, the indices R_j and z_j obey a uniform prior distribution in the intervals $[0,1]$ and $[1, z_m]$, respectively. Using the results of § 3.4, we can write the formulas for obtaining these estimates:

$$\hat{R}_j = \frac{1}{\beta_j} \int_1^{z_m} \frac{a_j(z)dz}{[b_j(z)+2]^{d_j+1}}, \tag{7.29}$$

and

$$\hat{z}_j = \frac{1}{\beta_j} \int_1^{z_m} \frac{z a_j(z)dz}{[b_j(z)+1]^{d_j+1}},$$

where

$$\beta_j = \int_1^{z_m} \frac{a_j(z)dz}{[b_j(z)+1]^{d_j+1}}.$$

Estimates (7.29) have at least two advantages in comparison to corresponding maximum likelihood estimates. To obtain the last ones we have to solve a complicated system of transcendental equations for the general case. Otherwise, if we use the formulas in (7.29), we need only to apply the methods of numerical integration for sufficiently smooth functions. Moreover, the maximum likelihood estimates for highly reliable devices give us for $d_j = 0$, $\hat{R}_j = 1$, $\hat{z}_j = 1$, i.e., formulas (7.27) and (7.28) don't work in this case.

7.2.5 *The Weibull distribution*

The present model is almost identical to the previous one. We apply the results of §3.5 for the description of this method. For the Weibull parametric family with the cumulative distribution function $F(t;\lambda,\alpha) = 1 - \exp(-\lambda t^{\alpha})$, we introduce a new parameterization (r,α), represented by the relation (3.66). Then the likelihood function is written in the form (3.67). Leaving the intermediate calculations, we write only the resulting formula for TTF estimates, $R(t_0)$.

For the case when the form of the parameter a is known, we have

$$\hat{R}_e^*(t_0) = \frac{\sum_{j=1}^{N} n_j \hat{R}_j^{\omega_N(\alpha)+1} |\ln \hat{R}_j|^{d_N}}{\sum_{j=1}^{N} n_j \hat{R}_j^{\omega_N(\alpha)} |\ln \hat{R}_j|^{d_N}}, \tag{7.30}$$

$$\sigma_{\hat{R}_e^*(t_0)} = \frac{\sum_{j=1}^{N} n_j \hat{R}_j^{\omega_N(\alpha)+2} |\ln \hat{R}_j|^{d_N}}{\sum_{j=1}^{N} n_j \hat{R}_j^{\omega_N(\alpha)} |\ln \hat{R}_j|^{d_N}} - \hat{R}_e^{*2}(t_0), \tag{7.31}$$

and

$$\hat{R}_j = \left[1 - \frac{1}{\omega_j + 2}\right]^{d_j+1}, \quad \omega_j(\alpha) = \sum_{i=1}^{n_j} \left(\frac{\tau_i^{(j)}}{t_0}\right)^{\alpha}.$$

Now, we shall consider the case when the form of the parameter α is unknown. We will assume that the maximal value $\alpha_m > \alpha$ is given and α is distributed uniformly in the interval $[1, \alpha_m]$. For almost all practical situations $\alpha < 5$, therefore we may certainly put $\alpha_m = 5$. The resulting estimate of the TTF is given by:

$$\hat{R}_e^*(t_0) = \frac{\sum_{j=1}^{N} n_j \hat{\alpha}_j^{d_N} \mu_N^{\hat{\alpha}_j - 1} \hat{R}_j^{\omega_N(\hat{\alpha}_j)+1} |\ln \hat{R}_j|^{d_N}}{\sum_{j=1}^{N} n_j \hat{\alpha}_j^{d_N} \mu_N^{\hat{\alpha}_j - 1} \hat{R}_j^{\omega_N(\hat{\alpha}_j)} |\ln \hat{R}_j|^{d_N}}, \tag{7.32}$$

and

$$\sigma^2_{\hat{R}_e^*(t_0)} = \frac{\sum_{j=1}^{N} n_j \hat{\alpha}_j^{d_N} \mu_N^{\hat{\alpha}_j - 1} \hat{R}_j^{\omega_N(\hat{\alpha}_j)+2} |\ln \hat{R}_j|^{d_N}}{\sum_{j=1}^{N} n_j \hat{\alpha}_j^{d_N} \mu_N^{\hat{\alpha}_j - 1} \hat{R}_j^{\omega_N(\hat{\alpha}_j)} |\ln \hat{R}_j|^{d_N}} - \hat{R}_e^{*2}(t_0), \tag{7.33}$$

where

$$\hat{R}_j = \frac{1}{\beta_j} \int_1^{\alpha_m} x^{d_j} \mu_j^{x-1} \frac{dx}{[\omega_j(x) + 1]^{d_j+1}},$$

$$\hat{\alpha}_j = \frac{1}{\beta_j} \int_1^{\alpha_m} x^{d_j+1} \mu_j^{x-1} \frac{dx}{\omega_j(x)^{d_j+1}}.$$

$$\beta_j = \int_1^{\alpha_m} x^{d_j} \mu_j^{x-1} \frac{dx}{\omega_j(x)^{d_j+1}}, \quad \mu = \prod_{i=1}^{d_j} \frac{t^{*(j)}}{t_0},$$

$$\omega_j(x) = \sum_{i=1}^{n_j} \left(\frac{\tau^{(j)}}{t_0}\right)^x.$$

7.3 Nonparametric empirical Bayes estimates of reliability under the condition of data accumulation

7.3.1 *Description of the problem*

Development of in-house databases is one of the most important aspects of an industrial complex. This cumulative information is analyzed, systematized and prepared in a desirable format to be easily accessible to the users. One extremely important use of this information is to develop reliability models to measure the quality of product-oriented industries, see Belyaev [15].

Belyaev obtains a new type of multiple estimates of a TTF under the conditions of accumulation of uniform data, i.e., under the assumption that experimental data of each new portion obey the same distribution law.

Below we attempt to estimate a TTF with the help of nonuniform data, denoted by $D_1, D_2, \ldots, D_N$. The solution of the problem is based on the empirical Bayes approach (see scheme in Fig. 7.2).

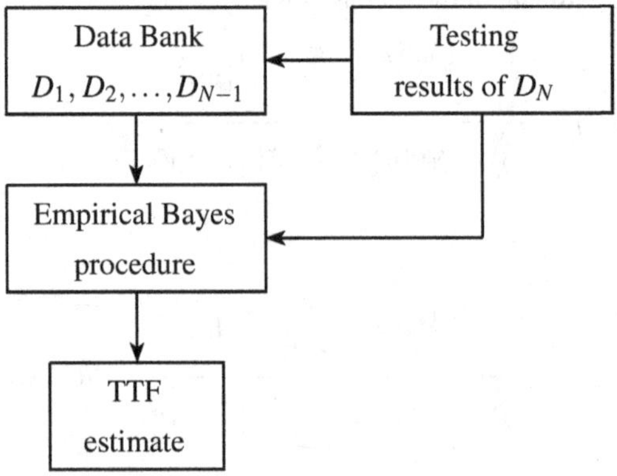

Fig. 7.2 Solution scheme.

Suppose that we have a problem of estimating the device TTF using the experimental results of its testing, D_{dev}. The designer operates with adatabase which contains the failure results of the device that is being tested. Using the empirical Bayes approach, we will find the TTF estimate by the experimental results, D_{dev}, taking into consideration a priori information stored in this database. In accordance with the number of given database observations, we will denote them by $D_N = D_{\text{dev}}$; the observations storedin the database will be enumerated in accordance with the sequence of their appearance, $D_1, D_2, \ldots, D_{N-1}$. The problem is to find the estimate of TTF, $\hat{R}_e^* = \hat{R}_e^*(D_1, D_2, \ldots, D_{N-1})$. Consider a possible form of representation of the observations. In [15] one proposes to represent the data D_j for the censored samples of the testing durations in the following form:

$$D_j = \begin{bmatrix} s_1^{(j)} & s_2^{(j)} & \cdots & s_{n_j}^{(j)} \\ d_1^{(j)} & d_2^{(j)} & \cdots & d_{n_j}^{(j)} \\ k_1^{(j)} & k_2^{(j)} & \cdots & k_{n_j}^{(j)} \end{bmatrix}.$$

The first row contains the testing durations, fixed in the experimental operating time, and written in increasing order; $s_j^{(j)}$ may be either the mean lifetime or operating time during which the system has the capacity to be operable, and thereafter the testing has been terminated. In the second row j-th column represents the number of failures corresponding to the operating time $s_i^{(j)}$. In the i-th column of the third row, we have the number of devices which have been tested at the time $s_i^{(j)}$ before the failure occurs. Later on such a generalized representation form of the censored sample will be used for investigations.

In addition to this method of representation of information about reliability, another approach may be used, corresponding to the case when the database contains directly the reliability estimates. Denote by C_j the j-th observations of the data. The contents of C_j are two numbers: either the pointwise TTF estimate of j-th analog $\hat{R}_j$ and the error of its estimate $\sigma_{\hat{R}_j}$ or the union of $\hat{R}_j$ and lower confidence limit $\underline{R}_{j\gamma}$. Let us assume that $C_j = (\hat{R}_j, \sigma_{\hat{R}_j})$. The scheme of obtaining the estimate $\hat{R}_e^*$ for this case will be slightly changed (see Fig. 7.3). It is clear that the passing $D_N \to C_N$ is connected with the loss of information.

The problem of obtaining a TTF estimate will be solved under the assumption that the distribution function of the time to failure, $F(t)$, belongs to the class of failure rate distributions S_0. The idea of obtaining the estimate lies in the construction of a suitable change of the function $F(t)$ with the help of the distribution function $\widetilde{F}(t) \in S_0$.

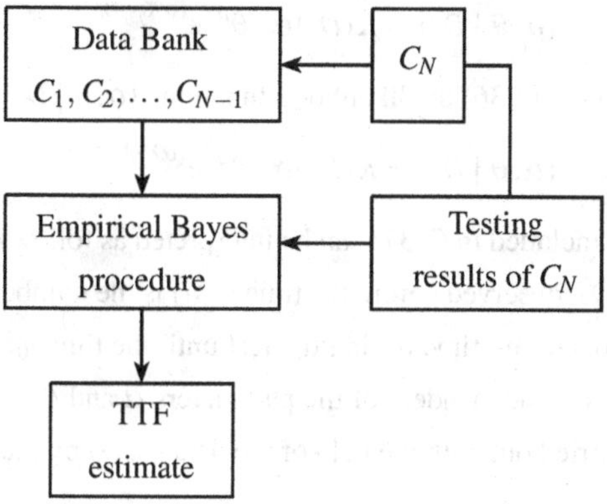

Fig. 7.3 Improved solution scheme.

7.3.2 *Solution of the problem for form D data representation*

We will use the following approximation of the unknown distribution function $F(t)$ with the help of a two parametric piecewise linear approximation of the resource function $\Lambda(t) =$

$-\ln[1-F(t)]$, that is,

$$\widetilde{\Lambda}(t) = \chi(t_0 - t)\alpha t + \chi(t - t_0)[\theta t - (\theta - \alpha)t_0] \tag{7.34}$$

where t_0 is the time for which we determine the TTF estimate, and θ and α are parameters. The form of approximation $\widetilde{\Lambda}(t;\alpha,\theta)$ is shown in Fig. 5.1. The parameters α and θ are defined by the following conditions:

1) At the point t_0, for which the TTF estimate is evaluated, the function $F(t)$ and $\widetilde{F}(t) = 1-\exp[-\widetilde{\Lambda}(t)]$ coincide;
2) The approximate distribution function, $\widetilde{F}(t) = 1-\exp[-\widetilde{\Lambda}(t)]$, belongs to the class of failure rate distributions.

Similarly, as in § 5.1 we consider the following conditions on the parameters α and θ:

$$\alpha = -\frac{1}{t_0}\ln R, \tag{7.35}$$

where $R = 1 - F(t_0)$ is the unknown value of TTF and

$$\theta \geqslant \alpha. \tag{7.36}$$

Using the equation (7.36) above we can write the likelihood function $\ell(\alpha,\theta \mid D_j)$ as:

$$\ell(\alpha,\theta \mid D_j) = K(D_j)\alpha^{r_j}\theta^{u_j}\,\mathrm{e}^{(\alpha K_j + \theta\mu_j)} \tag{7.37}$$

With the help of expression (7.36) the likelihood function $\ell(\alpha,\theta \mid D_j)$ may be written as

$$\ell(\alpha,\theta \mid D_j) = K(D_j)\alpha^{r_j}\theta^{u_j}\,\mathrm{e}^{(\alpha K_j + \theta\mu_j)} \tag{7.38}$$

The sufficient statistics included in (7.37) can be interpreted as follows: r_j is the number of failures in the data set D_j, observed before the time t_0, u_j is the number of failures after the time t_0, K_j is the total operating time during the test until the time t_0, u_j is the same as K_j after t_0, $K(D_j)$ is a statistic independent of the parameters α and θ. The calculation of the indicated statistics is carried out with the help of the data set D_j by the following formulas:

$$r_j = \sum_{i=1}^{m_j} d_i^{(j)} \quad \text{and} \quad \sum_{i=m_j+1}^{n_j} d_i^{(j)} \tag{7.39}$$

$$K_j = \sum_{i=1}^{m_j} \left(d_i^{(j)} + k_i^{(j)}\right)s_i^{(j)} + t_0 \sum_{i=m_j+1}^{n_j} \left(d_i^{(j)} + k_i^{(j)}\right), \tag{7.40}$$

and

$$\mu_j = \sum_{i=m_j+1}^{n_j} \left(d_i^{(j)} + k_i^{(j)}\right)\left(s_i^{(j)} - t_0\right), \tag{7.41}$$

where m_j is the number of elements in the sample $s_1^{(j)}, s_2^{(j)}, \ldots, s_{n_j}^{(j)}$ satisfying the conditions $s_i^{(j)} \leqslant t_0$ to, defined by the formula

$$m_j = \sum_{i=1}^{n_j} \chi\left(t_0 - s_i^{(j)}\right).$$

Now, having obtained the completely defined likelihood kernel (7.37), we may find the empirical Bayes estimate of a TTF following the general approach given in the preceding section. The function, $R = R(t_0)$, will be expressed with the help of $\widetilde{\Lambda}(t;\alpha,\theta)$; by substituting the value $t = t_0$ into (7.34) we get

$$R = R(t_0) = \exp[-\widetilde{\Lambda}(t_0;\alpha,\theta)] = \mathrm{e}^{-\alpha t_0}. \tag{7.42}$$

With the help of (7.15) and (7.16) the formula for TTF estimates takes on the form

$$\hat{R}_e^* = \frac{1}{B}\sum_{j=1}^{N} n_j \alpha_j^{r_N} \theta_j^{u_N} \mathrm{e}^{-[\hat{\alpha}_j(K_N+t_0)+\hat{\theta}_j\mu_N]}, \tag{7.43}$$

and

$$\sigma_{\hat{R}_e^*}^2 = \frac{1}{B}\sum_{j=1}^{N} n_j \alpha_j^{r_N} \theta_j^{u_N} \mathrm{e}^{-[\hat{\alpha}_j(K_N+t_0)+\hat{\theta}_j\mu_N]} - \hat{R}_e^{*2}, \tag{7.44}$$

where

$$B = \sum_{j=1}^{N} n_j \alpha_j^{r_N} \theta_j^{u_N} \mathrm{e}^{-(\hat{\alpha}_j K_N+\hat{\theta}_j\mu_N)}. \tag{7.45}$$

For application of the expressions (7.42)-(7.44), it is necessary to know the estimate $(\hat{\alpha}_j, \hat{\theta}_j)$ obtained with the help of the data D_j. In the preceding section, it was mentioned that the likelihood estimate cannot be used for this purpose. Under these circumstances we recommend using the Bayes estimate corresponding to the noninformative prior probability distribution. Let us use this recommendation to obtain the estimates $(\hat{\alpha}_j, \hat{\theta}_j)$, $j = 1, 2, \ldots, N$. To find the noninformative prior probability distribution for the parameters α and θ, we assume that $R = \exp(-\alpha t_0)$ is uniformly distributed in the interval $[0,1]$. With the help of the transformation (7.35), we can write the marginal prior density, $h_1(\alpha)$, of the parameter α as follows:

$$h_1(\alpha) = t_0 \mathrm{e}^{-\alpha t_0}, \quad 0 \leqslant \alpha < \infty. \tag{7.46}$$

This expression is a particular case of (5.30) with $R_\ell = 0$ and $R_u = 1$. We now define the conditional prior density, $h_2(\theta \mid \alpha)$, taking into account the inequality (7.36), and assuming that, $h_2(\theta \mid \alpha)$, as well as $h_1(\alpha)$ belongs to the class of exponential probability distributions:

$$h_2(\theta \mid \alpha) = t_0 \mathrm{e}^{-(\theta-\alpha)t_0}, \quad \alpha \leqslant \theta < \infty.$$

Now, we can easily write the joint prior density of the parameters α and θ:

$$h(\alpha,\theta) = h_1(\alpha)h_2(\theta \mid \alpha) = t_0^2\,\mathrm{e}^{-\theta t_0}, \quad 0 \leqslant \alpha < \infty, \quad \alpha \leqslant \theta < \infty. \tag{7.47}$$

Using expressions (7.37) and (7.46), we obtain the posterior probability distribution of the parameters α and θ with data D_j:

$$\hbar(\alpha,\theta \mid D_j) = \frac{1}{\beta_j}\alpha^{r_j}\theta^{u_j}\,\mathrm{e}^{-[\alpha K_j+\theta(\mu_j+t_0)]}, \quad 0 \leqslant \alpha < \infty, \quad \alpha \leqslant \theta < \infty, \tag{7.48}$$

where

$$\beta_j = \int_0^\infty \int_2^\infty \alpha^{r_j}\theta^{u_j}\exp\{-[\alpha K_j+\theta(\mu_j+t_0)]\}d\theta\,d\alpha. \tag{7.49}$$

Thus, the Bayes pointwise estimates $\hat{\theta}$ and $\hat{\alpha}$ are given by

$$\hat{\alpha}_j = \int_0^\infty \int_\alpha^\infty \alpha\hbar(\alpha,\theta \mid D_j)d\theta\,d\alpha \quad \text{and} \quad \hat{\theta}_j = \int_0^\infty \int_\alpha^\infty \theta\hbar(\alpha,\theta \mid D_j)d\theta\,d\alpha. \tag{7.50}$$

Having derived the integrals (7.49) for the function $\hbar(\alpha,\theta \mid D_j)$ of the form(7.47) and integral (7.48), we can write the resulting formulas for the desired estimates:

$$\hat{\alpha}_j = \frac{1}{t_0\beta_j}\sum_{i=0}^{u_j}\frac{(u_j+r_j+1-i)!}{(u_j-i)!}\cdot\frac{1}{(\omega_{1j}+1)^{i+1}(\omega_j+1)^{u_j+r_j+2-i}}, \tag{7.51}$$

$$\hat{\theta}_j = \frac{u_j+1}{t_0\beta_j}\sum_{i=0}^{u_j+1}\frac{(u_j+r_j+1-i)!}{(u_j+1-i)!}\cdot\frac{1}{(\omega_{1j}+1)^{i+1}(\omega_j+1)^{u_j+r_j+2-i}}, \tag{7.52}$$

and

$$\beta_j = \sum_{i=1}^{u_j}\frac{(u_j+r_j-i)!}{(u_j-i)!}\cdot\frac{1}{(\omega_{1j}+1)^{i+1}(\omega_j+1)^{u_j+r_j+1-i}}. \tag{7.53}$$

Let us note in conclusion that in practice we may meet a case when a scientist, carrying out the statistical analysis of each series of tests which possesses nontrivial prior information, i.e., he can find an interval of an uncertain prior indeterminacy $[R_{\ell_j},R_{u_j}]$ such that $R_j \in [R_{\ell_j},R_{u_j}]$, $j = 1,2,\ldots,N$. Such a set of data should be completed by two numbers R_{ℓ_j} and R_{u_j}. (It is clear that in some cases $R_{\ell_j} = 0$, $R_{u_j} = 1$, i.e., there is no a priori information.) In this general case the expressions for the estimates $\hat{\alpha}_j$ and $\hat{\theta}_j$' have the following form:

$$\hat{\alpha}_j = \frac{1}{t_0\beta_j}\sum_{i=1}^{u_j}\frac{1}{(u_j-i)!}\cdot\frac{1}{(\omega_{1j}+1)^{i+1}}\sum_{k=0}^{u_j+r_j+1-i}\frac{(u_j+r_j+1-i)!}{(u_j+r_j+1-i-k!)}\cdot\frac{1}{(\omega_j+1)^{k+1}}$$
$$\times\left(R_{u_j}^{\omega_j+1}|\ln R_{u_j}|^{u_j+r_j+1-i-k} - R_{\ell j}^{\omega_{j+1}}|\ln R_{\ell j}|^{u_j+r_j+1-i-k}\right), \tag{7.54}$$

$$\hat{\theta}_j = \frac{u_j+1}{t_0\beta_j}\sum_{i=0}^{u_j+1}\frac{1}{(u_j+1-i)!}\cdot\frac{1}{(\omega_{1j}+1)^{i+1}}\sum_{k=0}^{u_j+r_j+1-i}\frac{(u_j+r_j+1-i)!}{(u_j+r_j+1-i-k!)}\cdot\frac{1}{(\omega_j+1)^{k+1}}$$
$$\times\left(R_{u_j}^{\omega_j+1}|\ln R_{u_j}|^{u_j+r_j+1-i-k} - R_{\ell j}^{\omega_{j+1}}|\ln R_{\ell j}|^{u_j+r_j+1-i-k}\right), \tag{7.55}$$

and

$$\beta_j = \sum_{i=0}^{u_j} \frac{1}{(u_j-i)!} \cdot \frac{1}{(\omega_{1j}+1)^{i+1}} \sum_{k=0}^{u_j+r_j-i} \frac{(u_j+r_j+1-i)!}{(u_j+r_j-i-k!)} \cdot \frac{1}{(\omega_j+1)^{k+1}}$$
$$\times \left(R_{u_j}^{\omega_j+1} |\ln R_{u_j}|^{u_j+r_j-i-k} - R_{\ell j}^{\omega_{j+1}} |\ln R_{\ell j}|^{u_j+r_j-i-k}\right), \tag{7.56}$$

where ω_{1j} and ω_j denote the dimensionless statistics and $\omega_{1j} = \mu_j/t_0$ and $\omega_j = (K_j + \mu_j)/t_0$, which can be interpreted as the cumulative relative operable time in j-th series after time t_0, and total operable time, respectively. The expressions (7.50)-(7.52), obtained earlier, can be derived by (7.53)–(7.55) if one sets in the latter $R_{\ell j} = 0$ and $R_{uj} = 1$, respectively.

7.3.3 *Solution of the problem for the form of data representation*

Since the information contained in C_j touches directly upon the reliabilityfunction, R_j, we need to develop the empirical Bayes procedure, using a random parameter the unknown value R_j. We start with the following formula for a joint prior probability density $h(\alpha,\theta)$:

$$h(\alpha,\theta) = h_1(\alpha)h_2(\theta \mid \alpha) = h_1(\alpha)t_0\,\mathrm{e}^{-(\theta-\alpha)t_0}, \quad 0 \leqslant \alpha < \infty, \quad \alpha \leqslant \theta < \infty,$$

assuming that $h_1(\alpha)$ is unknown. Using the likelihood function of (7.37) and Bayes theorem we write the posterior probability density of these parameters:

$$\hbar(\alpha,\theta \mid D_j) \sim \alpha^{r_j}\theta^{u_j}\,\mathrm{e}^{-(\alpha K_j+\theta\mu_j)} h_1(\alpha)\,\mathrm{e}^{-(\theta-\alpha)t_0}. \tag{7.57}$$

Thereafter, we take into account the fact that unknown TTF $R = R(t_0) = \exp(-\alpha t_0)$, is defined only by the parameter α. Then from the expression for the joint probability density $\hbar(\alpha,\theta \mid D_j)$, we obtain the marginal posterior density

$$\hbar(\alpha \mid D_j) = \int_\alpha^\infty \hbar(\alpha,\theta \mid D_j)d\theta$$
$$\sim \alpha^{r_j}\,\mathrm{e}^{-\alpha(K_j+\mu_j)} \sum_{i=0}^{u_j} \frac{1}{(\mu_j-i)!} \cdot \frac{\alpha^{u_j-i}}{(\mu_j+t_0)^{i+1}} h_1(\alpha), \quad 0 \leqslant \alpha < \infty, \tag{7.58}$$

and then, we find the posterior probability density of unknown TTF, R, using the relation $\alpha(R) = -\ln R/t_0$;

$$\hbar_R(x \mid D_j) = \hbar(\alpha(x) \mid D_j)|\alpha'(x)| \sim [\alpha(x)]^{r_j}\,\mathrm{e}^{-\alpha(x)(K_j+\mu_j)}$$
$$\times \sum_{i=0}^{u_j} \frac{1}{(u_j-i)!} \cdot \frac{[\alpha(x)]^{u_j-i}}{(\mu_j+t_0)^{i+1}} \{h_1(\alpha(x))|\alpha'(x)|\}. \tag{7.59}$$

The expression enclosed in brackets in (7.59) is, by definition, the marginal prior probability density, $h_R(x)$, of the reliability function R, which is unknown. After simplification, we have

$$\hbar_R(x \mid D_j) \sim h_R(x)x^{\omega_j} \sum_{i=0}^{u_j} \frac{1}{(u_j-i)!} \cdot \frac{[\ln x]^{r_j+u_j-i}}{(\omega_{1j}+1)^{i+1}}. \tag{7.60}$$

The expression for the posterior probability density (7.59) of the N-th test series with the data set D_N enables us to write the desired pointwise TTF estimate in the form

$$\hat{R}_e^* = \frac{\sum\limits_{j=1}^{N} n_j \hat{R}_j \ell_0\left(\hat{R}_j; r_N; u_N, \omega_N, \omega_{1N}\right)}{\sum\limits_{j=1}^{N} n_j \ell_0\left(\hat{R}_j; r_N; u_N, \omega_N, \omega_{1N}\right)},$$

where

$$\ell_0(x; r, u, \omega, \omega_1) = x^{\omega} \sum_{i=0}^{u} \frac{1}{(u-i)!} \cdot \frac{|\ln x|^{r+u-i}}{(\omega_1+1)^{i+1}}. \tag{7.61}$$

When we use the formula for $\hat{R}_e^*$, two questions remain open: what do we use as an estimate $\hat{R}_N$ and how should we substitute the unknown sample sizes n_j participating in the procedure of obtaining the estimates $\hat{R}_j$ ($j = 1, 2, \ldots, N-1$). To answer the first question we will apply, as before, the recommendations of § 7.2. Choose as $\hat{R}_N$ the Bayes estimate of TTF, obtained with the help of the known data D_N, and use the posterior probability density (7.59). If we assume that the interval of an uncertain prior, $\left[R_{\ell N}, R_{uN}\right]$, is given, then the estimates $\hat{R}_N$ and $\sigma_{\hat{R}_N}$ may be found with the help of the formulas analogous to (5.73) and (5.74):

$$\hat{R}_N = \frac{I_1(\omega_N, \omega_{1N}, r_N+u_N, u_N)}{I_0(\omega_N, \omega_{1N}, r_N+u_N, u_N)}, \tag{7.62}$$

and

$$\sigma_{\hat{R}_N}^2 = \frac{I_1(\omega_N, \omega_{1N}, r_N+u_N, u_N)}{I_0(\omega_N, \omega_{1N}, r_N+u_N, u_N)} - \hat{R}_N^2 \tag{7.63}$$

where

$$I_m(\omega, \omega_1, n, k) = \sum_{i=0}^{k} \frac{(n-i)!}{k-i)!} \cdot \frac{1}{(\omega_1+1)^{i+1}} \sum_{j=0}^{n-i} \frac{1}{(n-i-j)!}$$
$$\times \frac{1}{(\omega+m+1)^{j+1}} \left(R_{uN}^{\omega+m+1} |\ln R_{uN}|^{n+i+j} - R_{\ell N}^{\omega+m+1} |\ln R_{\ell N}|^{n+i+j}\right). \tag{7.64}$$

In a simpler case, when there is no *a priori* information in the form of the interval $\left[R_{\ell N}, R_{uN}\right]$, the function $I_m(\omega, \omega_1, n, k)$ has the form

$$I_m(\omega, \omega_1, n, k) = \sum_{i=0}^{k} \frac{(n-i)!}{k-i)!} \cdot \frac{1}{(\omega_1+1)^{i+1}} \cdot \frac{1}{(\omega+m+1)^{n-i+1}}. \tag{7.65}$$

The calculation of the estimates $\hat{R}_N$ and $\sigma_{\hat{R}_N}$ should be carried out, as before, with the formulas (7.61) and (7.62), but for this purpose we use the function (7.64).

Consider now the second question touching upon the needed replacement of the sample sizes n_j. Recall that these quantities have been introduced in the general Bayes empirical procedure as weight coefficients reflecting the significance of each estimate under approximation of the posterior probability distribution. It is assumed that increasing the sample size used for the estimate implies a significant increase. Since the exactness of the obtained estimate appears to be, in some sense, an equivalence, we will use as characteristic of the significance of the j-th estimate the following quantity:

$$\nu_j = \frac{1/\sigma_{\hat{R}_j}}{\frac{1}{\sigma_{\hat{R}_1}} + \frac{1}{\sigma_{\hat{R}_2}} + \cdots + \frac{1}{\sigma_{\hat{R}_N}}}, \quad j = 1, 2, \ldots, N. \tag{7.66}$$

Such a choice may be explained, for example, by the fact that for most of the estimates $\sigma_{\hat{R}_j} \sim n_j^{-1}$.

The resulting expressions for the empirical Bayes TTF estimate have the following form:

$$\hat{R}_e^* = \frac{\sum_{j=1}^N \nu_j \hat{R}_j \ell_0(\hat{R}_j; r_N, r_N, \omega_N, \omega_{1N})}{\sum_{j=1}^N \nu_j \ell_0(\hat{R}_j; r_N, u_N, \omega_N, \omega_{1N})}, \tag{7.67}$$

and

$$\sigma_{\hat{R}_e^*}^2 = \frac{\sum_{j=1}^N \nu_j \hat{R}_j^2 \ell_0(\hat{R}_j; r_N, u_N, \omega_N, \omega_{1N})}{\sum_{j=1}^N \nu_j \ell_0(\hat{R}_j; r_N, u_N, \omega_N, \omega_{1N})} - \hat{R}_e^{*2}, \tag{7.68}$$

where $\ell_0(x; r, u, \omega, \omega_1)$ is given by the formula (7.60).

7.3.4 *Comparative analysis of estimates*

It is clear that the estimate, found in accordance with the second scheme, is more general, since the data D_j may be reduced to the data C_j with the help of formulas (7.61) and (7.62) by letting $N = j$. Use of this transformation allows us to estimate TTF for the mixed scheme when the database contains both data's D_j and C_j.The point is that the TTF estimate for some j-th device may not always be found with the help of D_j; we may need another source of information. Thereby, the second scheme allows a joint processing of reliability data, obtained with the help of different schemes. We should note also another important aspect. If one constructs a procedure by the second scheme, then it is possible to use the continuous approximation of the prior probability density, $h_R(x)$, by using Parzen's formula (7.7). This allows us, in turn, to find the lower confidence limit of TTF in accordance with equation (7.9). The construction of the scheme of defining the lower confidence limit of TTF is a further development of the proposed method.

7.3.5 *Investigation of the accuracy of TTF estimates*

Accuracy of the estimate $\hat{R}_e^*$, obtained by the proposed method, will be studied using statistical simulations. Let us simulate 5 samples of sizes 20, 40, 60, 80 and 100 from a random

Table 7.1 Comparison of the Bayes estimate of TTF with a true value and non-homogeneous a priori data.

$\alpha_N = 1; R(t_0) = 0.7516$					
N	$n_N = 20$	$n_N = 40$	$n_N = 60$	$n_N = 80$	$n_N = 100$
2	0.7139	0.7415	0.7328	0.7509	0.7524
4	0.7318	0.7418	0.7240	0.7418	0.7449
6	0.7094	0.7218	0.7443	0.7530	0.7518
8	0.6988	0.7610	0.7415	0.7488	0.7557
$\alpha_N = 2; R(t_0) = 0.9216$					
2	0.9248	0.9251	0.9230	0.9209	0.9219
4	0.9236	0.9249	0.9235	0.9187	0.9207
6	0.9254	0.9263	0.9224	0.9238	0.9230
8	0.927	0.9259	0.9244	0.9244	0.9238
$\alpha_N = 3; R(t_0) = 0.9769$					
2	0.9731	0.9740	0.9779	0.9744	0.9773
4	0.9729	0.9735	0.9735	0.9731	0.9261
6	0.9722	0.9746	0.9760	0.9753	0.9762
8	0.9754	0.979	0.9722	0.9733	0.9752

variable with the Weibull distribution

$$F(t) = F(t;\sigma,\alpha) = 1 - \exp\left[-\left(\frac{t}{\sigma}\right)^{\alpha}\right] \tag{7.69}$$

where parameter $\alpha = \alpha_N$ is fixed. Censoring to the right is carried out by the random number having the uniform distribution in the interval $[k_1\sigma,\, k_2\sigma]$.The observations are represented in the format D_N. For obtaining data sets $C_j = (\hat{R}_j, \sigma_{\hat{R}_j})$, $j = 1,2,\ldots,N-1$, similar samples of 40 sizes for different values of the shape parameter α_j are simulated. This parameter is chosen randomly in the interval $[0.8\alpha_N, 1.2\alpha_N]$.

Thus, we ensure the second scheme as the result of transformation of the first one for nonuniform data $D_1, D_2, \ldots, D_N$. The results of modeling with $t_0 = 100s$, $\sigma = 350s$, $k_1 = 0.75$, $k_2 = 2.0$ for different N are represented in Table 7.1. Comparison of the empirical pointwise Bayes estimate $\hat{R}_e^*$ with the exact value of TTF lets us draw the following conclusions:

1) With the increasing of the sample size n_N, the estimate $\hat{R}_e^*$ approaches the exact value of TTF;
2) With the increasing of the past data, the distance of the estimate $\hat{R}_e^*$ to the exact value decreases.

In Table 7.2 we represent the results of modeling for the case when the data $C_1, C_2, \ldots, C_{N-1}$ are generated by simulating homogeneous samples, i.e., the parameter

Table 7.2 Comparison of Bayes estimate of TTF with the true value and homogeneous a priori data.

$\alpha_N = 1; R(t_0) = 0.7516$					
N	$n_N = 20$	$n_N = 40$	$n_N = 60$	$n_N = 80$	$n_N = 100$
2	0.7229	0.7433	0.7324	0.7552	0.7508
4	0.7408	0.7441	0.7380	0.7499	0.7510
6	0.7551	0.7480	0.7421	0.7508	0.7512
8	0.7499	0.7500	0.7498	0.7521	0.7509
$\alpha_N = 2; R(t_0) = 0.9216$					
2	0.9241	0.9188	0.9234	0.9229	0.9201
4	0.9244	0.9212	0.9231	0.9215	0.9220
6	0.9230	0.9209	0.9212	0.9210	0.9*221
8	0.9209	0.9219	0.9208	0.9218	0.9213
$\alpha_N = 3; R(t_0) = 0.9769$					
2	0.9740	0.9751	0.9788	0.9753	0.9761
4	0.9737	0.9744	0.9760	0.9780	0.9772
6	0.9777	0.9754	0.9774	0.9761	0.9766
8	0.9752	0.9766	0.9772	0.9767	0.9773

Table 7.3 Comparison of Bayes estimate $\hat{R}^*_\varepsilon$ without a priori information ($N = 0$) for Weilbull distributions with $\alpha_N = 3$ ($R(t_0) = 0.9769$).

N	n_N				
	20	40	60	80	100
Homogeneous data					
0	0.9732	0.9740	0.9753	0.9787	0.9755
2	0.9740	0.9751	0.9788	0.9753	0.9761
4	0.9737	0.9744	0.9760	0.9780	0.9772
Nonhomogeneous data					
0	0.9732	0.9740	0.9753	0.9787	0.9755
2	0.9731	0.9740	0.9779	0.9744	0.9773
4	0.9729	0.9749	0.9735	0.9731	0.9761

α during the simulation of the data $D_1, D_2, \ldots, D_N$ is constant. Here we observe a property opposite to that one in the conclusion (2): with the increasing of N, the accuracy of estimating the exact value of the TTF increases.

The specific features mentioned above are in full accordance with the qualitative information about the properties of empirical Bayes estimates.

In reality, since the prior information is very influential under the small sample sizes, during the process of nonuniform data we encounter distortion of the posterior probability distribution. At the same time, if the past data and D_N are homogeneous, the completion of the sample D_N occurs which implies an increase in the accuracy of the estimate.

An illustration of this fact is that in the first and second cases a priori information allows us to increase the accuracy of the estimate obtained in comparison with the situation when TTF estimating is carried out only with the help of the sample D_N.

The conclusions we have made confirm the workability of the proposed method of empirical Bayes estimates and reinforce the quality of the estimate because of the use of the prior data.

Theoretical analysis of the quality of empirical Bayes estimates in accordance with the properties of prior data is impeded by the complicated form of the procedure of construction of nonparametric estimates. During the process of extensive statistical experimentation, we find that using a prior nonhomogeneous data portions can lead to a bias in the empirical Bayes estimates. This bias increases with an increase in the testing size for the tested device while the structure of the data about similar tests does not change.

Chapter 8

Theoretical Model for Engineering Reliability

8.1 Setting of the problem

In this and later chapters we shall investigate the methods of calculating the TTF of a technical device with the help of parametric models. The essence of this model is a formalization of the conditions of a normal (without failures) functioning of the device by the functional inequalities of the form

$$Z_j(\zeta,t) = \phi\left(X_1(\zeta,t),\ldots,X_N(\zeta,t)\right)(\zeta,t),\ldots,X_N(\zeta,t) > 0, \quad j = 1,2,\ldots,M, \tag{8.1}$$

where $Z_j(\zeta,t)$ is the initial random variable, depending on multivariate coordinate ζ and time t; Z_j is a status variable, $\phi_j(\cdot)$ is an efficiency function. For the reliability function, R, in the general case we will use the probability expression given by

$$R = R(\tau) = P\{Z_j(\zeta,t) > 0, \ j = 1,2,\ldots,M, \ \zeta \in R^k, \ 0 \leqslant t \leqslant \tau\}. \tag{8.2}$$

A lot of works are devoted to the application of such an approach for the investigation of technical devices [26, 32, 89, 112, 135, 173, 260]. The results of Chapters 8–10 represent the development of traditional methods of estimating TTF for technical devices under the condition of uncertainty with respect to initial data and the survival state model. In this chapter we will use a particular form of the reliability function (8.2), considering the object state in a fixed moment of time to and for a fixed point of the device ζ_0 with the most dangerous functioning conditions. In real practical situations for mechanical devices, the vector of initial variables $X = (X_1, X_2, \ldots, X_N)$ generates physical-mechanical characteristics, geometrical parameters and loading factors. Usually we have certain information about these variables which lets us find a probability density, $f_X(x;\theta)$, at least with an accuracy up to the parameter vector θ. Most commonly used in practice in the normal model when the parameter vector $\theta = (\theta_1, \theta_2, \ldots, \theta_k)$ consists of the expected values m_i, standard deviations σ_i and correlation coefficients ρ_{ij} $(i, j = 1, 2, \ldots, N, i < j)$. The point is that in real situations the error of the working capacity model (8.1) and initial data in the form of parameters $\theta_1, \theta_2, \ldots, \theta_k$ may be so large that the gain in strictly defining the TTF through the use of more exact (different from Gaussian) probability distributions gives us no positive effect. Thus, the authors choose another approach to improving existing methods. We shall proceed with the development of the error of the methods of estimating TTF, counting on all the possible initial data and the working capacity model and using the normal distribution for the approximation of the function $f_X(x;\theta)$. It is clear that the ideal way out of this situation is the solution of the problem of simultaneous consideration of all types of error that we mentioned. Unfortunately, such a problem takes on a very complicated and tedious form and, in most cases, is beyond the limits of engineering methods.

In this chapter we shall consider a simpler problem of estimating the device TTF with the help of uncertainty in assigning the initial data under the assumption that a working capacity model is free of error. Later on, we will touch upon a more general problem counting on both types of errors. We consider the Bayes approach as a methodological basis of solving the problem, and assume that only the experimental results are the actual information for the acceptance of decisions.

In accordance with the form of the working capacity model (8.1) and general expression (8.2), we rewrite the TTF in the form of the N-dimensional integral

$$R = R_X(\theta) = \int \overset{N}{\cdots} \int_{\substack{\phi(x)\geqslant 0\\ j=1,2,\ldots,M}} f_X(\mathbf{x};\theta)dx_1\cdots dx_N \tag{8.3}$$

There is another way of finding the reliability function, R, consisting of the following steps: we perform the transformation $\mathbf{X}\to\mathbf{Z}$ and find the probability density $f_Z(z;\vartheta)$ of the vector of state parameters, Z, where $\vartheta = (\vartheta_1, \vartheta_2, \ldots, \vartheta_\ell)$ is a vector of parameters, and evaluate the M-dimensional integral

$$R = R_Z(\vartheta) = \int_0^\infty \overset{M}{\cdots} \int_0^\infty f_Z(\mathbf{z};\vartheta)dz_1\cdots dz_M. \tag{8.4}$$

Since the transformation $f_X(\mathbf{x};\theta) \to f_Z(\mathbf{z};\vartheta)$ is univalent, the vector ϑ is determined uniquely by the vector θ. If the parameter θ or ϑ is given, the TTF is determined completely by the expressions (8.3) and (8.4). We will consider a problem of estimating TTF under the condition that the values of all or portion of the parameters are unknown; instead of the values of the parameters θ_i, their intervals of uncertainty $[\theta_i', \theta_i'']$ are given, or in a general case, a prior p.d.f. $h_\theta(\theta)$ is known.

8.1.1 *Setting of the problem*

The problem of obtaining TTF estimates is solved under the following assumptions:

(1) A working capacity model of the form (8.1) is known and appears to be ideal, i.e., it is free of errors;
(2) Given satisfactory, from the point of view of engineering exactness, expressions for the p.d.f.'s $f_X(\mathbf{x};\theta)$ and $f_Z(\mathbf{z};\vartheta)$, where the values of the parameters θ and ϑ are unknown;
(3) For a vector of parameters θ (or ϑ) given a prior p.d.f. $h_\theta(\theta)$ (or $h_\vartheta(\vartheta)$);
(4) During the tests, the values of the initial variables are fixed; the set of these variables will be denoted by $\underset{\sim}{\mathbf{x}} = \{x_{ij}\}$, where $i = 1, 2, \ldots, N$ is the variable number, $j = 1, 2, \ldots, n$ is the test number.

The phrase "are fixed during the tests" means that the parameter value may be measured in the test or it is a priori assumed that in the test the parameter takes on a certain value. The problem is to Bud the pointwise TTF Bayes estimate, $\hat{R}^*$, the posterior standard deviation, $\sigma_{\hat{R}^*}$, and Bayes lower confidence limit, $\underline{R}^*_\gamma$, under the given confidence level, γ. The general solution will cover two cases: in the first one, a prior p.d.f. $h_\theta(\theta)$ of the parameter vector of the initial variables **X**, in the second case, $h_\vartheta(\vartheta)$ for the vector of state variables **Z**.

8.1.2 *The solution algorithm in case one*

Let us write the likelihood function for the known p.d.f. $f_X(\mathbf{x};\theta)$ using the sample of results $\mathbf{x} = (x_1, x_2, \ldots, x_N)$. Since $\underset{\sim}{\mathbf{x}}$ are noncensored data, we have

$$\ell_X(\theta \mid \underset{\sim}{\mathbf{x}}) = \prod_{j=1}^{n} f_X(x_j;\theta). \tag{8.5}$$

Now we return to the traditional Bayes scheme. Using Bayes theorem, we obtain the posterior p.d.f. of the parameter θ

$$\hbar_0(\theta \mid \underset{\sim}{\mathbf{x}}) \sim h_\theta(\theta)\ell_X(\theta \mid \underset{\sim}{\mathbf{x}}).$$

Thereafter, in accordance with the standard Bayes scheme, we can find the pointwise estimate

$$\hat{\theta}^* = \arg\min_{\theta\in\Theta} \{G(\hat{\theta})\},$$

where $G(\hat{\theta})$ is the function of a mean posterior risk. In particular, if a mean square error loss function has been chosen, we have

$$\hat{\theta}_i^* = \int_\Theta \theta_i \hbar_\theta(\theta \mid \underset{\sim}{\mathbf{x}})d\theta, \quad i = 1, 2, \ldots, k. \tag{8.6}$$

Note that the Bayes estimate $\hat{\theta}^*$ is determined by the sample $\underset{\sim}{\mathbf{x}}$, a prior p.d.f., $h_\theta(\theta)$, and the form of the probability distribution $f_X(\mathbf{x};\theta)$. The Bayes TTF estimate may be found with the help of the obtained estimate (8.6) as $\hat{R}^* = R_X(\hat{\theta}^*)$ where the form of this dependence is defined with the help of the integral (8.3). The estimate $R_X(\hat{\theta}^*)$, generally speaking, may be biased. Therefore, the estimate of the form

$$\hat{R}^* = \arg\min_{\hat{R}} \int_{\Theta} L\big(R(\theta), \hat{R}\big)\hbar_\theta\big(\theta \mid \underset{\sim}{\mathbf{x}}\big)d\theta \tag{8.7}$$

is more preferable. Here $L\big(R(\theta), \hat{R}\big)$ represents a loss function. For a mean square error function we obtain

$$\hat{R}^* = \int_{\Theta} R_X(\theta)\hbar_\theta\big(\theta \mid \underset{\sim}{\mathbf{x}}\big)d\theta. \tag{8.8}$$

Comparing the expressions (8.8) and (8.3), we may draw the conclusion that the calculation of the estimate $\hat{R}^*$ is connected with the evaluation of the $(N+k)$-dimensional integral. The error in defining the estimate (8.8) may be represented in the form of the posterior mean-squared value of the function $R_X(\theta)$. This approach allows us to find the Bayes lower confidence limit $\underline{R}^*_\gamma$ for a TTF with a given confidence level γ. To do this we need to solve the equation

$$\int_{R_{X(\theta)} \geqslant \underline{R}^*_\gamma} \hbar\big(\theta \mid \underset{\sim}{\mathbf{x}}\big)d\theta = \gamma. \tag{8.9}$$

8.1.3 *The algorithm of the problem in case two*

Suppose that we are given a prior p.d.f. $h(\vartheta)$ of the status variable $\mathbf{Z} = (Z_1, Z_2, \ldots, Z_M)$. Having the system of working capacity functions $\phi_j(\cdot)$ (see assumption (1)) and sample $\underset{\sim}{\mathbf{x}}$, we may obtain the set of experimental values of the status variables $\{z_{ji}\} = (z_1, z_2, \ldots, z_N)$ (i is the test number, j is the variable number), where $z_{ji} = \phi_j(\mathbf{x}_i)$, $i = 1, 2, \ldots, n$; $j = 1, 2, \ldots, M$. The reasoning is similar to that for the first case. For the posterior probability density of the parameter ϑ we will have

$$\hbar\big(\vartheta \mid \underset{\sim}{\mathbf{z}}\big) \sim h(\vartheta)\ell_Z\big(\vartheta \mid \underset{\sim}{\mathbf{z}}\big), \tag{8.10}$$

where

$$\ell_Z\big(\vartheta \mid \underset{\sim}{\mathbf{z}}\big) = \prod_{i=1}^{n} f_Z(z_i; \theta) \tag{8.11}$$

For obtaining TTF estimates we should use the common integral (8.4). This may be done in the following two ways: with the help of the posterior estimate $\hat{\vartheta}^*$ or directly, by estimating the function $R_Z(\vartheta)$. With mean square error loss function in the first case we have $\hat{R}^* = R_Z(\vartheta^*)$, where

$$\hat{\vartheta}^*_j = \int_{\Theta_Z} \vartheta_j \hbar\big(\vartheta \mid \underset{\sim}{\mathbf{z}}\big)d\vartheta, \quad j = 1, 2, \ldots, \ell,$$

and Θ_Z is the domain of changing of the parameters ϑ. In the second case,

$$\hat{R}^* = \int_{\Theta_Z} R_Z(\vartheta)\hbar(\vartheta \mid \underset{\sim}{\mathbf{z}})d\vartheta = \int_{\Theta_Z} \hbar(\vartheta \mid \underset{\sim}{\mathbf{z}}) \int_0^\infty \overset{M}{\cdots} \int_0^\infty f_Z(\mathbf{z};\vartheta)dz. \tag{8.12}$$

The expression for the posterior variance of the TTF, which appears to be a characteristic of the accuracy of the estimate (8.12), may be represented in the form of an analogous integral:

$$\sigma^2_{\hat{R}^*} = \int_{\Theta_Z} R^2_Z(\vartheta)\hbar(\vartheta \mid \underset{\sim}{\mathbf{z}})d\vartheta = \hat{R}^{*2}. \tag{8.13}$$

The equation for obtaining the Bayes lower confidence limit in the case when the prior density $h(\vartheta)$ is given has a form similar to that for the equation (8.9):

$$\int_{R_Z(\vartheta)\geqslant \underline{R}^*_\gamma} \hbar(\vartheta \mid \underset{\sim}{\mathbf{z}})d\vartheta = \gamma. \tag{8.14}$$

Comparing these two cases we note that their corresponding estimates coincide only in the case when there is a correspondence between the $h_\theta(\theta)$, and $h(\vartheta)$ reflecting adequately the dependence $\vartheta = \vartheta(\theta)$. At the same time, these estimates differ between themselves if a priori information on parameters θ and ϑ are obtained independently, starting from different prior arguments. The question about the choice of the form ($h_\theta(\theta)$ or $h(\vartheta)$) of a prior distribution probably cannot be solved uniquely. On one hand, since $h_\theta(\theta)$ determines the prior distribution of the parameter, characterizing the initial variables, we have more various a priori information than information for $h(\vartheta)$. On the other hand, the calculation scheme which uses $h(\vartheta)$ will be simpler, since the dimension of the vector ϑ, as a rule, is much less than the one for the vector θ. We will prefer the second calculation scheme, assuming that the prior density $h(\theta)$ may be found with the help of the probability density $h_\theta(\vartheta)$.

In the last two sections we have solved the problem of estimating TTF for the technical device having a working capacity model represented by one inequality of the form (8.1) for the Gaussian distribution of a status variable. The solution is carried out in an ascending order, that is, at first we consider a simpler case of the known variance of a status variable Z, and thereafter, we investigate the general case when all parameters are unknown.

8.2 Reliability function estimates for the known variance of a status variable

Let a device TTF be defined by a single status variable, obeying a normal law with the p.d.f., $f_Z(z;m_Z,\sigma_Z)$.Then, in accordance with the general expression (8.2), we have

$$R = R(m_Z,\sigma_Z) = \Phi\left(\frac{m_Z}{\sigma_Z}\right), \tag{8.15}$$

where $\Phi(u)$ is the Laplace function. This case may serve as an approximate description of a one-dimensional model of survival time of the form $Z = \phi(X_1, X_2, \ldots, X_N) > 0$, when one uses a normal approximation of a probability distribution of the status variable Z, the parameters m_Z and σ_Z can be found approximately by the formulas

$$m_Z \cong \phi(m_X) + \frac{1}{2} \sum\sum_{1 \leqslant i \leqslant j \leqslant N} \frac{\vartheta^2 \phi(m_X)}{\vartheta m_i \vartheta m_j} \rho_{ij} \sigma_i \sigma_j, \tag{8.16}$$

and

$$\begin{aligned} \sigma_Z^2 &\cong [\phi(m_X) - m_Z]^2 \\ &+ \sum\sum_{1 \leqslant i \leqslant j \leqslant N} \left\{ \frac{\vartheta \phi(m_X)}{\vartheta m_i} \cdot \frac{\vartheta \phi(m_X)}{\vartheta m_j} + [\phi(m_X) - m_Z] \frac{\vartheta^2 \phi(m_X)}{\vartheta m_i \vartheta m_j} \rho_{ij} \sigma_i \sigma_j \right\}, \end{aligned} \tag{8.17}$$

where $m_X = (m_1, \ldots, m_N)$ is a vector of mean values of the initial variables $\mathbf{X}$, $\sigma_X = (\sigma_1, \ldots, \sigma_N)$ is a vector of the standard deviation values of $\mathbf{X}$, $\widetilde{\rho}_X = \{\rho_{ij}\}_{N \times N}$ is a matrix of correlation coefficients of the vector $\mathbf{X}$. The set $(m_X, \sigma_X, \widetilde{\rho}_X)$ generates the parameter vector θ.

Here we consider a particular case when the variance of a status variable is known, i.e., we assume that the parameter σ_Z is completely known, whereas for m_Z, we know the uncertainty interval $[\alpha_1, \alpha_2]$, on which the a priori distribution is defined with density $h(\vartheta)$. Often we meet the situation when it is difficult to substantiate the form of the density $h(\vartheta)$ in the interval $[\alpha_1, \alpha_2]$. Therefore, following Jeffrey's approach, we use a uniform prior distribution

$$h(\vartheta) = \begin{cases} \dfrac{1}{\alpha_2 - \alpha_1}, & \alpha_1 \leqslant \vartheta \leqslant \alpha_2, \\ 0, & \vartheta < \alpha_1, \ \vartheta > \alpha_2. \end{cases} \tag{8.18}$$

Now, since the parameter σ_Z is a priori fixed, the p.d.f. of the status variable Z is written as

$$f_Z(z; \vartheta) = \frac{1}{\sqrt{2\pi}\sigma_Z} e^{-(z-\vartheta)^2/\left(2\sigma_Z^2\right)}. \tag{8.19}$$

Let us use the general scheme described in 8.1.3. First we shall find the likelihood function. Suppose $\underset{\sim}{\mathbf{z}} = (z_1, z_2, \ldots, z_N)$ is the sample of results of independent tests. Moreover, in view of the assumptions (1) and (4), $z_i = \phi(x_i)$, $i = 1, 2, \ldots, n$. In accordance with the general expression (8.5) for the likelihood function,

$$\begin{aligned} \ell(\vartheta \mid \underset{\sim}{\mathbf{z}}) &= \frac{1}{(2\pi)^{n/2} \sigma_Z^n} \exp\left[-\frac{1}{2\sigma_Z^2} \left(n\nu_2 - 2n\nu_1 \vartheta + n\vartheta^2 \right) \right] \\ &\sim \exp\left[-\frac{1}{2\sigma_Z^2} \left(\vartheta^2 - 2n\nu_1 \vartheta \right) \right], \end{aligned} \tag{8.20}$$

where $v_k = \left(z_1^k + z_2^k + \cdots + z_N^k\right)/n$ is the k-th statistical initial moment. With the help of the relation (8.20) we can write the prior p.d.f. conjugate with a likelihood kernel as

$$h(\vartheta) = h(\vartheta; \alpha_1, \alpha_2) \sim \exp\left[-\frac{1}{2\sigma_Z^2}\left(\alpha_2 v^2 - \alpha_1 \vartheta\right)\right], \tag{8.21}$$

which depends on two parameters. Using the relations (8.20) and (8.21) together with the Bayes theorem for the posterior p.d.f. $\hbar(\vartheta \mid \underset{\sim}{\mathbf{z}})$, we obtain

$$\hbar(\vartheta \mid \underset{\sim}{\mathbf{z}}) \sim \exp\left[-\frac{1}{2\sigma_Z^2}\left(\alpha_2' v^2 - \alpha_1' \vartheta\right)\right], \tag{8.22}$$

where $\alpha_1' = \alpha_1 - 2v_1 n$, $\alpha_2' = \alpha_2 + n$. If we have chosen the uncertainty interval $[\alpha_1, \alpha_2]$ and put $\alpha_1 = \alpha_2 = 0$, then the prior density (8.21) is transformed into the uniform one (8.18) associated with the posterior probability density

$$\hbar(\vartheta \mid \underset{\sim}{\mathbf{z}}) \sim \exp\left[-\frac{n}{2\sigma_Z^2}\left(v^2 - 2v_1\vartheta\right)\right], \quad \alpha_1 \leqslant \vartheta \leqslant \alpha_2 \tag{8.23}$$

Let us note that for practical calculations it is better to use (8.23) than (8.22), because we can address serious difficulties connected with the choice of the parameters α_1, α_2.
Define the Bayes prior estimate $\hat{\vartheta}^*$ as the posterior mean value. The resulting expression will be obtained after certain transformations and results in the form

$$\hat{\vartheta}^* = v_1 + \frac{1}{\sqrt{2\pi}} \cdot \frac{\sigma_Z}{\sqrt{n}} \cdot \frac{\mathrm{e}^{-u_1^2/2} - \mathrm{e}^{-u_2^2/2}}{\Phi(u_2) - \Phi(u_1)} \tag{8.24}$$

where $u_k = (\alpha_k - v_1)\sqrt{n}/\sigma_Z$, $k = 1, 2$.
Let us study the obtained estimate. At first, $\hat{\vartheta}^* \to v_1$ as $n \to \infty$, i.e., the Bayes estimate converges asymptotically to the maximum likelihood estimate. Consider the symmetric prior interval $[\vartheta_0 - u,\ \vartheta_0 + u]$, where ϑ_0 is a center point. In this case, $u_1 = (\vartheta_0 - u - v_1)\sqrt{n}/\sigma_Z$, $u_2 = (\vartheta_0 + u - v_1)$. If the sample mean v_1 is near to ϑ_0, i.e., the test results are well-consistent with the prior information, then $|u_1| \cong |u_2|$ and $\hat{\vartheta}^* \cong v_1$. Suppose now $u \to \infty$, that corresponds to the case of absence of a prior information about the parameter ϑ. Then, for any n, we have $|u_k| \to \infty$. Consequently, $\hat{\vartheta}^* \to v_1$, i.e., the Bayes estimate coincides with the asymptotic sample mean value.
To find the posterior variance of the parameter ϑ, we apply the expression for the posterior probability density (8.23) and write

$$\sigma_{\hat{\vartheta}^*}^2 = \int_\Theta \vartheta^2 \hbar(\vartheta \mid \underset{\sim}{\mathbf{z}})\, d\vartheta - \hat{\vartheta}^*.$$

After the necessary calculations we finally get

$$\sigma_{\hat{\vartheta}^*}^2 = \frac{1}{\sqrt{2\pi}} \cdot \frac{\sigma_Z}{\sqrt{n}} \cdot \frac{1}{\Phi(u_2) - \Phi(u_1)} \left\{ \sqrt{2\pi}\left(v_1^2 + \frac{\sigma_Z^2}{n}\right)[\Phi(u_2) - \Phi(u_1)] \right.$$
$$\left. + 2v_1 \frac{\sigma_Z}{\sqrt{n}}\left(\mathrm{e}^{-u_1^2/2} - \mathrm{e}^{-u_2^2/2}\right) + \frac{\sigma_Z^2}{n}\left(u_1 \mathrm{e}^{-u_1^2/2} - u_2 \mathrm{e}^{-u_2^2/2}\right) \right\}. \tag{8.25}$$

Note that as $n \longrightarrow \infty$, $\sigma_{\hat{\vartheta}^*} \longrightarrow 0$.

The approximate pointwise TTF estimate and posterior variance of this estimate may be found with the help of Kramer's theorem [132]

$$\hat{R}^* = \Phi\left(\frac{\hat{\vartheta}^*}{\sigma_Z}\right) + O\left(\frac{1}{n}\right), \qquad \sigma_{\hat{R}^*} = \frac{1}{2\pi\sigma_Z^2}\exp\left(-\frac{\hat{\vartheta}^{*2}}{\sigma_Z^2}\right)\sigma_{\hat{\vartheta}^*}^2 + O\left(\frac{1}{n^{3/2}}\right). \qquad (8.26)$$

For practical use of the dependencies (8.26) one should omit the terms $O(1/n)$ and $O(1/n^{3/2})$, which, generally speaking, may be done only for large n.

The TTF estimates can be found exactly if we use the general expressions (8.12)–(8.14). The resulting expressions for $\hat{R}^*$ and $\sigma_{\hat{R}^*}^2$ have the form

$$\hat{R}^* = \frac{U_1}{\Phi(u_2) - \Phi(u_1)} \text{ and } \sigma_{\hat{R}^*}^2 = \frac{U_2}{\Phi(u_2) - \Phi(u_1)} - \hat{R}^{*2}, \qquad (8.27)$$

where

$$U_k = \frac{1}{\sqrt{2\pi}}\int_{u_1}^{u_2} \Phi^k\left(\frac{u}{\sqrt{n}} + \frac{v_1}{\sigma_Z}\right) e^{-u^2/2}\, du.$$

The given scheme has an obvious shortcoming. The integrals U_k cannot be represented in a finite form and, therefore, we have to apply methods of numerical integration. Numerous calculations emphasize the coincidence of exact and approximate formulas for $n \geqslant 20$.

Consider now the problem of obtaining a Bayes lower confidence limit of the TTF. Principally this problem can be reduced to the solution of the equation (8.14) for the prior density having the form (8.23). In view of the monotonicity of the Laplace function, this problem may be solved in the following way. Let us find the Bayes lower confidence limit $\underline{\vartheta}_\gamma$ of the parameter ϑ. To do this, it is necessary to solve the equation

$$\int_{\underline{\vartheta}_\gamma}^{\alpha_2} \hbar(\vartheta \mid \underset{\sim}{\mathbf{z}})\, d\vartheta - \gamma = 0,$$

which may be rewritten in the resulting form in the following way:

$$\Phi(u_2)(1-\gamma) + \gamma\Phi(u_1) - \Phi\left(\frac{\underline{\vartheta}_\gamma}{\sigma_Z/\sqrt{n}}\right) = 0. \qquad (8.28)$$

Now the desired estimate may be obtained with the help of the simple formula

$$\underline{R}_\gamma^* = \Phi\left(\frac{\underline{\vartheta}_\gamma}{\sigma_Z}\right) \qquad (8.29)$$

8.3 General estimates of the reliability function for a one-dimensional model

8.3.1 *Formulation of the problem*

In this paragraph we will give a generalization of the previous result for the case when a priori information about the parameters m_Z and σ_Z is uncertain. In accordance with the notations used in this chapter, we let $\vartheta_1 = m_Z$, $\vartheta_2 = \sigma_Z$, and represent each parameter as a sum $\vartheta_k = \vartheta_{k0} + \varepsilon_k$, $k = 1, 2$, where ϑ_{k0} can be interpreted as a theoretical value of the parameter, which is assumed to be given in the Bayes procedure and ε_k represents the deviations from the theoretical value. Suppose that prior p.d.f.'s $h_1(\varepsilon_1)$ and $h_2(\varepsilon_2)$ are known. For the purposes of practical application of this procedure, it is useful to use uniform prior probability distributions:

$$h_k(\varepsilon_k) = \begin{cases} \dfrac{1}{\varepsilon_k'' - \varepsilon_k'}, & \varepsilon_k' \leqslant \varepsilon_k \leqslant \varepsilon_k'', \\ 0, & \varepsilon_k < \varepsilon_k', \ \varepsilon_k > \varepsilon''. \end{cases} \tag{8.30}$$

Now we can formulate the problem of obtaining Bayes estimates of TTF in the following way. The TTF is represented in the form of a function depending on the quantities ε_1 and ε_2, that is,

$$R = R(\varepsilon_1, \varepsilon_2) = \Phi\left(\frac{\vartheta_{10} + \varepsilon_1}{\vartheta_{20} + \varepsilon_2}\right). \tag{8.31}$$

We are given a priori information about the parameters ε_1, ε_2 in the form of a prior p.d.f., $h(\varepsilon_1, \varepsilon_2)$. Also, n tests have been carried out. During these tests we determine directly or indirectly the values of a status variable Z. These values generate a sample $\underset{\sim}{\mathbf{z}} = (z_1, z_2, \ldots, z_N)$. The problem is to Bud the Bayes estimates of TTF in the form of a pointwise estimate $\hat{R}^*$, posterior value of the standard deviation, $\sigma_{\hat{R}^*}$ and Bayes lower confidence limit $\underline{R}_\gamma^*$. For the solution of the problem we use a standard Bayes procedure.

Let us write the likelihood function $\ell(\varepsilon_1, \varepsilon_2 \mid \underset{\sim}{\mathbf{z}})$. In accordance with the chosen parameterization, a p.d.f. of the status variable has the form

$$f(z; \varepsilon_1, \varepsilon_2) = \frac{1}{\sqrt{2\pi}(\vartheta_{20} + \varepsilon_2)} \exp\left[-\frac{(z - \vartheta_{10} - \varepsilon_1)^2}{2(\vartheta_{20} + \varepsilon_2)^2}\right]. \tag{8.32}$$

Using the general expression (8.11) we obtain

$$\begin{aligned} \ell(\varepsilon_1, \varepsilon_2 \mid \underset{\sim}{\mathbf{z}}) &= \frac{1}{(2\pi)^{n/2}} \cdot \frac{1}{(\vartheta_{20} + \varepsilon_2)^n} \\ &\times \exp\left\{\frac{n}{2(\vartheta_{20} + \varepsilon_2)^2}\left[\nu_2 - 2\nu_1(\vartheta_{10} + \varepsilon_1) + (\vartheta_{10} + \varepsilon_1)^2\right]\right\}. \end{aligned} \tag{8.33}$$

The obtained estimate of the TTF is based on the prior p.d.f.'s $h_1(\varepsilon_1)$ and $h_2(\varepsilon_2)$ of the form (8.30), i.e., we will assume that the set $E = [\varepsilon_1', \varepsilon_1''] \times [\varepsilon_2', \varepsilon_2'']$ appears to be the unknown domain of the parameters ε_1 and ε_2. In accordance with the Bayes theorem, for the posterior probability density of the parameters ε_1 and ε_2 the following relation holds:

$$\hbar(\varepsilon_1, \varepsilon_2 \mid \underset{\sim}{\mathbf{z}}) \sim \frac{1}{(\vartheta_{20} + \varepsilon_2)^n} \exp\left\{\frac{\nu_2 - 2\nu_1(\vartheta_{10} + \varepsilon_1) + (\vartheta_{10} + \varepsilon_1)^2}{2(\vartheta_{20} + \varepsilon_2)^2/n}\right\}$$

$$(\varepsilon_1, \varepsilon_2) \in E. \tag{8.34}$$

We will distinguish the simplified and main schemes of the solution of the problem. The choice of the scheme is connected with the type of loss function, used in the Bayes procedure. In accordance with the simplified scheme, the loss function is chosen with respect to each parameter separately. The complexity of the scheme depends on the choice of the loss function for TTF, $R(\varepsilon_1, \varepsilon_2)$.

8.3.2 *The simplified scheme of the solution*

This scheme starts with the finding of the parameters ε_1 and ε_2 which are used for obtaining TTF estimates. We will carry out the estimation of each parameter by minimization of the posterior risk function for the mean square error, i.e.

$$\hat{\varepsilon}_j^* = \arg\min_{\hat{\varepsilon}_j} \int_{\varepsilon_j'}^{\varepsilon_j''} (\varepsilon_j - \hat{\varepsilon}_j)^2 \hbar_j(\varepsilon_j \mid \underset{\sim}{\mathbf{z}})\, d\varepsilon_j, \quad j = 1, 2, \tag{8.35}$$

where the marginal posterior densities are obtained in the usual manner:

$$\hbar_1(\varepsilon_1 \mid \underset{\sim}{\mathbf{z}}) \sim \int_{\varepsilon_2'}^{\varepsilon_2''} \hbar(\varepsilon_1, \varepsilon_2)^2 \hbar(\varepsilon_1, \varepsilon_2 \mid \underset{\sim}{\mathbf{z}})\, d\varepsilon_2, \quad \varepsilon_1' \leqslant \varepsilon_1 \leqslant \varepsilon_1'' \tag{8.36}$$

and

$$\hbar_2(\varepsilon_2 \mid \underset{\sim}{\mathbf{z}}) \sim \int_{\varepsilon_1'}^{\varepsilon_1''} \hbar(\varepsilon_1, \varepsilon_2)^2 \hbar(\varepsilon_1, \varepsilon_2 \mid \underset{\sim}{\mathbf{z}})\, d\varepsilon_1, \quad \varepsilon_2' \leqslant \varepsilon_2 \leqslant \varepsilon_2''. \tag{8.37}$$

The solution of the problem (8.35) is known [202]:

$$\hat{\varepsilon}_j^* = \int_{\varepsilon_j'}^{\varepsilon_j''} \varepsilon_j \hbar(\varepsilon_j \mid \underset{\sim}{\mathbf{z}})\, d\varepsilon_j, \quad j = 1, 2. \tag{8.38}$$

The complicated form of the relation (8.34) doesn't allow us to hope that the final results will have a simple form. The reason is that the kernel of the posterior probability density $\hbar(\varepsilon_1, \varepsilon_2 \mid \underset{\sim}{\mathbf{z}})$, determined by the right-hand part of the relation (8.34), cannot be integrated in the final form with respect to any of the parameters. Use of the Laplace function $\Phi(u)$ lets us reduce the resulting expressions for the estimates to the one-dimensional integrals and represent them in the form

$$\begin{aligned}\hat{\varepsilon}_1^* = &\frac{1}{\beta} \int_{\vartheta_2'}^{\vartheta_2''} \frac{1}{y^{n-1}} \exp\left[-\frac{n(v_2 - v_1^2)}{2y^2}\right] \Bigl\{ [\Phi(u_2(y)) - \Phi(u_1(y))] \\ &\times (v_1 - \vartheta_{10}) + \frac{y}{\sqrt{2\pi n}} \left[\exp\left(-\frac{u_1^2(y)}{2}\right) - \exp\left(-\frac{u_2^2(y)}{2}\right)\right]\Bigr\} dy, \end{aligned} \tag{8.39}$$

and

$$\hat{\varepsilon}_2^* = \frac{1}{\beta} \int_{\vartheta_2'}^{\vartheta_2''} \frac{y - \vartheta_{20}}{y^{n-1}} \exp\left[-\frac{n(v_2 - v_1^2)}{2y^2}\right] [\Phi(u_2(y)) - \Phi(u_1(y))]\, dy \tag{8.40}$$

where

$$\beta = \int_{\vartheta_2'}^{\vartheta_2''} \frac{1}{y^{n-1}} \exp\left[-\frac{n\left(v_2 - v_1^2\right)}{2y^2}\right] \left[\Phi(u_2(y)) - \Phi(u_1(y))\right] dy,$$

$$\vartheta_2' = \vartheta_{20} + \varepsilon_2', \quad \vartheta_2'' = \vartheta_{20} + \varepsilon_2''$$

$$u_1(y) = \frac{\sqrt{n}}{y}\left(\vartheta_{10} + \varepsilon_1' + v_1\right) \text{ and } u_2(y) = \frac{\sqrt{n}}{y}\left(\vartheta_{10} + \varepsilon_1'' + v_1\right) \tag{8.41}$$

Analyzing the expression (8.39), we see that for $v_1 = \vartheta_{10}$ the Bayes estimate $\hat{\varepsilon}_1^*$ equals zero. This fact has a logical explanation. If a sample mean value v_1 coincides with the predicted theoretical value of the mean m_Z (the center of the interval of a prior information), then the value, whose role ε_1 plays, must equal zero.

Define now the posterior variances $\sigma^2_{\hat{\varepsilon}_1^*}$ and $\sigma^2_{\hat{\varepsilon}_2^*}$ of the parameters ε_1 and ε_2, respectively. Let us use the general expression

$$\sigma^2_{\hat{\varepsilon}_j^*} = \int\int_E \varepsilon_j^* \hbar(\varepsilon_1, \varepsilon_2 \mid \underset{\sim}{\mathbf{z}}) = d\varepsilon_1 d\varepsilon_2 - \hat{\sigma}_j^{*2}, \quad j = 1, 2.$$

The resulting expressions for the variances also may be written with the help of one-dimensional integrals, having the following complicated forms:

$$\begin{aligned}
\sigma^2_{\hat{\varepsilon}_1^2} = & \frac{1}{\beta} \int_{\vartheta_2'}^{\vartheta_2''} \frac{1}{y^{n-1}} \exp\left[-\frac{n\left(v_2 - v_1^2\right)}{2y^2}\right] \left\{\left[(v_1 - \vartheta_{10})^2 + \frac{y^2}{n}\right]\right. \\
& \times \left[\Phi(u_2(y)) - \Phi(u_1(y))\right] + \frac{\sqrt{2}y}{\sqrt{\pi n}} (v_1 - \vartheta_{10}) \left[\exp\left(-\frac{u_1^2(y)}{2}\right) - \exp\left(-\frac{u_2^2(y)}{2}\right)\right] \\
& \left. + \left[u_1(y) \exp\left(-\frac{u_1^2(y)}{2}\right) - u_2(y) \exp\left(-\frac{u_2^2(y)}{2}\right)\right]\right\} dy - \hat{\varepsilon}_1^{*2},
\end{aligned} \tag{8.42}$$

and

$$\sigma^2_{\hat{\varepsilon}_2^*} = \frac{1}{\beta} \int_{\vartheta_2'}^{\vartheta_2''} \frac{(y - \vartheta_{20})^2}{y^{n-1}} \times \exp\left[-\frac{n\left(v_2 - v_1^2\right)}{2y^2}\right] \left[\Phi(u_2(y)) - \Phi(u_1(y))\right] dy - \hat{\varepsilon}_2^{*2}. \tag{8.43}$$

The final goal of this procedure is obtaining the pointwise Bayes TTF estimate and posterior TTF variance $\sigma^2_{\hat{R}^*}$. To this end, we apply Kramer's theorem for the function of statistical estimates. In conformity to this case, Kramer's theorem has the form

$$\hat{R}^* = \Phi\left(\frac{\vartheta_{10} + \hat{\varepsilon}_1^*}{\vartheta_{20} + \hat{\varepsilon}_2^*}\right) + O\left(\frac{1}{n}\right) \tag{8.44}$$

and

$$\sigma^2_{\hat{R}^*} = \frac{1}{2\pi\left(\vartheta_{20} + \hat{\varepsilon}_2^*\right)} \exp\left[-\left(\frac{\vartheta_{10} + \hat{\varepsilon}_1^*}{\vartheta_{20} + \hat{\varepsilon}_2^*}\right)^2\right] \tag{8.45}$$

$$\left\{\sigma^2_{\hat{\varepsilon}_1^*} + \left(\frac{\vartheta_{10} + \hat{\varepsilon}_1^*}{\vartheta_{20} + \hat{\varepsilon}_2^*}\right) \sigma^2_{\hat{\varepsilon}_2^*} - 2\frac{\vartheta_{10} + \hat{\varepsilon}_1^*}{\left(\vartheta_{20} + \hat{\varepsilon}_2^*\right)^2} K_{\varepsilon_1 \varepsilon_2}\right\} + O\left(\frac{1}{n^{3/2}}\right), \tag{8.46}$$

where $K_{\varepsilon_1\varepsilon_2}$ is the posterior correlation between the random variables ε_1 and ε_2. The numerical characteristic is defined by the integral

$$K_{\varepsilon_1\varepsilon_2} \int\int_E \varepsilon_1\varepsilon_2 \hbar(\varepsilon_1,\varepsilon_2 \mid \underset{\sim}{\mathbf{z}})d\varepsilon_1 d\varepsilon_2 - \hat{\varepsilon}_1^*\hat{\varepsilon}_2^*.$$

Finally

$$K_{\varepsilon_1\varepsilon_2} = \frac{1}{\beta}\int_{\vartheta_2'}^{v_2''} \frac{y-\vartheta_{20}}{y^{n-1}} \exp\left[-\frac{n(v_2-v_1^2)}{2y^2}\right]\left\{[\Phi(u_2(y)) - \Phi(u_1(y))]\right.$$
$$\left.\times(v_1-\vartheta_{10}) + \frac{y}{\sqrt{2\pi n}}\left[\exp\left(-\frac{u_1^2(y)}{2}\right) - \exp\left(-\frac{u_1^2(y)}{2}\right)\right]\right\}dy. \tag{8.47}$$

Therefore, defining the estimates $\hat{R}^*$ and $\sigma_{\hat{R}^*}^2$ requires evaluating six one-dimensional integrals (8.39)–(8.43) and (8.46) by numerical methods. The value of the lower Bayes confidence limit can be found approximately, with the help of approximation of the posterior probability distribution of the TTF by a beta-distribution $Be(a,b)$ with the parameters

$$a = \hat{R}^*\left[\frac{\hat{R}^*(1-\hat{R}^*)}{\sigma_{\hat{R}^*}^2} - 1\right] \quad \text{and} \quad b = (1-\hat{R}^*)\left[\frac{\hat{R}^*(1-\hat{R}^*)}{\sigma_{\hat{R}^*}^2} - 1\right].$$

Later we will need to either solve the transcendental equation

$$\int_0^{\underline{R}_\gamma^*} x^{a-1}(1-x)^{b-1}dx = (1-\gamma)B(a,b),$$

or use the finite expression

$$\underline{R}_\gamma^* = \left(1 + \frac{b}{a}F_{1-\gamma};2b;2a\right)^{-1}.$$

where $F_{\alpha;\delta_1;\delta_2}$ is the α-th percentile of the F-distribution with δ_1 and δ_2 degrees of freedom. Note that the calculation procedure described above doesn't give us any difficulties since the numerical methods of one-dimensional integration and the solution of transcendental equations are well-developed for computer implementations.

8.3.3 *The main calculation scheme*

This scheme deals with the mean square error loss function $L(\hat{R},R) = \left[R(\varepsilon_1,\varepsilon_2) - \hat{R}\right]^2$ and gives the Bayes TTF estimate of the form

$$\hat{R}^* = \int\int_E R(\varepsilon_1,\varepsilon_2)\hbar(\varepsilon_1,\varepsilon_2 \mid \underset{\sim}{\mathbf{z}})d\varepsilon_1 d\varepsilon_2.$$

The handiest numerical representation of this integral has the form

$$\hat{R}^* = \frac{1}{\beta}\sqrt{\frac{n}{2\pi}}\int_{\vartheta_1'}^{\vartheta_1''}\int_{\vartheta_2'}^{\vartheta_2''} \Phi\left(\frac{x}{y}\right)\frac{1}{y^n}\exp\left(-\frac{v_2-2v_1x+x^2}{2y^2/n}\right)dx\,dy, \tag{8.48}$$

where $\vartheta_k' = \vartheta_{k0} + \varepsilon_k'$, $\vartheta_k'' = \vartheta_{k0} + \varepsilon_k''$, $k = 1, 2$. The posterior variance is determined by a similar integral

$$\sigma_{\hat{R}^*}^2 = \frac{1}{\beta}\sqrt{\frac{n}{2\pi}} \int_{\vartheta_1'}^{\vartheta_1''} \int_{\vartheta_2'}^{\vartheta_2''} \Phi^2\left(\frac{x}{y}\right) \frac{1}{y^n} \exp\left(-\frac{v_2 - 2v_1 x + x^2}{2y^2/n}\right) .dx\,dy - \hat{R}^{*2} \tag{8.49}$$

As seen from the expressions (8.47) and (8.48), for obtaining the Bayes estimates we, unfortunately, cannot avoid the double numerical integration. Only the fact that the integration intervals $[\vartheta_1', \vartheta_1'']$, $[\vartheta_2', \vartheta_2'']$ are small and the integrand on these intervals is sufficiently smooth is encouraging. Because of these properties we can use the simplest methods of numerical integration of the rectangular lattice. In the case of a large interval, we need to apply more complicated approximating formulas.

Evaluating the lower Bayes confidence limit, we run into serious calculation difficulties. To find $\underline{R}_\gamma^*$ we need to solve the following equation

$$\int_\Omega \int_{(\underline{R}_\gamma^*)} \hbar(\varepsilon_1, \varepsilon_2 \mid z) d\varepsilon_1\, d\varepsilon_2 - \gamma = 0, \tag{8.50}$$

where the integration domain $\Omega(\underline{R}_\gamma^*)$ is an intersection of the set $E = [\varepsilon_1', \varepsilon_2''] \times [\varepsilon_2', \varepsilon_2'']$ with the set of the parameters ε_1 and ε_2 for which the in-equality $R(\varepsilon_1, \varepsilon_2) \geqslant \underline{R}_\gamma^*$ holds, i.e., $\underline{R}_\gamma^*$ lies in the integration domain. With the help of the new variables $x = \vartheta_{10} + \varepsilon_1$ and $\hat{y} = \vartheta_{20} + \varepsilon_2$, (8.49) is given by

$$\iint\limits_{\Omega(\underline{R}_\gamma^*)} \frac{1}{y^n} \exp\left(-\frac{v_2 - 2v_1 x + x^2}{2y^2/n}\right) dx\,dy - \gamma\beta = 0. \tag{8.51}$$

The idea of solving the equation (8.50) based on using one of the standard numerical methods of solution of the equation $F(u) = 0$, where, for each value u, evaluation of the integral is carried out not over the whole rectangular $[\vartheta_1', \vartheta_1''] \times [\vartheta_2', \vartheta_2'']$ but over such a part of it that ensures the fulfilment of the condition $\Phi(x/y) \geqslant u$. Taking into account the monotonicity of the Laplace function, we resort to the following simplification. Instead of equation (8.50), we will solve the equation with respect to the quantile of a normal distribution, $v = \Phi^{-1}(\underline{R}_\gamma^*)$, which corresponds to the unknown probability $\underline{R}_\gamma^*$. Since the inequality $\Phi(x/y) \geqslant \Phi(v)$ implies the fulfillment of the inequality $x/y \geqslant v$, the equation (8.50) is equivalent to the following one:

$$\iint\limits_{\Omega(\underline{R}_\gamma^*)} \frac{1}{y^n} \exp\left(-\frac{v_2 - 2v_1 x + x^2}{2y^2/n}\right) dx\,dy - \gamma\beta = 0 \tag{8.52}$$

in which the integration domain $\Omega(v)$ represents by itself the intersection of the rectangular $[\vartheta_1', \vartheta_1''] \times [\vartheta_2', \vartheta_2'']$ with the domain of values of x and y satisfying the inequality $x \geqslant vy$

(see Fig. 8.1). Thereafter, we can rewrite the equation (8.51) in the formal form $F(v) = 0$ and solve it by one of the standard methods. In this approach, we should take into account the fact that the unknown value v lies in the interval $[\vartheta_1'/\vartheta_2'', \vartheta_1''/\vartheta_2']$. This fact is easy to verify (see Fig. 8.1). After the equation (8.51) has been solved, the desired estimate of $\underline{R}_\gamma^*$ may be obtained from the formula $\underline{R}_\gamma^* = \Phi(v)$.

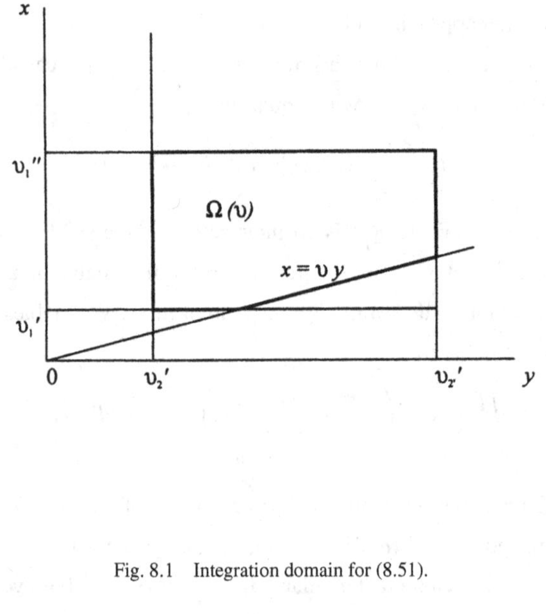

Fig. 8.1 Integration domain for (8.51).

8.4 Examples of calculation of the reliability estimates

In this section we give examples illustrating the particulars of estimating Bayes procedures of the TTF with undefined initial data.

8.4.1 *Calculation of TTF estimates of a carrier construction*

Consider the construction of a bar depicted in Fig. 8.2. We have chosen this construction because its working capacity model has a simple form and is, apparently, error free. Both bars have an angle profile and are made of steel. The relation of the acting forces is such that the first bar is expanded and the second one is contracted. The set of lifetime conditions includes [23]:

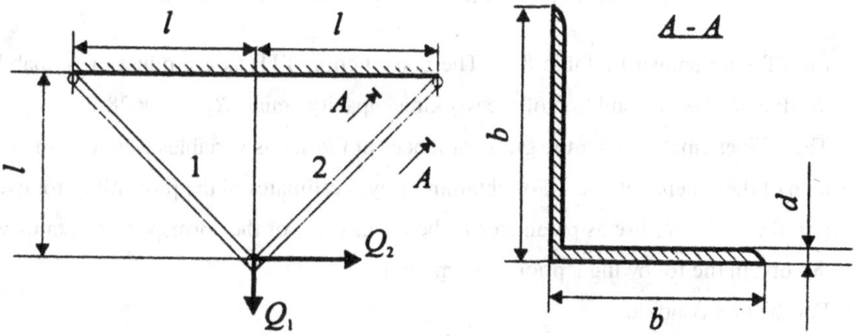

Fig. 8.2 An element of the construction under the static load.

The condition of durability of bar 1:

$$Z_1 = \phi_1(\sigma_T, F_1, Q_1, Q_2) = \sigma_T F_1 - \frac{Q_1 + Q_2}{\sqrt{2}} > 0; \tag{8.53}$$

the condition of global stability of bar 2:

$$Z_2 = \phi_2(\ell, E_2, J_2, Q_1, Q_2) = \frac{\pi^2 E_2 J_2}{\ell^2} - \frac{Q_2 - Q_1}{\sqrt{2}} > 0; \tag{8.54}$$

The condition of local stability of bar 2:

$$Z_3 = \phi_3(E_2, \mu_2, d_2, b_2, F_2, Q_1, Q_2) = \frac{3,6 \cdot E_2, F_2}{12 \cdot (1 - \mu_2^2)} \left(\frac{d_2}{b_2}\right)^2 - \frac{Q_2 - Q_1}{\sqrt{2}} > 0. \tag{8.55}$$

The inequalities (8.52)–(8.54) are used as follows: F represents the cross section area of the bar, J is the moment of inertia of the cross section, μ is the Poisson coefficient, E is the elasticity module; σ_T is the fluidity limit of the material, indices 1 and 2, correspond to the bar numbers. The calculation of the project (prior) value of the TTF has been carried out with the help of (8.15), where the numerical characteristics m_Z and σ_Z were obtained in accordance with the expressions (8.16) and (8.17). The initial data used for the evaluation of the construction reliability are given in Table 8.1. The arguments of the working capacity functions and status variables are assumed to be independent. The calculation results

Table 8.1 Results of evaluation for project TTF estimate.

Number of working conditions	$m_{z_j}\mathbf{H}$	$m_{z_j}\mathbf{H}$	R_j
1	$1.64\cdot 10^5$	$0.536\cdot 10^5$	0.999
2	$0.828\cdot 10^5$	$0.451\cdot 10^5$	0.9641
3	$2.48\cdot 10^5$	$0.738\cdot 10^5$	0.9997

for TTF are shown in Table 8.2. The construction TTF as a product of probabilities of fulfilment of each condition of the working capacity equals $R_c = 0.9628$

The TTF estimates under the given variances of the status variables were obtained with the help of the scheme of § 8.2. For obtaining Bayes estimates of the probability for every condition to hold, we use as parameter ϑ the mean value of the corresponding status variable. We obtain the following a priori information:

For the first condition:

$$\vartheta \in \left[1.58\cdot 10^5 H,\ 1.68\cdot 10^5 H\right],\ \sigma_Z = 0.536\cdot 10^5 H;$$

For the second condition:

$$\vartheta \in \left[0.880\cdot 10^5 H,\ 0.885\cdot 10^5 H\right],\ \sigma_Z = 0.451\cdot 10^5 H;$$

For the third condition:

$$\vartheta \in \left[2.35\cdot 10^5 H,\ 2.61\cdot 10^5 H\right],\ \sigma_Z = 0.738\cdot 10^5 H.$$

The values of the parameters of the working capacity function have been measured during the 12 independent tests. After this, we have obtained the statistic v_1. In Table 8.3 we present the experimental results in the form of the sufficient statistic v_1 with respect to each status variable. We have performed two calculations. The first one uses the method based on the formulas (8.24)–(8.26). The calculation results are presented in Table 8.3. The estimates of the lower Bayes confidence limits for the probability for each of the working capacity conditions to hold have been obtained with the help of approximation of the posterior p.d.f.'s by beta-distributions. The second calculation variant corresponds to the exact integral expressions (8.27)–(8.29). Numerical integration and solution of the transcendental equation (8.28) have been performed with the subroutines QUANC8 and ZEROIN [86]. The results of the calculations are presented in Table 8.4. It follows from the comparison of the data from Table 8.3 with those from Table 8.4, that the method of approximating and exact estimating gives us practically the same results. The calculation of a lower confidence limit of the construction of TTF has been performed with the help of the approach proposed in [247]. For the result, the estimate $\underline{R}^*_{0.9}$ was obtained.

Table 8.2 Bayes TTF estimates with known variance (approximate method).

Number of working conditions j	Statistics values v_1, H	$\hat{R}_j^*$	$\sigma_{\hat{R}_j^*}$	$\underline{\hat{R}}_{09j}^*$
1	$1.42 \cdot 10^5$	0.9987	0.000519	0.9984
2	$0.852 \cdot 10^5$	0.9668	0.002590	0.9633
3	$2.07 \cdot 10^5$	0.9995	0.000152	0.9993

Table 8.3 Bayes TTF estimates with known variance (exact method).

Number of working conditions j	Statistics values v_1, H	$\hat{R}_j^*$	$\sigma_{\hat{R}_j^*}$	$\underline{\hat{R}}_{09j}^*$
1	$1.42 \cdot 10^5$	0.9988	0.000592	0.9984
2	$0.852 \cdot 10^5$	0.9667	0.002540	0.9631
3	$2.07 \cdot 10^5$	0.9994	0.001460	0.9992

Table 8.4 A priori information for TTF evaluation.

Number of working conditions	v_{10}, H	$e_1' = -e_1$, H	v_{20}, H	$e_2' = -e_2$, H
1	$1.64 \cdot 10^5$	$1.3 \cdot 10^4$	$0.536 \cdot 10^5$	$1.5 \cdot 10^4$
2	$0.828 \cdot 10^5$	$2.7 \cdot 10^4$	$0.451 \cdot 10^5$	$4.2 \cdot 10^4$
3	$2.48 \cdot 10^5$	$1.3 \cdot 10^4$	$0.738 \cdot 10^5$	$2.5 \cdot 10^4$

The estimates of TTF, when the variance of a status variable is unknown, have been obtained with the help of the method discussed in § 8.3 in accordance with the simplified and main schemes. A priori information used in the calculations is given in Table 8.5. Experimental data in the form of statistics v_1 and v_2 are presented in Table 8.6. The results of the calculations are based on the simplified scheme which operates with the expressions (8.39)–(8.46) and are given in Table 8.6. The estimates of TTF, according to the main scheme, are given in Table 8.7. For evaluating the double integral, we performed the repeated calls of the subroutine QUANC8, mentioned above. As in the previous case, we observed a satisfactory coincidence of the results of the approximate and exact estimates. The value of the Bayes lower confidence limit for the subject construction was $\underline{R}_{0.9}^*$.
The numerical data demonstrate the evolution of the reliability estimate after the testing has been performed.

Table 8.5 Bayes TTF estimates with unknown variance of the status variable (simplified scheme).

Number of working conditions	v_1, H	$(v_2 - v_1^2)^{1/2}$, H	$\hat{R}_j^*$	$\sigma_{\hat{R}_j^*}$	$\underline{\hat{R}}_{09j}^*$
1	$1.023 \cdot 10^5$	$0.583 \cdot 10^5$	0.9970	0.000534	0.9964
2	$0.852 \cdot 10^5$	$0.458 \cdot 10^5$	0.9721	0.007200	0.9703
3	$2.07 \cdot 10^5$	$1.204 \cdot 10^5$	0.9996	0.000163	0.9992

Table 8.6 Bayes TTF estimates with unknown variance of the status variable (basic scheme).

Number of working conditions	$\hat{R}_j^*$	$\sigma_{\hat{R}_j^*}$	$\underline{\hat{R}}_{09j}^*$
1	0.9980	0.000495	0.9974
2	0.9708	0.006800	0.9605
3	0.9995	0.000179	0.9993

8.4.2 *Calculated case "loading—carrying capability" with unknown correlation coefficient*

Below we present the results of the work [98] devoted to the investigation of the TTF for the technical device with a working capacity model of the form "loading carrying capability". Customarily in many practical situations when estimating the device reliability, we do not have complete information about the correlation coefficient. At the same time, the correlation coefficient influences the TTF value.

Setting of the problem

Consider an element of construction with the carrying capability U and acting load S which obeys the Gaussian distribution with unknown correlation coefficient ρ. As TTF is used the following probability:

$$R = P\{U > S\}. \tag{8.56}$$

It is assumed that marginal numerical characteristics of the variables U and S are given. It enables us to represent the probability (8.55) in the form of a function depending on the correlation coefficient:

$$R = R(\rho) = \Phi\left(\frac{\eta - 1}{\sqrt{v_U^2 \eta_2 + v_S^2 - 2\rho v_U v_S \eta}}\right), \tag{8.57}$$

where v_U and v_S are the variation coefficients of the carrying capability and loading, respectively, with $\eta = m_U/m_S$ being the coefficient margin of safety.
We will assume that we are given an interval of a prior uncertainty $[a,b]$ such that $\rho \in [a,b]$. Often in practice it is possible to establish that if the correlation coefficient appears to be either positive or negative, then we may put correspondingly $\rho \in [0,1]$ and $\rho \in [-1,0]$. If it is known that there exists a weak stochastic dependence between U and S, we may suppose that $\rho \in [-0.5,0.5]$. Let us choose a uniform p.d.f. $h(\rho)$ on $[a,b]$.
The problem is to obtain the Bayes estimate R^* for the probability (8.56) with the given prior probability density $h(\rho)$, defined on $[a,b]$.

Bayes TTF estimates

Following the general scheme of Bayes estimating, the pointwise prior TTF estimate may be written in the form

$$R^* = \frac{1}{b-a}\int_a^b R(\rho)d\rho. \tag{8.58}$$

Here we can obtain the resulting formula in the analytical form

$$R^* = \frac{(\eta-1)^2}{(b-a)\eta v_U v_S}(F(v) - F(w)), \tag{8.59}$$

where

$$v = \frac{\eta - 1}{\left(v_U^2\eta^2 + v_S^2 - a v_U v_S \eta\right)^{1/2}}, \qquad w = \frac{\eta - 1}{\left(v_U^2\eta^2 + v_S^2 - 2b v_U v_S \eta\right)^{1/2}},$$

and

$$F(x) = \frac{1}{2x^2}\Phi(x) + \frac{1}{2x}K(x) - \frac{1}{2}(1 - \Phi(x)),$$

with

$$K(x) = \frac{1}{\sqrt{2\pi}} e^{x^2/2}.$$

The posterior TTF estimate R* for the uniform prior distribution law is written as

$$\hat{R}^* = \frac{1}{\beta}\int_a^b \frac{R(\rho)}{(1-\rho^2)^{n/2}} \exp\left\{-\frac{1}{2(1-\rho^2)}\left[\frac{\omega_U^2}{\sigma_U^2} - 2\rho\frac{\omega_{US}}{\sigma_U\sigma_S} + \frac{\omega_S^2}{\sigma_S^2}\right]\right\} dp, \tag{8.60}$$

where β is a constant coefficient having the form

$$\beta = \int_a^b \frac{1}{(1-x^2)^{n/2}} \exp\left\{-\frac{1}{2(1-x^2)}\left[\frac{\omega_U^2}{\sigma_U^2} - 2x\frac{\omega_{US}}{\sigma_U\sigma_S} + \frac{\omega_S^2}{\sigma_S^2}\right]\right\} dx.$$

The probability $R(\rho)$ is defined by the formula (8.56), and sufficient statistics ω_U^2, ω_S^2 and ω_{US} by the following expressions:

$$\omega_U^2 = \sum_{i=1}^{n} (u_i - m_U)^2, \quad \omega_S^2 = \sum_{i=1}^{n} (s_i - m_S)^2,$$

and

$$\omega_{US} = (u_i - m_U)(s_i - m_S),$$

where (u_i, s_i) is the set of pairs of experimental values of U and S.

In contrast to the analytical procedure of evaluating a prior TTF estimate (8.58), the posterior estimate (8.59) may be found approximately with the help of the methods of numerical integration.

Comparative analysis of different estimates

In practice for obtaining a prior TTF estimate, one often uses the following formulas:

$$R_0 = \Phi\left(\frac{\eta - 1}{\sqrt{v_U^2 \eta^2 + v_S^2}}\right), \tag{8.61}$$

and

$$R_{cK} = \Phi\left(\frac{\eta - 1}{\sqrt{v_U^2 \eta^2 + v_S^2 - 2\rho_{cK} v_U v_S \eta}}\right). \tag{8.62}$$

For obtaining the estimate R_0, we put $\rho = 0$; the estimate R_{cK} have been obtained under the assumption that the correlation coefficient equals the midpoint of the segment of prior uncertainty: $\rho = \rho_{cK} = (a+b)/2$. In [98] a numerical comparison of the estimates R_0 and R_{cK} with a prior Bayes estimate of TTF R^* of the form (8.58) has been carried out. The calculations have been performed for $v_U = v_S = 0.1$, different coefficients of a margin of safety $\eta = 1.1,\ 1.2,\ 1.3,\ 1.4$ and different lengths of uncertainty coefficients $J = b - a = 0, 0.2, 0.4, \ldots, 1.8, 2.0$.

In Fig. 8.3, it is shown that the dependence of the relative difference of a prior Bayes estimate on the TTF estimate with zero correlation $(R^* - R_0/R_0)$ for the uncertainty segment $[-a, a]$, when R_0 and R_{cK} coincide. By increasing the coefficient of a margin of safety η, this relative quantity decreases substantially. For example, for the maximal interval of uncertainty ($J = 2$) $(R^* - R_0)/R_0$ it reaches $\approx 4.3\%$, for the uncertainty interval having the length which is half smaller ($j = 1$) is 0.7%. We note also one additional important

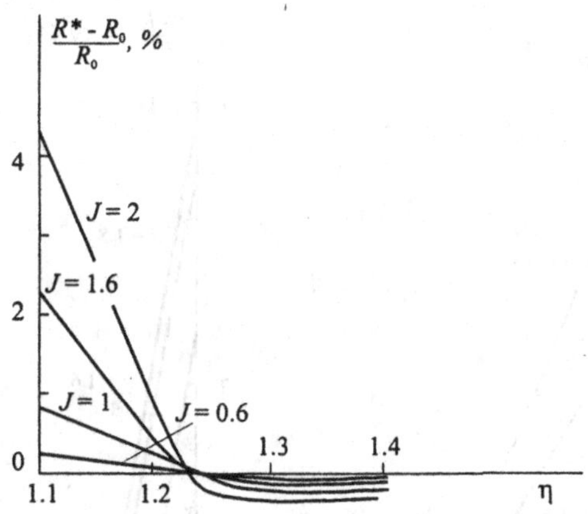

Fig. 8.3 The Relative Difference Between R^* and $R_0 = R_{cK}$. With Symmetric Interval of Uncertainty.

property: if $\eta < 1.25$, then for all J the Bayes estimate R^* is always greater than R_0, and if $\eta < 1.25$, then $R^* < R_0$.

In Fig. 8.4 we represent the patterns of change of relative difference for all three TTF estimates for the asymmetric interval of uncertainty when the upper limit of the segment is fixed ($b = 1$). As seen from the graphs, the roughest TTF estimate is R_0, which can be used only for large margin of safety ($\eta > 1.4$). The estimate R_{cK} approaches near to R^*, beginning already with $\eta = 1.3$.

The posterior Bayes estimates have been illustrated with the help of the numerical example in [98]. As initial data, the following values of dimensionless coefficients were chosen: $v_U = v_S = 0.1$, $\eta = 1.3$, and $\rho \in [-0.8, 0.8]$. In this case, the Bayes prior estimate of TTF equals $R^* = 0.906214$.

If one defines the posterior estimate (8.59), it is desirable to choose the following statistics: $\varepsilon_U^2 = \omega_U^2/\sigma_U^2$, $\varepsilon_S^2 = \omega_S^2/\sigma_S^2$, and $\varepsilon_{US} = \omega_{US}/\sigma_S$.The calculations have been done for the following hypothetical testing results. Ten tests have been carried out. During these tests we have measured the values U and S. Moreover, the test results are such that the corresponding marginal statistics $\varepsilon_U^2 = 9.5$ and $\varepsilon_S^2 = 10.2$. Three cases have been considered: $\varepsilon_{US}^{+} = 5$ (positive correlation), $\varepsilon_{US}^{(0)} = 0$ (absence of correlation), $\varepsilon_{US}^{(-)} = -5$ (negative correlation). For these cases, in Fig. 8.5 the posterior densities $\hbar_+(\rho)$, $\hbar_0(\rho)$ and $\hbar_-(\rho)$ have

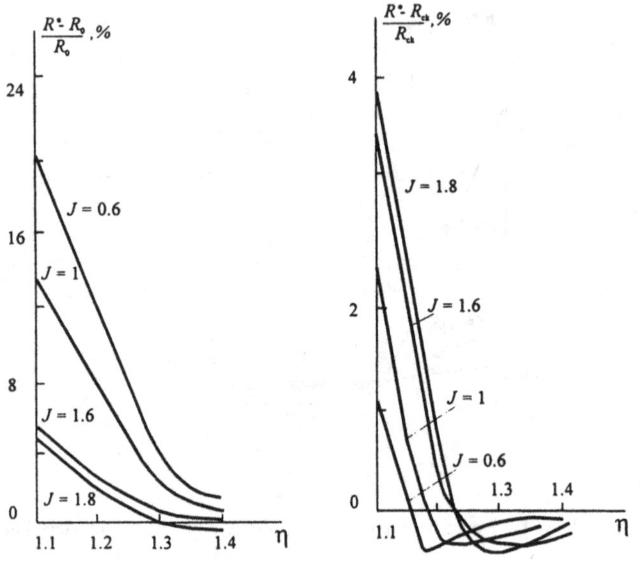

Fig. 8.4 The Relative Difference Between R^* and R_0; (a) and in Addition Between R^* and R_{cK}; (b) with Asymmetric Interval of Uncertainty.

been constructed. As seen from Fig. 8.5, for the positive correlation the density biases to the right, for $\varepsilon_{US}^{(-)}$ vice-versa, to the left. Corresponding posterior Bayes TTF estimates equal $\hat{R}_+^* = 0.902966$, $\hat{R}_0^* = 0.90016$ and $\hat{R}_-^* = 0.89694$.

The result given above lets us more correctly (in comparison to the existing approaches) establish the prior Bayes estimate of the TTF probability under the conditions of uncertainty with respect to the correlation between the loading and carrying capability, and correct this estimate by the testing results

8.5 The statistical design optimization based on the Bayes approach

The settings of the solutions of the problems of probability optimal projection are well-known [112, 120, 173, 193]. The distinctive characteristic of the proposed problem setting is that the optimization process deals not only with the project reliability estimates, but also with the results of the consequent experiments. Project contents itself is in favor of such an

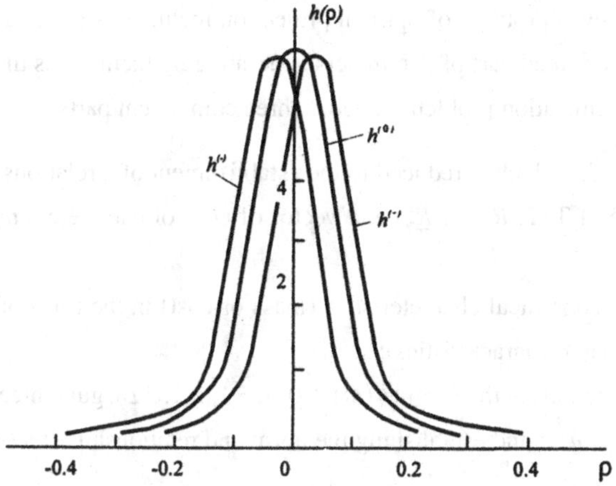

Fig. 8.5 Posterior p.d.f.'s for different correlation coefficients.

approach. Project parameters are chosen with the help of existing working capacity models of the type (8.1), engineering experience and a priori statistical information about the loadings, physical-mechanical characteristics and geometrical parameters. Thereafter, one carries out an experiment which confirms the principal working capacity of the device, the reliability estimates are defined more exactly, and innovations are put into the project to satisfy reliability requirements. The union of a project (prior) and experimental information is among the most important elements of this chain of measures. To this end, we recommend using the Bayes approach. Below we give one of the possible ways of the Bayes statistical optimization.

8.5.1 *Formulation of the problem*

Suppose the device structure is defined and the problem is to choose the values of controlled parameters generating a vector ω which ensures the extreme value of some parameter of quality. It is usual that the nominal values (or mean values) and dispersions (or mean-squared values) of some geometrical parameters play the role of controlled parameters. For the sake of simplicity throughout what follows, we will assume that the designer cannot vary the loadings, and data are chosen for more general reasons. In practice we often meet the situation when a designer can choose nominal values of geometrical parameters which have given dispersions determined by technical documentation (GOST, industrial standards and norms). Thereby, a problem of optimal projection includes as a rule a choice of mean values of some determined part of parameters generating by themselves the vector ω.

The considered optimization problem includes three component parts:

1) A reliability model which is reduced to the establishment of a relationship between the Bayes estimate of TTF, R^* (or $\underline{R}_\gamma^*$) and vector of control parameters ω. Later we will write $\hat{R}^*(\omega)$;
2) Technical and economical characteristics (mass or cost) in the form of a function $S = S(\omega)$ (or set of such characteristics);
3) Additional restrictions of the form $\psi_\ell(\omega) \leqslant 0$ $(\ell = 1, 2, \ldots, L)$, guaranteeing the physical reliability of a project and establishing the norm and relationship of a projection.

The problem may be formulated in two different ways when one optimization criterion is chosen:

Direct problem:

$$\begin{aligned} &\hat{R}^*(\omega) \to \max, \\ &S(\omega) \leqslant S_0, \\ &\psi_\ell(\omega) \leqslant 0, \qquad \ell = 1, 2, \ldots, L; \end{aligned} \tag{8.63}$$

Inverse problem:

$$\begin{aligned} &S(\omega) \to \min, \\ &\hat{R}^*(\omega) \geqslant R_{\text{req}}, \\ &\psi_\ell(\omega) \leqslant 0, \qquad \ell = 1, 2, \ldots, L. \end{aligned} \tag{8.64}$$

Considering a direct problem, we assume that a threshold value of the characteristic S_0 is given, whereas in the inverse problem a required R_{req}, by the technical documentation, TTF value is known. The technical-economical characteristic is usually chosen in the form of a cost, sometimes in the form of an object mass, and the representation of the function (ω) doesn't present any difficulties. The main obstacle in this action is obtaining the dependence of $\hat{R}^*$ from a vector ω. Let us investigate the following question: in what way can the parameter ω be introduced into the Bayes scheme (for example, as described in § 8.3)? From the arguments of § 8.1, we conclude that a Bayes TTF estimate is defined by:

1) a sample of testing results $\underset{\sim}{\mathbf{x}}$ in the form of a vector of initial variables $\mathbf{X}$;
2) a form of a p.d.f. $f_X(\mathbf{x};\theta)$;

3) a form of a working capacity function $\phi_j(\cdot)$, $j = 1, 2, \ldots, M$;

4) a prior probability density $h(\theta)$ of the parameter vector θ.

A vector of controlled parameters ω is naturally included in the Bayes scheme in connection with a prior density $h(\theta)$ as some subset of the set α_θ with the help of which a prior density $h(\theta; \alpha_\theta)$, $\alpha_\theta \in A$ is parameterized. Suppose, for example, that a vector parameter θ consists of mean values m_i of all (in practice only some of them) initial variables, i.e., $\theta = (m_1, m_2, \ldots, m_N)$. A prior distribution density $h(\theta; \alpha_0)$ appears to be uniform. Moreover, each of the parameters $\theta_i = m_i$ is distributed inside of the interval $\mu_i = [m_i', m_i'']$, $i = 1, 2, \ldots, N$. The interval μ_i is determined by the mean value m_{i0} and relative length χ_i so that $m_i' = m_{i0}(1 - \chi_i/2)$, $m_i'' = m_{i0}(1 + \chi_i/2)$. The set m_{i0}, χ_i ($i = 1, 2, \ldots, N$) forms a vector of parameters α_θ. The quantity χ_i determines the degree of uncertainty, impossibility to ensure a theoretical value m_{i0} in practice. At the same time m_{i0} is such a new value of the i-th initial variable (as was mentioned, of a geometrical parameter) which should be chosen by a designer in the process of a solution of the optimization problem, i.e., $\omega = \left(m_{10}, m_{20}, \ldots, m_{N0}\right)$. Including ω as a subset of α_θ into the Bayes procedure, we obtain the relationships between the TTF estimates, $\hat{R}^*$ or $\underline{R}_\gamma^*$, and a vector of controlling parameters ω.

The algorithm for the solution of the optimization problem consists of the following steps. At first, before the testing, the problem (8.62) is solved under the assumption of absence of experimental data. Thereafter, while the data $\underset{\sim}{\mathbf{x}}$ are accumulated, we repeat the problem solution. This enables us to correct the value of the vector of controlled parameters ω, obtained a priori.

8.5.2 *An example of solving the optimization problem*

Consider a problem of a choice of optimal project parameters for a cylindrical shell having a wafer type (see Fig. 8.6). As controlled parameters three mean values of the following initial variables have been chosen: δ', δ, c, b.The shell is loaded by the axis compressible force T, a bending moment M and abundant pressure p.

The mass of the shell is chosen as a goal function

$$S(\omega) = S\left(\delta_0', \delta_0, c_0, b_0\right) = \rho\left\{2\pi r\left[\alpha\delta_0 + c_0 h N_k\right] + N_\pi c_0 h\left(h - c_0 N_k\right)\right\}$$

where ρ is a material density, the index 0 denotes a mean value $h = \delta_0' - \delta_0$, $N_k = [L/(b_0 + c_0)]$, $N_\pi = [2\pi r/(b_0 + c_0)]$, $[A]$ denotes the integral part of A.

The reliability function is determined as the probability that the following set of working

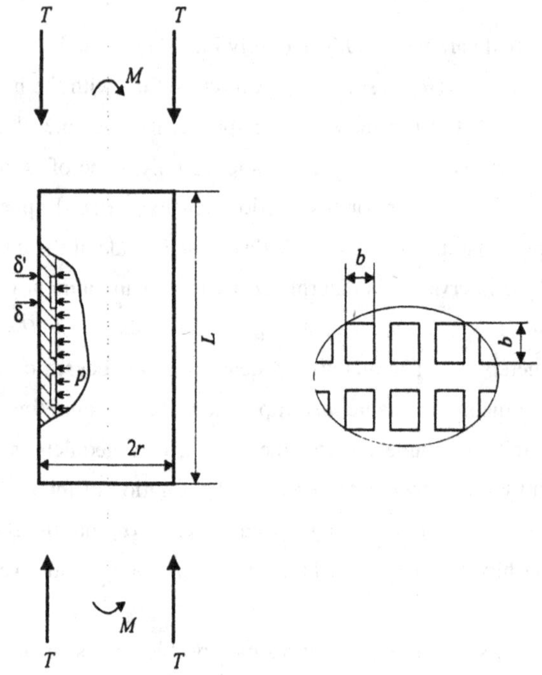

Fig. 8.6 Loaded cylindrical shell.

capacity conditions [151]: the durability condition

$$Z_1 = \sigma_U - \frac{\pi r N}{\delta + c(\delta' - \delta)/b} > 0, \quad N = T + \frac{M}{2r} - \pi r^2 p,$$

the condition of a global stability

$$Z_2 = 2\pi k E \delta^2 \left[1 + \phi'(\psi' - 1)^2 \left(\frac{0.4}{\sqrt[3]{\phi'}} + \frac{1.3}{\sqrt{\psi'}} - 0.54 \right) \right] N > 0,$$

and local stability

$$Z_3 = 12\pi E \frac{r^2 \delta^3}{b - c} \left[1 + 0.16\phi'(\psi' - 1) \right] - N > 0,$$

where $\phi' = 2\pi c/\delta$, $\psi' = \delta'/\delta$, k is the stability coefficient, σ_U is the durability limit, E is the resiliency coefficient. It follows from the working capacity model described above, the vector of initial variables is formed by the quantities $(M, T, p, r, L, \delta', \delta, c, b, \sigma_U, E, k)$.

For evaluation of TTF estimate, $\hat{R}^*$, we apply a linearization of the working capacity function. The results of optimization based on using the project TTF estimate in problem (8.62) consists of the following: from the initial point $\omega_0 = (8,3,100,4)$ mm corresponding to the mass $S(\omega_0) = 330.2$kg and $R(\omega_0) = 0.9983$, the searching trajectory leads into the point $\omega_* = (7.3;2.8,150,3.1)$ mm for which $S(\omega_0) = 291$ kg when $R_{\text{req}} = 0.99$. Note that if a value of a project TTF estimate is chosen as R_{req}, i.e., $R_{\text{req}} = R(\omega_0) = 0.9983$, then $S(\omega_0) = 319.4$ kg. It is seen that the optimization mass gain is more than 10 kg.

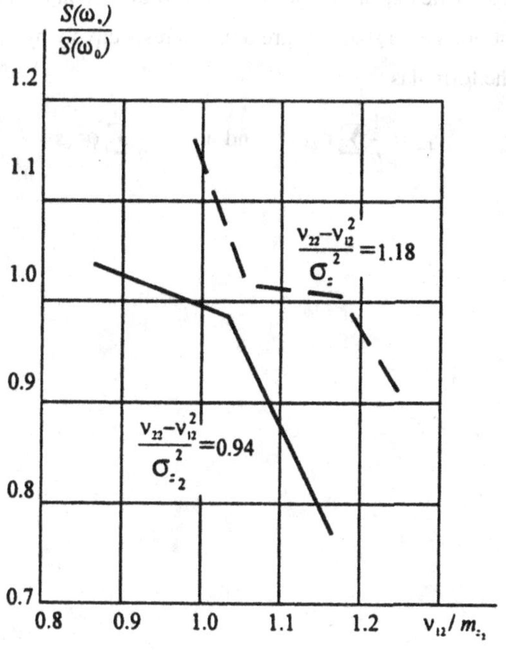

Fig. 8.7 Dependence of optimal mass on testing results.

The statistical optimization is carried out in accordance with the method of evaluation of $\hat{R}^*(\omega)$ (see § 8.3) under the condition that uncertainty intervals form a 5% segment with respect to the project values m_{z_j} and σ_{z_j}. The experimental results are modeled on the computer in accordance with the chosen distribution laws of initial variables. Fig. 8.7 shows the dependencies of $S(\omega_0)$ on testing results represented by sufficient statistics ν_1

and v_2. The following conclusions may be stated: (1) when the statistic v_{2j} (the sample variance) increases, the estimate $\underline{R}_\gamma^*$ decreases, which implies the decreasing of $S(\omega^*)$; (2) if the statistic v_{1j} exceeds m_{zj}, then $S(\omega^*)$ is less than the values of the goal function during the project optimization, otherwise, vice-versa, the value of the goal function increases. We have applied for optimization an algorithm of random searching together with a method of continuous penalty functions. An optimization problem for one sample $\underset{\sim}{\mathbf{x}}$ has been solved on the EC-1045 computer during a period of two hours. It is found that the second working capacity condition appears to be the most dangerous so that the shell TTF is completely determined by the probability for the second condition to hold. Due to this circumstance, only the sufficient statistics v_1 and v_2 with respect to the second status variable affect the results of optimization. These statistics are denoted respectively by v_{12} and v_{22} in Fig. 8.7, and are given by the formulas

$$v_{12} = \frac{1}{n}\sum_{i=1}^{n} \phi_2(\mathbf{x}_i) \quad \text{and} \quad v_{22} = \frac{1}{n}\sum_{i=1}^{n} \phi_2^2(\mathbf{x}_i).$$

Chapter 9

Statistical Reliability Analysis Prior Bayes Estimates

9.1 Traditional and Bayes interpretations of the error of the working capacity model

This chapter is a continuous development of the previous chapter, and we consider a more general situation when a theoretical working capacity model contains the error stipulated by the defects of physical theories used for its construction. Such a situation appears quite often in many technical devices or systems which are based on experimental data processing. In this chapter we propose a method of statistical Bayes analysis for technical devices directed to the estimation of the TTF for these devices and errors which are used in mathematical calculations. The chapter includes the problem setting, its description and the solution of the problem for the stage prior to the experimental elaboration and analysis of the system.

The real *working capacity model* is based on mathematical models in the form of finite analytical expressions and sets of differential equations used in the corresponding field of knowledge. Any mathematical model is either more or less than a complete formalized description of the processes and phenomena originated from the examined technical system. Due to this fact, a working capacity model necessarily contains the error that produces eventually a methodological mistake in estimating TTF.

Very often a designer of a technical system has available only tentative information about the model error. In particular, for the projection of carrying construction elements and some other technical systems, one uses the so-called *safety coefficients* solving a two-sided problem. In the opinion of Korolev [127], a safety coefficient includes, on one hand, a random scatter, and on the other hand, it has to compensate for the defects of the calculation method, and consequently, of a working capacity model. If we use for the analysis of the system working capacity a representation of its parameters in the form of random variables or processes, then the first aspect of the safety coefficient will not be necessary. At the same time, the second one remains and, apparently, completely determines the accuracy of the working capacity model.

The value of the safety coefficient is chosen so as to overstate a calculation load or, equivalently, to understate the system functional capability obtained theoretically. As a result, the developed constructions often have extremely large weights and are very cumbersome. The current method of estimating model error uses information about this error (in the form of a safety coefficient) which is unchangeable during the system lifetime cycle. At the same time for the system projecting and exploitation one carries out the tests which give information (direct or indirect) about its real functional capability. This information may be used as the basis for the reconsideration of the approved prior representation of the model error. Coming from the logic and intention of the process of design and exploitation of technical systems, the error estimate of the model of functioning and working capacity must have a dynamic nature, i.e., it must change in accordance with the new obtained experimental information. It is clear also that the TTF estimate must "superintend" the evolution of representation about the working capacity model error. At the initial stage of the system lifetime cycle, when we have no experimental data, the TTF is estimated with the help of a priori representation about the model error. This representation may have a very approximate nature. During the process of experimental data processing this representation changes and appears to be more complete which implies the increasing of accuracy of the TTF estimate.

The scheme considered above is adequate to the Bayes procedure of obtaining a statistical conclusion. Use of the Bayes approach for the problem solution enables us to overcome all specific shortcomings to the traditional method of the model error accounting mentioned above. In view of the optimality of the Bayes decision rules, TTF estimates obtained with the help of such an approach will be the best in the sense of maximization of some usefulness function, and use of complete available information.

In this and following chapters we propose a method of TTF estimation for the technical device which uses the error of its survival state model and a method of statistical estimation of the error in accordance with the existing testing results and a priori information. All arguments that we will use touch upon the case when a survival state model represents one functional inequality. Such a simplification has been chosen for the following reasons. First, this simplification is not very restrictive and serves the purposes of a clearer understanding of the method, free of the complicated mathematical constructions. Second, such an approach lets us investigate working capacity models consisting of many uncorrelated working capacity conditions. The assumption about noncorrelatedness may be justified since, if rough (inexact) working capacity models are used, it's unlikely to take into account their "acute" properties as a correlation.

Let us give the Bayes definition of the error for a survival state model and investigate in what way it differs from the traditional one. Assume that a working capacity model has the form

$$\phi\,(X_1, X_2, \ldots, X_N) > 0, \tag{9.1}$$

where $\mathbf{X} = (X_1, X_2, \ldots, X_N)$ is a vector of an initial variable which may be random variables, processes or fields. A working capacity function $\phi(\cdot)$ is, as a rule, written in a special way as a final result of the solution of a model problem which describes the process of a normal functioning of the system. For example, for the thin-walled bar of the length ℓ with a minimal momentum of inertia of the cross-section J, subjected to the action of the axis compressible force T, the theoretical working capacity model of the form (9.1) can be written as

$$\frac{\pi^2 EJ}{\mu^2 \ell^2} - T > 0, \tag{9.2}$$

where E is the material resiliency module, μ is a constant depending on the bar fixing. The quantity

$$T_{\text{cr}} = \frac{\pi^2 EJ}{\mu^2 \ell^2} \tag{9.3}$$

is called a critical force of the stability loss (by Euler) and characterizes a functional capability of the bar to withstand the load T. The vector of initial variables $\mathbf{X}$ is composed of T, E, J, ℓ. Since the initial variables are random, the condition (9.1) for some realization $\mathbf{X}$ cannot be fulfilled. This event is considered a failure. The probability of fulfilment of the inequality (9.1) during the given time interval τ (or at the given time instance t) is classified as a time to failure probability.

For the research connected with calculations of the parameters of the construction elements which don't touch upon the probability representations, one introduces the safety coefficient η compensating for the error of the theoretical model. For the considered example, in particular, calculation of the parameters is carried out for the force ηT as $\eta > 1$, i.e., under the condition $T_{\text{cr}} = \eta T$.The working capacity condition is written as

$$\frac{T_{\text{cr}}}{\eta} - T > 0. \tag{9.4}$$

This survival state model takes into account, in contrast to (9.2), the error that appeared because of the inaccuracy of the formula (9.3).

The form of representation of the working capacity model (9.4) may be considered as conditional in a definite sense. We can introduce just as well instead of the coefficient η, $\zeta = \eta^{-1}$ that brings a change of the inequality (9.4). For further analysis we need (it seems), to order the method of representation of the model error with the help of the quantity ε, linear with respect to the right-hand part of the inequality (9.1). The essence of error accounting does not change in this case, and the method of construction of the statistical estimates of the model error and TTF is simplified.

In accordance with our assumption, instead of the working capacity condition we will write

$$\phi(\mathbf{X}) + \varepsilon > 0 \tag{9.5}$$

The quantity ε is termed an *additive error* of the working capacity model. This quantity appears to be an aggregate representation of the large number of random and nonrandom unaccounted factors in the theoretical model. Due to this reason we will assume that ε is a random variable.

With the help of this example, we show the equivalence of the additive error of the model and the safety coefficient. Since the last one is, by definition, nonrandom, we will use it in the testing instead of ε only its possible limit value which, as usual, cannot be exceeded in real situations. In Mathematical Statistics one uses for these purposes a quantile ε_p of the distribution $f_\varepsilon(\varepsilon)$, represented by the expression

$$\int_{-\infty}^{\varepsilon_p} f_\varepsilon(\varepsilon)\,d\varepsilon = p,$$

which corresponds to the large probability p. Using ε_p, from the inequality (9.5) we pass to the corresponding (but nonequivalent, generally speaking) nonrandom inequality

$$\phi\left(\mathbf{m}_X\right) + \varepsilon_p > 0. \tag{9.6}$$

where $\mathbf{m}_X$ is a mean value of a random vector. For the working capacity condition (9.2), inequality (9.6) takes on the form

$$T_{\mathrm{cr}} - T + \varepsilon_p > 0. \tag{9.7}$$

Transforming the working capacity condition (9.4) written with the safety coefficient η to the equivalent form

$$(T_{\mathrm{cr}} - T) - T_{\mathrm{cr}}\frac{\eta - 1}{\eta} > 0,$$

we see that ε_p is determined uniquely with the help of η:

$$\varepsilon_p = -T_{\mathrm{cr}}\frac{\eta - 1}{\eta} \tag{9.8}$$

It is important to note that, since $\eta > 1$, from the equality (9.8) there follows $\varepsilon_p < 0$, i.e., the additive error, as well as the safety coefficient, understates the capability of the construction element, obtained theoretically with the help of the Euler formula.

Let us discuss the possible ways of assignment of ε_p. If a choice of the safety coefficient is strictly substantiated, ε_p is determined uniquely, for example, by the formula of the type (9.8). But the point is that η is often chosen under more general arguments which are, generally speaking, far from the real relationships between the real and theoretical values of the working capacity of the concrete investigated object. Representation of the error of a theoretical model has, as a rule, an undetermined nature. For example, we often know only that a calculated value exceeds or, vice versa, understates the real value of the functional capability. Sometimes we may say that the maximal error equals some percent of the calculated value and may be either positive or negative. Therefore it seems reasonable in the general case to represent the error ε_p not in the form of the in determined value as it was in (9.8), but in the form of some interval $E_\varepsilon = [a_\varepsilon, b_\varepsilon]$, assuming that $\varepsilon_p \varepsilon E_\varepsilon$. Thus, as was done earlier, we use, based on the safety coefficient and relations of the form (9.8), the categorical statement of the type: the limit error ε_p equals $-12H$, but now we assume that it is possible to make a more undetermined (and at the same time more flexible) statement, for example, ε_p lies in the interval $[-12H, 0]$. A designer may have, coming from his own experience, access to more "thin" information characterizing the chances of ε_p lying in different intervals in E_ε.

Later, using the terminology of the Bayes approach, we will say: analyzing the error of a working capacity model, a designer assigns a prior probability distribution $h(\varepsilon_p)$, $\varepsilon_p \varepsilon E_\varepsilon$. Due to this reason, instead of a given number for ε_p, using the Bayes methodology, we have some of its neighborhood ("smearing" representation of the number). The points of this neighborhood may have different probability significance, corresponding to a prior p.d.f., $h(\varepsilon_p)$. Note that the determined form of representation of ε_p as ε_p' is a limiting case of the Bayes form, when a probability significance $\varepsilon_p' \varepsilon E_\varepsilon$ equals unity, and a prior p.d.f., $h(\varepsilon_p)$, degenerates into a delta-function.

The Bayes form of representation of the error of a survival state model has several preferences. First, it corresponds in a stronger form to give information about the model error, i.e., to the unspecified nature of the model. Secondly, when one assigns the values of E_ε and $h(\varepsilon_p)$, its responsibility decreases. Responsibility is understood in the following sense. On one hand, the object must be reliable enough; on the other hand, its construction must be non-overweight or superfluous in details because of its super-reliability. Usually that responsibility deals with only the first aspect, forgetting about the second one.

The third, most important, advantage of the Bayes form of error representation lies in the possibility of correction of this representation as experimental data are obtained. The scheme of this correction assumes the use of the Bayes theorem.

Finally, the Bayes methodology is attractive in the following sense. The resulting TTF estimate with regard to the working capacity error will always be optimal from the point-of-view of the minimum of the chosen loss function. In other words, choosing in the corresponding way the loss function, we can achieve the desired quality of the TTF estimate. For example, if the object failure is connected with human victims or losses of expensive equipment, then for the reliability estimate of this object, the most pessimistic estimate should be used. This corresponds to the loss function possessing the property that overstating is worse than understating. In conclusion, we note that estimating of the additive model error with the help of only one numerical characteristic of a situation in capacity of which the quantile ε_p has been used is a very rough approximation of the desired result. A more complete solution of the problem assumes that other numerical characteristics should be used. Later we will consider calculation cases based on two characteristics corresponding to two parameters of the p.d.f. of the additive error ε.

9.2 The problem of estimation of the additive error of the working capacity model attached to estimation of the reliability function

We will assume that the object's working capacity is represented by the working capacity model with an additive error ε of the following form:

$$\psi(\mathbf{X},\varepsilon) = \phi(\mathbf{X}) + \varepsilon > 0, \tag{9.9}$$

where $\phi(\cdot)$ is a theoretical working capacity function, and $\psi(\cdot)$ is called a *generalized working capacity function.* Analogously to a status variable $Z = \phi(\mathbf{X})$, $W = \psi(\mathbf{X},\varepsilon)$ will be called a *generalized status variable.*The relationship between W and Z is given by the linear transformation

$$W = Z + \varepsilon. \tag{9.10}$$

The variables W and Z may be random fields, processes and variables. For the description of the additive error ε, we choose a model as a random variable and further on will assume that ε obeys some distribution with a probability density $f_\varepsilon(\varepsilon) = f_\varepsilon(\varepsilon;\theta)$, where θ is a vector of parameters.

If Z is a random variable, then TTF will be defined by the probability statement

$$R_0 = P\{W > 0\}. \tag{9.11}$$

This expression will be used as a reliability characteristic of the object in the initial or some fixed time, corresponding to extremal exploitation conditions.

In the more general case, Z is a random process, and the probability

$$R_\tau = R(\tau) = P\{W(t) > 0,\ 0 \leqslant t \leqslant \tau\} \tag{9.12}$$

is used as a TTF. The general problem is the estimation of the error ε and TTF of the form (9.11) or (9.12) under the following assumptions:

(1) The theoretical working capacity function $\phi(\mathbf{X})$ is assumed to be given.

(2) We are given the values of the set of numerical characteristics k_X of the vector of initial variables $\mathbf{X}$. If the vector $\mathbf{X}$, consists of only random variables, then K_X is formed by mean values, mean-squared values, correlative coefficients and, possibly, numerical characteristics of moments of higher order. Provided that some components of the vector $\mathbf{X}$ are random processes, K_X contains additionally the parameters of corresponding correlative functions.

(3) We are given the form of probability characteristics necessary for the TTF evaluation. In particular, for the evaluation of R_0 we need to know the form of the p.d.f. or cumulative distribution function of the status variable Z. For calculation of R_τ, generally speaking, we have to know an infinite dimensional distribution density of the coordinates of the process $Z(t)$. Under the assumption that $Z(t)$ is Gaussian and stationary and the flux of intersection of the process $W(t)$ of the zero-level is Poisson, it suffices to know a one-dimensional density of the distribution of the coordinates of the process $Z(t)$ and correlation function of the process.

(4) We are given a p.d.f. $f_\varepsilon(\varepsilon;\theta)$ of the additive error ε and given a prior p.d.f. $h(\theta)$ of the parameter vector θ.

(5) We may have carried out the testing, given the information (direct or indirect) with respect to the values of the additive model error ε. These tests may have two different forms. The first one is based on the establishment of the real levels of functional capabilities of the model. We fix the values of the status variable Z at the failure time (when $W = 0$), whence empirical values of the quantity ε are found. The second form consists of functional tests which are carried out under the exploitation conditions near to them. After these tests, one can obtain censored data for ε, since not all tests are ended by the event $W = 0$.

Under the assumptions (1)–(4), the problem of obtaining a prior estimate is solved. The general scheme of the problem solution can be represented by the following three steps.

Step 1. Determination of the conditional TTF, $R = R(\theta)$, depending on the parameter vector which characterizes the additive error ε. This step uses the assumptions (1)–(4).

Step 2. Determination of a prior TTF estimate with the help of a prior p.d.f., $h(\theta)$, and some loss function $L\left(\hat{R}, R\right)$. Assumption (4) will be methodologically fundamental for this step. A TTF estimate is sought in the form of a pointwise estimate, R^*, minimizing a prior Bayes risk and a lower prior confidence limit, $\underline{R}_\gamma^*$, under the given confidence level γ.

Step 3. Determination of the posterior TTF estimate by the results of the experiment mentioned in assumption (5). Here we use the Bayes theorem which enables us to find a posterior density of the distribution of the vector θ. As discussed earlier, information about TTF is formed by the pointwise posterior estimate, $\hat{R}^*$, minimizing posterior Bayes risk, and posterior lower confidence limit, $\underline{R}_\gamma^*$.

Note that the first step is free of the use of principles of the Bayes methodology. We will consider it in § 9.3; Steps 2 and 3 will be investigated in §§ 9.4, 10.2.

9.3 The conditional estimates of the reliability function

In this section we touch upon the questions of obtaining TTF estimates which depend on unknown parameters $\theta = (\theta_1, \theta_2)$ of the distribution of additive error. Later these estimates will be called conditional, i.e., known, if the parameters are given. At first we introduce and substantiate two calculation cases for the probability distribution of the error ε, and thereafter for each case we will write the corresponding TTF estimates of the form (9.11) and (9.12).

9.3.1 *Calculation case of a generalized exponential error*

This case is given by a p.d.f. $f_\varepsilon(\varepsilon;\theta)$ of the form:

$$f_\varepsilon(\varepsilon;\theta_1,\theta_2) = \begin{cases} \dfrac{1}{\theta_2-\theta_1}\exp\left(-\dfrac{\varepsilon}{\theta_1}\right), & \varepsilon < 0, \\ \dfrac{1}{\theta_2-\theta_1}\exp\left(-\dfrac{\varepsilon}{\theta_2}\right), & \varepsilon \geqslant 0 \quad (\theta_1 \leqslant 0,\ \theta_2 \geqslant 0). \end{cases} \tag{9.13}$$

The choice of the density (9.13) as a probability characteristic of the error ε is prompted by the following reasons. The p.d.f. (9.13) corresponds to a situation when a theoretical working capacity model may induce either decreasing or increasing of the working capacity of the system. We assume also that our theoretical model doesn't have a systematic error. Due to this circumstance, we choose as $f_\varepsilon(\varepsilon)$ a p.d.f. which has a mode at the point $\varepsilon = 0$. The p.d.f. (9.13) in a general case is not symmetric which enables us, with the help of the parameters θ_1 and θ_2, to characterize the corresponding significance of negative and positive errors of the model. The p.d.f. (9.13) has a form depicted in Fig. 9.1, a.

Partial cases of the p.d.f. (9.13) describe unilateral estimates (see Fig. 9.1, b, c). That is, for the partial case of a negative additive error $\theta_2 = 0$, the p.d.f. $f_\varepsilon(\varepsilon)$ becomes one-parametric and takes on the form

$$f_\varepsilon(\varepsilon;\theta) = \begin{cases} -\dfrac{1}{\theta}\exp\left(-\dfrac{\varepsilon}{\theta}\right), & \varepsilon \leqslant 0, \\ 0, & \varepsilon > 0 \;\; (\theta = \theta_1 \leqslant 0). \end{cases} \tag{9.14}$$

The probability distribution (9.14) should be used only in the case when it is a priori known that a theoretical model overstates the real functional capability of the system. The exponential nature of the p.d.f. of ε conveys that the functional form of the theoretical model approximates well the real properties of the system, since the probability of the error ε being in the domain of small, in magnitude, values are greater than in the domain of greater values. For the opposite case, when it is known a priori that the theoretical working capacity model understates the real functional capability of the system, the p.d.f. $f_\varepsilon(\varepsilon)$ has the form

$$f_\varepsilon(\varepsilon;\theta) = \begin{cases} 0, & \varepsilon < 0, \\ \dfrac{1}{\theta}\exp\left(-\dfrac{\varepsilon}{\theta}\right), & \varepsilon \geqslant 0 \;\; (\theta = \theta_2 \geqslant 0). \end{cases} \tag{9.15}$$

9.3.2 *Calculation of the Gaussian error*

This calculation is determined by the p.d.f. $f_\varepsilon(\varepsilon)$ of the form

$$f_\varepsilon(\varepsilon;\varepsilon_0,\sigma_\varepsilon) = \frac{1}{\sqrt{2\pi}\,\sigma_\varepsilon}\exp\left(-\frac{\varepsilon-\varepsilon_0}{2\sigma_\varepsilon^2}\right). \tag{9.16}$$

The use of this calculation case is substantiated under the conditions of a great number of unaccounted factors of a theoretical model which act by the additive scheme. In this situation we apply the central limit theorem leading to the normal probability distribution of the error. The p.d.f. (9.16) assumes the existence of a systematic error ε_0. If there is no such error, we set $\varepsilon_0 = 0$ in (9.16), which guarantees that the error ε possesses a Gaussian property of symmetry.

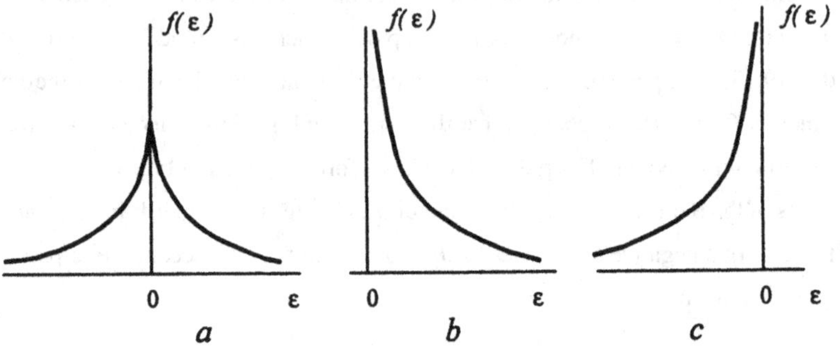

Fig. 9.1 Probability Density Function of the Generalized Exponential Error.

9.3.3 *Conditional TTF estimates for a fixed time*

Starting from assumptions (3) and (4), we suppose that the p.d.f. of the status probability variable Z and additive error of the model ε are given, i.e., the forms of the densities $F_z(z;K_z)$ and $f_\varepsilon(\varepsilon;\theta)$ are given, where the vector θ is unknown, and parameters contained in the set K_z may be found because of the assumptions (1) and (2). The problem of approximate determination of K_z is considered below in Subsection 9.3.4.

Assuming that the state variable Z and error ε are independent, the sought-after probability, R_0, in the general case will be written with the help of the integral

$$R_0 = P\{Z+\varepsilon > 0\} = \iint_{(z+\varepsilon>0)} f_z(z;K_z) f_\varepsilon(\varepsilon;\theta)\,dz\,d\varepsilon. \tag{9.17}$$

Below we will consider the case of the Gaussian distribution of the status variable Z, in accordance with which the set k_z consists of a mean value $m_Z = E[Z]$ and standard deviation $\sigma_Z = E\left[(Z = m_Z)^2\right]^{1/2}$. Since, under the assumption, m_Z and σ_Z are known, later we will emphasize the dependence of a TTF only on θ. Suppose at first that the error ε appears to be a generalized exponential. Let us rewrite the integral (9.17) in the form

$$R_0 = \iint_{\omega_1} f_z(z) f_\varepsilon(\varepsilon)\,dz\,d\varepsilon + \iint_{\omega_2} f_z(z) f_\varepsilon(\varepsilon)\,dz\,d\varepsilon, \tag{9.18}$$

where $\omega_1 = \{0 \leqslant z < \infty, -z \leqslant \varepsilon \leqslant 0\}$ and $\omega_2 = \{(0 < z < \infty, 0 \leqslant \varepsilon < 0 < \infty \cup (-\infty < z < 0, -z \leqslant \varepsilon < \infty))\}$. After the substitution of (9.13) into (9.18) and integration for the Gaussian density $f_z(z)$ we finally have

$$R_0 = R_0(\theta_1,\theta_2) = \Phi\left(\frac{m_Z}{\sigma_Z}\right) + \Delta R_1(\theta_1,\theta_2) + \Delta R_2(\theta_1,\theta_2), \tag{9.19}$$

where

$$\Delta R_1(\theta_1,\theta_2) = \frac{\theta_1}{\theta_2-\theta_1}\Phi\left(\frac{m_Z+\frac{\sigma_Z^2}{\theta_1}}{\sigma_Z}\right)\exp\left(\frac{m_Z}{\theta_1}+\frac{\sigma_Z^2}{2\theta_1^2}\right) \leqslant 0, \tag{9.20}$$

and

$$\Delta R_2(\theta_1,\theta_2) = \frac{\theta_2}{\theta_2-\theta_1}\left[1-\Phi\left(\frac{m_Z+\frac{\sigma_Z^2}{\theta_2}}{\sigma_Z}\right)\right]\exp\left(\frac{m_Z}{\theta_2}+\frac{\sigma_Z^2}{2\theta_2^2}\right) \geqslant 0, \tag{9.21}$$

Let us investigate the obtained expression (9.19). First, as $\theta_1 = 0$, we have $\Delta R_1 = 0$, and the expression (9.19) corresponds to the case of a positive additive error. Analogously, as $\theta_2 = 0$, we obtain $\Delta R_2 = 0$, and (9.19) characterizes the case of a negative additive error. Second, using the limit passing, we found that, as $|\theta_1| \to \infty$ and for all θ_2, $\Delta R_1 \to \Phi(m_Z\sigma_Z)$ and $\Delta R_2 \to 0$, i.e., in this case $R_0 = 0$, and infinite negative error leads to a zero TTF value. Analogously, as $\theta_2 \to \infty$ and for all θ_1, we get $\Delta R_1 = 0$ and $\Delta R_2 \to \Phi(m_Z\sigma_Z)$, whence $R_0 = 1$, i.e., infinite positive error leads to absolute reliability. Drawn conclusions can be easily interpreted in the range of the considered model. Moreover, they convince us that θ_1 and θ_2 in (9.19) play the role of significance characteristics corresponding to negative and positive errors. This, however, doesn't mean that for $|\theta_1| = |\theta_2|$ we will obtain $R_0 = \Phi(m_Z\sigma_Z)$. The cause is that the fact of having a random additive error leads to an increasing of the variance of a status variable, i.e., $\sigma_W > \sigma_Z$, whence follows $R_0 < \Phi(m_Z\sigma_Z)$.

For the calculation of the Gaussian additive error, it is easy to obtain an expression for the conditional TTF estimate, since in the case of the normal probability distribution of Z and ε, a generalized status variable W also has the Gaussian p.d.f. with the parameters $m_W = m_Z + \varepsilon_0$ and $\sigma_W^2 = \sigma_Z^2 + \sigma_\varepsilon^2$. Consequently, the resulting expression for R_0 may be written as follows:

$$R_0 = P\{W > 0\} = \Phi\left(\frac{m_Z+\varepsilon_0}{\sqrt{\sigma_Z^2+\sigma_\varepsilon^2}}\right). \tag{9.22}$$

For many theoretical working capacity models, we may a priori assume that there is no systematic error. Then

$$R_0 = \Phi\left(\frac{m_Z}{\sqrt{\sigma_Z^2+\sigma_\varepsilon^2}}\right). \tag{9.23}$$

It follows from (9.23), even in the case of symmetric error ε an approximate reliability estimate is less than the theoretical one. They coincide only in the case $\sigma_\varepsilon = 0$.

9.3.4 *The problem of determining m_Z and σ_Z*

The solution of this problem is guaranteed by the assumptions (1) and (2). In the general case the function $\phi(\cdot)$ is nonlinear, which impedes obtaining exact values of numerical characteristics of the status variable Z. A regular approximate solution may be found with the help of an approximate representation of the function.$\phi(\cdot)$. One of the possible ways is based on the following procedure. To determine $m_Z = E[\phi(\mathbf{X})]$, we approximate the function $\phi(\mathbf{X})$ by the use of Taylor series. If one restricts himself to the smallest second-order term, then an approximate formula for m_Z may be written as

$$m_Z \cong \phi(\mathbf{m}_X) + \frac{1}{2} \sum_{1 \leqslant i \leqslant j \leqslant N} \sum \frac{\partial^2 \phi}{\partial m_i \partial m_j} \rho_{ij} \sigma_i \sigma_j, \tag{9.24}$$

where

$$\mathbf{m}_X = (m_1, m_2, \ldots m_N), \quad m_i = E[X_i]$$
$$\sigma_i^2 = E[X_i^2 - m_i^2]$$

and

$$\rho_{ij} = \frac{E[X_i X_j] - m_i m_j}{\sigma_i \sigma_j}.$$

These quantities, under the assumption, form a priori information. To determine σ_Z^2 we replace a function $(\phi(\mathbf{X}) - m_Z)^2$ by a segment of the Taylor series. If one restricts himself to the smallest of the second order terms, inclusively, the expression for the variance of the status variable is written as

$$\sigma_Z^2 = [\phi(\mathbf{m}_X) - m_Z]^2 + 2 \sum_{1 \leqslant i \leqslant j \leqslant N} \sum \left[\frac{\partial \phi}{\partial m_i} \cdot \frac{\partial^2 \phi}{\partial m_j} \right] + (\phi(\mathbf{m}_X) - m_Z)^2 \frac{\partial \phi}{\partial m_i \partial m_j} \rho_{ij} \sigma_i \sigma_j. \tag{9.25}$$

The detailed examination of the question of obtaining numerical characteristics of the state variable with the help of different approximations of the working capacity function is given in [173].

9.3.5 *Conditional TTF estimates for variable time*

Consider the problem of determining a TTF, R_τ, of the form (9.12), assuming that the status variable $Z(t)$ is a stationary random process, and $W(t)$ lies out of the zero level are rare events, i.e., the reliability of a system is high enough. Many practical situations, when a system is being subjected for a short time to random stationary loadings under the nonchangeable value of carrying capability, lead to this problem.

The problem of determination of the conditional TTF estimate, $R_\tau = R_\tau(\theta)$, in a general case may be solved by the following scheme. At first we fix the value of an additive model error ε, i.e., it is assumed to be nonrandom, and find the probability of $r_\tau(\varepsilon)$ not being out of the level $(-\varepsilon)$, that is,

$$r_\tau(\varepsilon) = P\{Z(t) > -\varepsilon,\ 0 \leqslant t \leqslant \tau\}. \tag{9.26}$$

For determination of $r_\tau(\varepsilon)$ we will use the method based on an approximate determination of the probability of the nonfrequent exceeding observations of the stationary process $Z(t)$ out of the level $(-\varepsilon)$ with the help of the mean number of rejected observations per unit time $v(\varepsilon)$ [26]. If one denotes by $q_\tau^{(k)}(\varepsilon)$ the probability of k intersections to the one side (i.e., whether with a positive or negative derivative) of the level $(-\varepsilon)$, then the probability of at least one exceeding (rejected) point is written as:

$$q_\tau(\varepsilon) = \sum_{k=1}^{\infty} q_\tau^{(k)}(\varepsilon). \tag{9.27}$$

The mean number of exceeding observations per time τ may be represented as a mean value of a discrete random variable of the number of exceeding observations:

$$N_\tau(\varepsilon) = \sum_{k=1}^{\infty} k q_\tau^{(k)}(\varepsilon). \tag{9.28}$$

The assumption about a nonfrequent exceeding observation of the process $Z(t)$ is equivalent to the assumption that the probability of two or more exceeding observations is negligibly small in comparison to the probability of one exceeding observation. Whence, neglecting in formulas (9.27) and (9.28) all terms beginning with the second one, we will have $q_\tau(\varepsilon) = q_\tau^{(1)}(\varepsilon)$ and $N_\tau(\varepsilon) = q_\tau^{(1)}(\varepsilon)$ or $q_\tau(\varepsilon) = N_\tau(\varepsilon)$. Thereafter, for the probability (9.26) we will write

$$r_\tau(\varepsilon) = 1 - q_\tau(\varepsilon) = 1 - N_\tau(\varepsilon).$$

Since the stochastic process $Z(t)$ is stationary, the mean number of exceeding observations per unit of time $v(\varepsilon)$ is independent of the current time, i.e., $N_\tau(\varepsilon) = \tau v(\varepsilon)$. Because of this fact, for the probability $r_\tau(\varepsilon)$the following approximate expression holds:

$$r_\tau(\varepsilon) \cong 1 - v(\varepsilon)\tau. \tag{9.29}$$

As seen from (9.28), $N_\tau(\varepsilon) \geqslant q_\tau(\varepsilon)$, whence, $r_\tau(\varepsilon) \geqslant 1 - v(\varepsilon)\tau$, i.e., the quantity $1 - v(\varepsilon)\tau$ for $r_\tau(\varepsilon)$ is a lower estimate. This fact emphasizes the practical use of the approximate expression (9.29), which is made possible with the help of the conclusions that may be added to the "reliability potential".

In order to determine the mean number of exceeding observations of the stochastic process $Z(t)$ out of the level $(-\varepsilon)$ per unit of time, we apply the Rise formula [133]. Restricting ourselves to a Gauss stationary random process, we will write the expression for $v(\varepsilon)$:

$$v(\varepsilon) = \frac{a_Z}{\sigma_Z} \exp\left[-\frac{(-\varepsilon - m_Z)^2}{2\sigma_Z^2}\right], \tag{9.30}$$

where

$$a_Z = \frac{1}{2\pi}\sqrt{-\frac{d^2K_z(\tau)}{d\tau^2}\bigg|_{\tau=0}}. \tag{9.31}$$

The correlation function of the status variable $K_z(\tau)$ is determined starting from the initial assumptions (1) and (2), as it was for m_Z and σ_Z. Substituting the expression (9.30) into (9.29), we will write the resulting expression for the probability of the stochastic process $Z(t)$ not being out of the level $(-\varepsilon)$:

$$r_\tau(\varepsilon) = 1 - \frac{a_Z\tau}{\sigma_Z}\exp\left[-\frac{(\varepsilon+m_Z)^2}{2\sigma_Z^2}\right]. \tag{9.32}$$

Returning to the initial situation when the additive error is assumed to be random, we determine the desired conditional TTF estimate, $R_\tau(\theta)$, having evaluated the mean value, $r_\tau(\varepsilon)$ over the set of possible values of the variable $\varepsilon \in E$:

$$R_\tau(\theta) = \int_E r_\tau(\varepsilon) f_\varepsilon(\varepsilon;\theta) d_\varepsilon,$$

or, more explicitly,

$$R_\tau(\theta) = 1 - \frac{a_Z\tau}{\sigma_Z}\int_E f_\varepsilon(\varepsilon;\theta)\exp\left[-\frac{(\varepsilon+m_Z)^2}{2\sigma_Z^2}\right] d_\varepsilon. \tag{9.33}$$

The case of a generalized error ε is reduced to the substitution of the p.d.f. (9.13) into the integral of the expression (9.33), which leads to the following expression:

$$R_\tau(\theta_1,\theta_2) = 1 - \frac{a_Z\tau}{\sigma_Z}\left\{\frac{1}{\theta_2-\theta_1}\int_{-\infty}^{0}\exp\left[-\frac{\varepsilon}{\theta_1}-\frac{(\varepsilon+m_Z)^2}{2\sigma_Z^2}\right]d\varepsilon \right.$$
$$\left. + \frac{1}{\theta_2-\theta_1}\int_{0}^{\infty}\exp\left[-\frac{\varepsilon}{\theta_2}-\frac{(\varepsilon+m_Z)^2}{2\sigma_Z^2}\right]d\varepsilon\right\}, \tag{9.34}$$

With the help of direct calculations, we can verify the validity of the following expressions:

$$\int_{-\infty}^{0}\exp\left[-\frac{\varepsilon}{\theta_1}-\frac{(\varepsilon+m_Z)^2}{2\sigma_Z^2}\right]d\varepsilon = \sqrt{2\pi}\sigma_Z\exp\left(\frac{m_Z}{\theta_1}+\frac{\sigma_Z^2}{2\theta_1^2}\right)\Phi\left(\frac{m_Z+\frac{\sigma_Z^2}{\theta_1}}{\sigma_Z}\right),$$

and

$$\int_{-\infty}^{0}\exp\left[-\frac{\varepsilon}{\theta_2}-\frac{(\varepsilon+m_Z)^2}{2\sigma_Z^2}\right]d\varepsilon = \sqrt{2\pi}\sigma_Z\exp\left(\frac{m_Z}{\theta_2}-\frac{\sigma_Z^2}{2\theta_2^2}\right)\left[1-\Phi\left(\frac{m_Z+\frac{\sigma_Z^2}{\theta_2}}{\sigma_Z}\right)\right].$$

Substituting these integrals into the expression (9.34), we write the resultant formula for $E_\tau(\theta_1,\theta_2)$:

$$R_\tau(\theta_1,\theta_2) = 1 - \frac{2\pi a_Z\tau}{\theta_2-\theta_1}\left\{\exp\left(\frac{m_Z}{\theta_1}+\frac{\sigma_Z^2}{2\sigma_1^2}\right)\Phi\left(\frac{m_Z+\frac{\sigma_Z^2}{\theta_1}}{\sigma_Z}\right)\right.$$
$$\left. +\exp\left(\frac{m_Z}{\theta_2}+\frac{\sigma_Z^2}{2\sigma_2^2}\right)\left[1-\Phi\left(\frac{m_Z+\frac{\sigma_Z^2}{\theta_1}}{\sigma_Z}\right)\right]\right\}. \tag{9.35}$$

Let us investigate (9.35). At first, as $\theta_2 \to 0^+$, we have

$$\exp\left(\frac{m_Z}{\theta_2}+\frac{\sigma_Z^2}{2\sigma_2^2}\right)\left[1-\Phi\left(\frac{m_Z+\frac{\sigma_Z^2}{\theta_2}}{\sigma_Z}\right)\right]\to 0,$$

whence it follows that TTF estimate for the case of negative additive error of a model, that is,

$$R_\tau(\theta_1,0)=1+\frac{\sqrt{2\pi}a_Z\tau}{\theta_1}\exp\left(\frac{m_Z}{\theta_2}+\frac{\sigma_Z^2}{2\sigma_1^2}\right)\Phi\left(\frac{m_Z+\frac{\sigma_Z^2}{\theta_1}}{\sigma_Z}\right). \tag{9.36}$$

For the positive error we analogously obtain

$$R_\tau(0,\theta_2)=1-\frac{\sqrt{2\pi}a_Z\tau}{\theta_2}\exp\left(\frac{m_Z}{\theta_2}+\frac{\sigma_Z^2}{2\sigma_2^2}\right)\left[1-\Phi\left(\frac{m_Z+\frac{\sigma_Z^2}{\theta_2}}{\sigma_Z}\right)\right]. \tag{9.37}$$

Secondly, it is necessary to investigate the area of applicability of the expression (9.36). The reason it that it is approximate, and is valid only in the case when exceeding observation of the process is a rare event. At the same time, as $|\theta_1|$ increases, this property may be broken. We can represent (9.36) in the form

$$R_\tau(\theta_1,0)=\left(1-\frac{a_Z\tau}{\sigma_Z}e^{-\frac{m_Z^2}{2\sigma_Z^2}}\right)=\Delta R_\tau(\theta_1), \tag{9.38}$$

where the expression in the parentheses is the theoretical probability of nonexceeding observation under the assumption of zero error, and $\Delta R_\tau(\theta_1)$ is a correction caused by the existence of the additive error in the working capacity model,

$$\Delta R_\tau(\theta_1)=a_Z\tau\left[\frac{1}{\sigma_Z}\exp\left(-\frac{m_Z^2}{2\sigma_Z^2}\right)+\frac{\sqrt{2\pi}}{\theta_1}\exp\left(\frac{m_Z}{\theta_1}+\frac{\sigma_Z^2}{2\theta_1^2}\right)\Phi\left(\frac{m_Z+\frac{\sigma_Z^2}{\theta_1}}{\sigma_Z}\right)\right]. \tag{9.39}$$

Let us investigate the correction $\Delta R_\tau(\theta_1)$. Find the limit of $\Delta R_\tau(\theta_1)$ as $\theta_1 \to 0^-$. At first, in order to find the limit of the first term $y(\theta_1)$ we apply the L'Hospital rule:

$$\begin{aligned}\lim_{\theta_1\to 0^-} y(\theta_1) &= \lim_{\theta_1\to 0^-}\frac{\sqrt{2\pi}}{\theta_1}\exp\left(\frac{m_Z}{\theta_1}+\frac{\sigma_Z^2}{2\theta_1^2}\right)\Phi\left(\frac{m_Z+\frac{\sigma_Z^2}{\theta_1}}{\sigma_Z}\right)\\ &= -\frac{1}{\sigma_Z}\exp\left(-\frac{m_Z^2}{2\theta_1^2}\right).\end{aligned}$$

Comparing the obtained limit value with the first summand of the formula (9.39), we observe that $\Delta R_\tau(\theta_1)\to 0$ as $\theta_1 \to 0^-$ This fact can be interpreted in the following way: if a mean value of the error tends to zero, then the conditional TTF estimate tends to its theoretical value R_τ. At the same time, as $\theta \to -\infty$ we have $y(\theta_1)\to 0$ and $R_\tau(\theta_1)\to 1$. We arrive at the contradiction: the increasing of the absolute value of a mean error in this case must imply the decreasing of TTF estimate, which in the limit form takes on zero value. The cause of this contradiction is explained by the approximate nature of the formula (9.32), which may be used (we bear in mind the assumptions imposed on it) for the calculation of large probabilities ($R_\tau(\theta_1) \geqslant 0.9$).

Let us find the range of the parameter θ_1 for the possibility of using formulas (9.35) and (9.36). Taking into account the fact that for known m_Z and σ_Z the absolute value of the error ε satisfies the condition $r_\tau(\varepsilon) \geqslant 0.9$, or, using (9.32)

$$\frac{a_Z\tau}{\sigma_Z}\exp\left[-\frac{(\varepsilon+m_Z)^2}{2\sigma_Z^2}\right] \leqslant 0.1.$$

Solving this inequality for the case of intersection of the stochastic process $Z(t)$ with the level $(-\varepsilon)$, we obtain

$$\varepsilon \geqslant -m_Z+\sigma_Z\sqrt{-2\ln\frac{0.1\sigma_Z}{a_Z\tau}} = \varepsilon_*.$$

The limit value for θ_1 we find under the condition that the probability that this inequality holds, coincides in practice with the probability of the certain event, i.e.,

$$\int_{\varepsilon_*}^{0} -\frac{1}{\theta_1}e^{-\varepsilon/\theta_1}\,d\varepsilon = 0.99 \Rightarrow \theta_{1_*} = \frac{\varepsilon_*}{\ln 0.01}.$$

Finally, the interval of the values θ_1, for which the formulas (9.35) and (9.36) may be used, has the form

$$\frac{-m_Z+\sigma_Z\sqrt{-2\ln\frac{0.1\sigma_Z}{a_Z\tau}}}{\ln 0.01} \leqslant \theta_1 \leqslant 0.$$

This condition should be taken into account, when one chooses a prior probability distribution for θ_1. The case of a *Gaussian additive error* is easier. The conditional TTF estimate depends in this case on the parameters ε_0 and σ_ε (the systematic error and mean square value of the error, respectively). For determination of R_τ $(\varepsilon_0,\sigma_\varepsilon)$ we will use not the common expression (9.33), but a more simple argument. Since $R_\tau(\varepsilon_0,\sigma_\varepsilon) = P\{Z(t)+\varepsilon > 0, 0 \leqslant t \leqslant \tau\}$, for the Gaussian distribution of $Z(t)$ and ε their sum has also a Gaussian distribution with the mean value $m_Z+\varepsilon_0$ and correlation function $K_W(\tau) = \sigma_\varepsilon^2 + K_z(\tau)$, where $K_z(\tau)$ is the correlation function of the process $Z(t)$. Repeating the scheme applied for (9.32) for determining the probability $R_\tau(\varepsilon_0,\sigma_\varepsilon) = P\{W(t) > 0, 0 \leqslant t \leqslant \tau\}$, we get

$$R_\tau(\varepsilon_0,\sigma_\varepsilon) = 1-\frac{\alpha_W\tau}{\sigma_W}\exp\left(-\frac{m_W^2}{2\sigma_W^2}\right),$$

where

$$\alpha_W = \frac{1}{2\pi}\sqrt{-\frac{d^2K_W(\tau)}{d\tau^2}\bigg|_{\tau=0}}.$$

It is easy to check that $a_Z = \alpha_W$.Therefore, the resulting expression for $R_\tau(\varepsilon_0, \sigma_\varepsilon)$ is written as

$$R_\tau(\varepsilon_0, \sigma_\varepsilon) = 1 - \frac{a_Z \tau}{\sqrt{\sigma_Z^2 + \sigma_\varepsilon^2}} \exp\left[-\frac{(m_Z + \varepsilon_0)^2}{2(\sigma_Z^2 + \sigma_\varepsilon^2)}\right]. \qquad (9.40)$$

9.3.6 *The method of determination of the numerical characteristics of mz, sz and az*

Here, we use the assumptions (1) and (2). We represent the vector of initial variables **X** as random processes $\xi(t) = \{\xi_1(t), \ldots, \xi_k(t)\}$ and random variables $\zeta = \{\zeta_1, \ldots, \zeta_\ell\}$, $K + L = N$. Let us restrict ourselves to the case when only loadings acting on the system are random processes and physical-mechanical characteristics are independent of time. Analysis of a great number of working capacity conditions imposed on the carrying constructions and mechanical type systems shows that loading factors appear additively in the working capacity function as some generalized loading $S(t) = \alpha_1 \xi_1(t) + \cdots + \alpha_k \xi_k(t)$, where α_j are nonrandom constants. Moreover, any working capacity function may be represented in the form

$$\phi(\xi(t), \zeta) = Q(\zeta) - S(\xi(t)), \qquad (9.41)$$

where Q depends only on physical-mechanical characteristics and geometrical parameters of the system, and is called a *carrying capability.* The theoretical model of the device is reduced, in essence, to the establishment of the dependence $Q(\zeta)$. Let, in accordance with the assumption (2), there be given the numerical characteristics for the vector of initial variables whose order is restricted by the frames of Linear Correlation Theory. For the random vector ζ we are given the mean values m_{ζ_i}, mean square values (standard deviation) σ_{ζ_i} and correlation matrix $\bar{\rho}_\zeta = \rho_{ij}$, $i = 1, 2, \ldots, L$; $j = 1, 2, \ldots, L$. For the vector random process $\xi(t)$ we are given the mean values m_{ξ_i}, and the correlation functions $(K_{ij}(\tau))$, $i = 1, 2, \ldots, K$, where $K_{ii}(\tau) = K_i(\tau)$. The problem of obtaining m_Z, σ_Z and a_Z with the help of the mentioned set of initial data can be solved in the form of the following sequence.

Step 1. We determine a mean value m_Q and mean square value σ_Q of a carrying capability Q. To this end, we apply formulas (9.24) and (9.25) for $\phi = Q$.

Step 2. We determine a mean value m_S and correlation function $K_S(\tau)$ of the generalized loading $S(t)$:

$$m_S = \sum_{i=1}^{K} a_i m_{\xi_i}, \quad K_S(\tau) = \sum_{i=1}^{K} a_i^2 K_i(\tau) + 2 \sum_{1 \leqslant i < j \leqslant K} \sum a_i a_j K_{ij}(\tau) \qquad (9.42)$$

These formulas are given in [200].

Step 3. Using (9.41) we find a mean value $m_Z = m_Q - m_S$ and correlation function $K_z(t)$ of the status variable $Z(t) = Q - S(t)$:

$$K_z(\tau) = \sigma_Q^2 + K_S(\tau). \tag{9.43}$$

The following reasoning gives us the formula (9.43). By the definition of the correlation function we have

$$K_z(\tau) = E\left[(Z(t) - m_Z)(Z(t+\tau) - m_Z)\right] = \left[E\left(Q^\circ - S^\circ(t)\right)\left(Q^\circ - S^\circ(t+\tau)\right)\right],$$

where $Q^\circ = Q - m_Q$ and $S^\circ(t) = S(t) - m_S$. Taking into account the independence of Q and $S(t)$, we obtain

$$K_z(\tau) = E\left[E^{\circ 2}\right] + \left[S^\circ(t)S^\circ(t+\tau)\right] = \sigma_Q^2 + K_S(\tau).$$

The variance of the stochastic process $Z(t)$, by the definition, equals

$$\sigma_Z^2 = K_z(0) = \sigma_Q^2 + K_S(0) = \sigma_Q^2 + \sigma_S^2.$$

Step 4. Starting from the formula (9.31), we find, in view of (9.43),

$$a_z = \frac{1}{2\pi}\sqrt{-K_z''(0)} = \frac{1}{2\pi}\sqrt{-K_S''(0)}.$$

this being the final step of the proposed procedure.

9.4 Bayes estimation of the reliability functions under the lack of experimental data

9.4.1 *General procedure of Bayes estimation*

The essence of Bayes estimating in conformity to the given problem is that we assign to the unknown parameter θ some additive error ε of some prior p.d.f. $h(\theta)$ which characterizes the degree of uncertainty of the information about a model error. For realization of the Bayes procedure of obtaining a TTF estimate we need to have:

a) A prior probability density of the distribution, $h(\theta)$, $\theta \in \Theta$;
b) A functional relation connecting the parameter vector θ and TTF in the form, $R = R(\theta)$;
c) A loss function $L(\hat{R}, R)$ which, in essence, characterizes the losses which appear because of the replacement of the real TTF value by its estimate, $\hat{R}$.

In accordance with the setting of the problem, we are interested in pointwise estimate R^* and Bayes lower confidence limit $\underline{R}_\gamma^*$ of the TTF with a confidence level γ. The pointwise estimate is determined by minimization of the function of the mean prior risk:

$$R^* = \arg\min_{\hat{R}} \int_\Theta L\left(\hat{R}, R(\theta)\right) h(\theta)\, d\theta. \tag{9.44}$$

To obtain E we need to solve the following equation:

$$\int_{\underline{R}_\gamma^* \leqslant R(\theta \leqslant 1)} h(\theta)\, d\theta = \gamma. \tag{9.45}$$

The choice of the loss function $L(R,R)$ will be made in accordance with a rule broadly used in Reliability Theory: overstating of the estimated parameter is worse than its understating. The following loss function, introduced in [217], may be chosen as an example of this rule in the theory of Bayes estimation:

$$L\left(\hat{R},R(\theta)\right) = \begin{cases} K_1\left(\hat{R}-R(\theta)\right)^2, & \text{if } \hat{R} \leqslant R(\theta), \\ K_1\left(\hat{R}-R(\theta)\right)^2 + K_2\left(\hat{R}-R(\theta)\right)^2, & \text{if } \hat{R} > R(\theta). \end{cases} \tag{9.46}$$

The loss function (9.46) is very handy for practical calculations, and possesses several merits. Given relations between the coefficients K_1 and K_2, we can control the degree of overestimating or underestimating the real TTF by $\hat{R}$. For example, with $K_1 = 0$ and $K_2 = 1$, overstating of the TTF estimate of its real value is excluded. With $K_2 = 0$, the loss function (9.46) transforms into a mean square loss function.

With respect to the choice of the prior p.d.f., $h(\theta)$, we must consider three different forms:

a) Prior distributions based on previous empirical data;

b) Subjective prior ones based on the designer's experience;

c) Prior distributions describing a lack of knowledge about the parameter.

Clearly, the first form of a prior distribution is more preferable than the others, since it is based on real data, characterizing existing information about the parameters of error of a theoretical model. However, for a large volume of data about the deviation between the real and theoretical working capacity models, a designer modifies the theoretical model with the help of different empirical coefficients in order to bring it nearer to the real model. After this, the necessity of construction of a prior distribution $h(\theta)$ based on these data drops out. Unfortunately, this situation so desirable is rare.

In most cases, a designer possesses a very small amount of data about the working capacity model error, i.e., such samples with the help of which obtaining a certain estimate of a prior distribution is impossible. However, these data form some of his opinions about a working capacity model which he attempts to express quantitatively, in particular, with the help of a safety coefficient. Namely, this situation makes possible construction of a prior distribution. Let us investigate peculiarities of construction of a prior distribution in the following example with a working capacity condition (9.7). For the sake of convenience of further arguments, we rewrite it in the dimensionless form

$$\left(\frac{T_{\text{cr}}(\mathbf{X})}{A} - \frac{T}{A}\right) + \frac{\varepsilon}{A} > 0,$$

where $A = E\left[T_{\rm cr}(\mathbf{X})\right]$ is a nonrandom value of a mean carrying capability. Throughout what follows we will assume that the general form of a working capacity condition

$$\phi(\mathbf{X}) + \varepsilon > 0$$

has a dimensionless nature, and ε is the relative error of the theoretical model.

Suppose that a designer is convinced that a limit value of a safety coefficient equals η. In accordance with (9.8), the corresponding quantile of the relative estimate is $\varepsilon_p = (\eta-1)/\eta$. Representation of an interval of a prior uncertainty for the safety coefficient in the form $[1,\eta]$ corresponds more closely to a given state of information, in other words, a statement has a less categorical nature: a safety coefficient takes on some value from an interval. The corresponding interval for the quantile ε_p is $E_\varepsilon = \left[-(\eta-1)/\eta, 0\right]$. Now we can use more exact information. A designer has to estimate the chances of an error value having one or other values from the interval E_ε, i.e., he must represent a prior distribution $h(\theta)$ in one of the three forms given in Fig. 9.2. In the first case, we have a uniform prior distribution; in the second one, we prefer to choose such values of the parameter error which are near the limit one, in the third case, we choose values near to the mean. Let us emphasize again that construction of a prior density in the general case is followed by nonformal representations by the designer.

In the considered situation $\eta > 1$, which corresponds to a negative additive error ε, a distribution density (9.14) with the parameter θ_1, having a natural mean error, has been used. Now we can easily pass from $h(\varepsilon_p)$ to $h(\theta_1)$, taking into account a linear dependence between these characteristics:

$$\theta_1 = k\varepsilon_p,$$

in which the coefficient k is determined by the condition

$$\int_{-\varepsilon_p}^{0} f_\varepsilon(\varepsilon;\theta_1)d\varepsilon = p \Rightarrow k = -\frac{1}{\ln(1-p)}.$$

In particular, if $\eta = 1, 2$, and in accordance with it a uniform distribution for ε_p the interval $E_\varepsilon = [-0.01667; 0]$ is chosen, then for $p = 0.99$, θ_1 is distributed uniformly in the interval $E_\theta = [-0.0362; 0]$, i.e., the limit value of a mean relative negative model error equals 3.62%.

A designer who has no information about the characteristic of error may carry out some tests for the construction of a prior distribution during which values of errors $\varepsilon_1, \varepsilon_2, \ldots, \varepsilon_m$ are fixed. Even for a small m, it is possible to find a non biased estimate of a mean error $\hat{\theta}_1$ and choose it as a base value for the construction of a prior density $h(\theta_1)$. We may choose as interval E_ε a confidence interval for θ_1 and determine on it a uniform prior distribution. Note that with such an approach a choice of a prior distribution is formalized and a designer may not approve a strict decision.

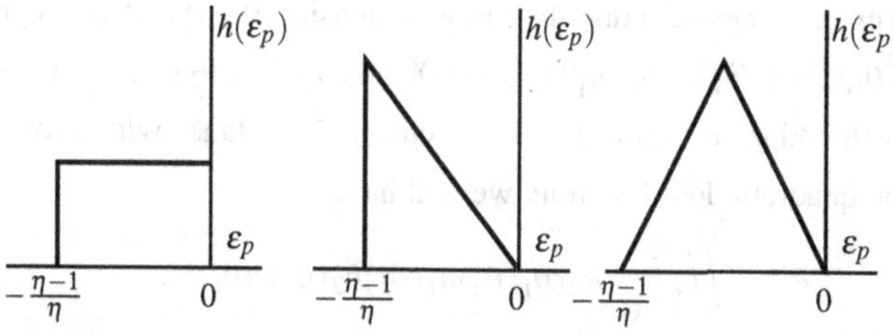

Fig. 9.2 Prior Probability Density of the Quartiles of the Additive Error.

In conclusion of this question, we investigate a possibility of using nonformal (or improper) prior distributions, characterizing a complete lack of knowledge about an error value. For a noninformative prior density the following relation holds [114]:

$$\int_\Theta h(\theta)d\theta = \infty.$$

Investigate a possibility of obtaining a meaningful conclusion about a TTF for the case of a Gaussian additive error with a zero systematic component, when we have only σ_ε as a parameter and conditional TTF estimate has the form (9.23). In accordance with Jeffrey's' approach [114], an absolute lack of information about σ_ε is determined by the p.d.f.

$$h(\sigma_\varepsilon) \sim \frac{1}{\sigma_\varepsilon}, \quad 0 \leqslant \sigma_\varepsilon < \infty.$$

The use of a mean square error loss function in this case gives us the following Bayes TTF estimate:

$$R^* = \frac{\displaystyle\int_0^\infty \phi\left(\frac{m_Z}{\sqrt{\sigma_Z^2+\sigma_\varepsilon^2}}\right)\frac{d\sigma_\varepsilon}{\sigma_\varepsilon}}{\displaystyle\int_0^\infty \frac{d\sigma_\varepsilon}{\sigma_\varepsilon}}.$$

Analysis of this expression shows that the quantity R^* is reduced to the indeterminate form ∞/∞. Consequently, the use of noninformative prior distributions gives us an undetermined inference about the TTF. The conclusion does not mean, however, that improper prior distributions cannot be used for obtaining a meaningful conclusion about the reliability in the presence of experimental data.

9.4.2 *TTF estimates for a fixed time*

Consideration of this question will be carried out separately for the generalized exponential and Gaussian errors of the working capacity model.

Suppose that the error ε obeys the distribution with density (9.13) and given prior distribution densities $h_1(\theta_1)$, $\theta_1 \in \Theta_1 = [\theta_1', \theta_1''] \subset (-\infty, 0]$, and $h_2(\theta_2)$, $\theta_2 \in \Theta_2 = [\theta_2', \theta_2''] \subset [0, \infty)$; it is assumed that θ_1 and θ_2 are a priori independent. In accordance with a common expression (9.44) for the quadratic loss function, we will have

$$R_0^* = \iint_{\Theta_1 \times \Theta_2} R_0(\theta_1, \theta_2) h_1(\theta_1) h_2(\theta_2)\, d\theta_1\, d\theta_2. \tag{9.47}$$

Denote by

$$u = u(x) = \frac{1}{\sigma_Z}\left(m_Z + \frac{\sigma_Z^2}{x}\right) \quad \text{and} \quad v = v(x) = \frac{m_Z}{x} + \frac{\sigma_Z^2}{2x^2}, \tag{9.48}$$

and rewrite integral (9.47) in the form

$$R_0^* = \Phi\left(\frac{m_Z}{\sigma_Z}\right) + \int_{\Theta_1} \theta_1 \Phi(u)(\theta_1) e^{v(\theta_1)} U_1(\theta_1) h_1(\theta_1) d\theta_1$$
$$+ \int_{\Theta_2} \theta_2 [1 - \Phi(u(\theta_2))] e^{v(\theta_2)} U_2(\theta_2) h_2(\theta_2) d\theta_2, \tag{9.49}$$

where

$$U_1(\theta_1) = \int_{\Theta_2} \frac{h_2(\theta_2)}{\theta_2 - \theta_1} d\theta_2 \quad \text{and} \quad U_2(\theta_2) = \int_{\Theta_1} \frac{h_1(\theta_1)}{\theta_2 - \theta_1} d\theta_1\,. \tag{9.50}$$

Formula (9.49) is used in the calculating algorithm. The functions $U_1(\theta_1)$ and $U_2(\theta_2)$ may be easily written with the help of analytical expressions for any prior densities considered earlier. In particular, for the uniform $h_1(\theta_1)$ and $h_2(\theta_2)$ we get

$$U_1(\theta_1) = \ln \frac{\theta_2'' - \theta_1}{\theta_2' - \theta_1} \geqslant 0, \quad \theta_1 \in \Theta_1, \tag{9.51}$$

and

$$U_2(\theta_2) = \ln \frac{\theta_2 - \theta_1'}{\theta_2 - \theta_1''} \geqslant 0, \quad \theta_2 \in \Theta_2, \tag{9.52}$$

the functions $U_1(\theta_1)$ and $U_2(\theta_2)$ vanish, if correspondingly, $h_2(\theta_2)$ and $h_1(\theta_1)$ degenerate. It gives us a zero value of the corresponding term in (9.49).

A procedure of evaluating R_0^* for the loss function (9.46) is more complicated, and may be reduced to the following problem:

$$R^* = \arg\min_{\hat{R}} \iint_{\Theta_1 \times \Theta_2} F\left(\theta_1, \theta_2; \hat{R}\right) d\theta_1\, d\theta_2, \tag{9.53}$$

where

$$F(\theta_1,\theta_2;x)=\begin{cases} K_1\left(x-R_0(\theta_1,\theta_2)\right)^2 h_1(\theta_1)h_2(\theta_2), & x\leqslant R_0(\theta_1,\theta_2),\\ \left[K_1\left(x-R_0(\theta_1,\theta_2)\right)^2\right. & \\ \quad \left.+K_2\left(x-R_0(\theta_1,\theta_2)\right)\right]h_1(\theta_1)h_2(\theta_2), & x>R_0(\theta_1,\theta_2), \end{cases} \tag{9.54}$$

and $R_0(\theta_1,\theta_2)$ is determined by the relation (9.19). We cannot get rid of the double integration in this case. The integration procedure is simplified by the fact that the integration domain $\Theta_1\times\Theta_2$ is a rectangle whose sides are not large.

For evaluating $\underline{R}^*_{0\gamma}$ we don't use the common equation (9.45), since in the given case it gives us a very complicated calculating procedure. Let us apply the following simple arguments. Find values and $\theta_2\in\Theta_2$, such that

$$P\{\theta_1>\underline{\theta}_1,\theta_2>\underline{\theta}_2\}=\int_{\underline{\theta}_1}^{\theta_1''}\int_{\underline{\theta}_2}^{\theta_2''} h_1(\theta_1)h_2\theta_2 d\theta_1 d\theta_2=\gamma \tag{9.55}$$

where γ is a confidence probability. Since $R_0(\theta_1,\theta_2)$ in view of (9.19) is a monotonically increasing function of both arguments, we get

$$P\{R_0(\theta_1,\theta_2)>R_0\left(\underline{\theta}_1,\underline{\theta}_2\right)\}=P\{\theta_1>\underline{\theta}_1,\ \theta_2>\underline{\theta}_2\}.$$

Thus, if the values of $\underline{\theta}_1,\underline{\theta}_2$ are given, the lower Bayes confidence limit $\underline{R}^*_{0\gamma}$ may be determined as

$$\underline{R}^*_{0\gamma}=R_0\left(\underline{\theta}_1,\underline{\theta}_2\right). \tag{9.56}$$

condition (9.55) does not give us a possibility of finding the values $\underline{\theta}_1$ and $\underline{\theta}_2$. Let us assign an equal positive probability for the events $\{\theta_1>\underline{\theta}_1\}$ and $\{\theta_2>\underline{\theta}_2\}$:

$$\int_{\underline{\theta}_1}^{\theta_1''} h_1(\theta_1)d\theta_1=\int_{\underline{\theta}_2}^{\theta_2''} h_2(\theta_2)d\theta_2. \tag{9.57}$$

Having considered (9.55) and (9.57) mutually, we find

$$\int_{\underline{\theta}_1}^{\theta_1''} h_1(\theta_1)d\theta_1=\gamma^{1/2},\quad \int_{\underline{\theta}_2}^{\theta_2''} h_2(\theta_2)d\theta_2=\gamma^{1/2}. \tag{9.58}$$

Finally, we obtain $\underline{\theta}_1$ and $\underline{\theta}_2$ are quantiles of the probability $1-\gamma^{1/2}$ of prior distributions with densities $h_1(\theta_1)$ and $h_2(\theta_2)$ we have the following simple formula for $\underline{\theta}_1$ and $\underline{\theta}_2$:

$$\underline{\theta}_k=\theta_k''-\gamma^{1/2}(\theta_k''-\theta_k'),\quad k=1,2. \tag{9.59}$$

Thus, the procedure for obtaining $\underline{R}^*_{0\gamma}$ is reduced to the calculation of the function (9.19) for the values $\underline{\theta}_1$ and $\underline{\theta}_2$, determined by the relations (9.58), or in the particular case, by (9.59).

For the case of a Gaussian model error ε, all the arguments used above remain valid. We need only to put $\theta_1=\varepsilon_0$ and $\theta_2=\sigma_\varepsilon$, and instead of $R_0(\theta_1,\theta_2)$ one should use $R_0\left(\varepsilon_0,\sigma_\varepsilon\right)$, determined by the formula (9.22). In all further reasoning, we have a similar picture. Therefore, we restrict ourselves only to the consideration of the first model of additive error ε.

9.4.3 *TTF estimates during the time τ*

Here all assumptions with respect to a prior density $h(\theta_1,\theta_2)=h_1(\theta_1)h_2(\theta_2)$, $\theta_1\in\Theta_1$, $\theta_2\in\Theta_2$ remain in force. The expression for the pointwise TTF estimate R_γ^* will be written in accordance with a common approach (9.44) for the conditional TTF estimate of the form (9.35). Under the assumption of a mean square error loss function, we have,

$$R_\gamma^*=1-\sqrt{2\pi}a_Z\tau\iint\limits_{\Theta_1\times\Theta_2}\left\{\Phi(u(\theta_1))\mathrm{e}^{\nu(\theta_1)}+[1-\Phi(u(\theta_2))]\right\}\frac{h_1(\theta_1)h_2(\theta_2)}{\theta_2-\theta_1}d\theta_1 d\theta_2. \quad (9.60)$$

The use of the functions $U_1(\theta_1)$ and $U_2(\theta_2)$, introduced by the expression (9.50), lets us write R_γ^* with the help of a one-dimensional integral

$$R_\gamma^*=1-\sqrt{2\pi}a_Z\tau\left\{\int_{\Theta_1}\Phi(u(\theta_1))\mathrm{e}^{\nu(\theta_1)}h_1(\theta_1)U_1(\theta_1)\,d\theta_1\right.$$
$$\left.+\int_{\Theta_2}\Phi(u(\theta_2))\mathrm{e}^{\nu(\theta_2)}h_2(\theta_2)U_2(\theta_2)d\theta_2\right\}. \quad (9.61)$$

Taking into account the smallness of the domains Θ_1 and Θ_2 we can obtain an approximate formula. To this end, we use the following approximation:

$$F(\theta_1,\theta_2)=\frac{1}{\theta_2\theta_1}\left\{\Phi(u(\theta_1))\mathrm{e}^{\nu(\theta_1)}+[1-\Phi(u(\theta_2))]\,\mathrm{e}^{\nu(\theta_2)}\right\}$$
$$\cong F(\theta_{10},\theta_{20})+F'_{\theta_1}(\theta_{10},\theta_{20})(\theta_1-\theta_{10})+F(\theta_{10},\theta_{20})+F'_{\theta_2}(\theta_{10},\theta_{20})(\theta_2-\theta_{20}),$$

where θ_{i0} is a prior mean value of the parameter θ_i. With the help of it we will write

$$R_\gamma^*\cong 1-\frac{\sqrt{2\pi}a_Z\tau}{\theta_{20}-\theta_{10}}\left\{\Phi(u(\theta_1))\mathrm{e}^{\nu(\theta_1)}+[1-\Phi(u(\theta_{20}))]\,\mathrm{e}^{\nu(\theta_{20})}\right\}. \quad (9.62)$$

We may conclude, taking into account the form of the expression (9.62), that the obtained approximate estimate depends on prior mean values θ_{10} and θ_{20} of the parameters θ_1 and θ_2, respectively. Formula (9.62), as well as a pointwise expression (9.61), has a correct interpretation: $|\theta_{10}|\uparrow\to R_\gamma^*\downarrow$, $\theta_{20}\uparrow\to R_\gamma^*\uparrow$.

For the loss function of the form (9.46), the procedure of estimation of a TTF will be more complicated:

$$R_\gamma^*=\arg\min_{\hat{R}}\iint_{\Theta_1\times\Theta_2}Y\left(\theta_1,\theta_2;\hat{R}\right)d\theta_1 d\theta_2,$$

where

$$Y(\theta_1,\theta_2;y)=\begin{cases}K_1\left[y-R_\tau(\theta_1,\theta_2)\right]^2h_1(\theta_1)h_2(\theta_2), & y\leqslant R_\tau(\theta_1,\theta_2),\\ \left[K_1\left(y-R_\tau(\theta_1,\theta_2)\right)^2\right.\\ \quad\left.+K_2\left(y-R_\tau(\theta_1,\theta_2)\right)\right]h_1(\theta_1)h_2(\theta_2), & y>R_\tau(\theta_1,\theta_2).\end{cases}$$

For obtaining a lower Bayes confidence TTF limit, we use the approach of 9.4.2. In accordance with it,

$$\underline{R}_{\tau\gamma}^*=R_\tau\left(\underline{\theta}_1,\underline{\theta}_2\right),$$

where $\underline{\theta}_1$ and $\underline{\theta}_2$ are determined by the expressions (9.58), and for the case of uniform prior distributions, by the finite formula (9.59).

9.4.4 *Bayes TTF estimates considering uncertainty of the initial data*

As follows from the expressions given in 9.4.2, the Bayes TTF estimates for the fixed moment of time depend on m_Z and σ_Z, which are parameters of the distribution of the status variable Z, and are determined by the set of numerical characteristics K_X of the vector of initial variables $\mathbf{X}$ by the formulas (9.24) and (9.25). In practice we often deal with the initial data which include the element of uncertainty. In particular, if in the frames of Linear Correlation Theory, K_X consists of mean values of the initial variables (characterizing nominal values), mean squared values (characterizing scatterings) and correlation coefficients (characterizing relationships among the variables), then with respect to the last ones we are given, as a rule, very approximate values. For example, we may often only as certain that a correlation coefficient is positive, and there is no additional information. An analogous situation may take place also for the scattering characteristics. Intervals of uncertainty $\mathcal{K}_i$ with prior distributions $h(K_i)$ on them may be considered as adequate forms of representation of indicated initial data. Moreover, $h(K_i)$ are, as a rule, prior densities. If the value of some parameter K_k is determined uniquely and equals $K_k^{(0)}$, then we choose for it a prior probability density in the form of a delta-function $h_k(K_k) = \delta\left(K_k + K_k^{(0)}\right)$; the interval $\mathcal{K}_k$ degenerates into a point $K_k^{(0)}$. Thus, the form of representation of the set K_X with the help of prior distributions is common for the strictly determined and undetermined initial data. Below we present a method which takes into account the uncertainty of initial data during the estimating of the TTF with respect to the working capacity model with additive error. Expressions obtained in 9.4.2 for the Bayes estimate of a TTF depend on mean value m_Z and mean squared value $\sigma_Z : R_0 = R_0(m_Z, \sigma_Z)$. In turn, by the formulas (9.24) and (9.25) we have

$$m_Z = p(K_X) \text{ and } \sigma_Z = q(K_X) \tag{9.63}$$

We will assume that a prior density $h_i(K_i)$ is given for each numerical characteristic $K_i \in \mathcal{K}_i$. In practical situations, for the intervals $\mathcal{K}_i$ not degenerating into a point, we may assume that prior densities $h_i(K_i)$ are uniform. We will suppose also that K_i are mutually independent, i.e,

$$h(K_X) = \prod_{i=1}^{m} h_i(K_i), \quad K_X \in \mathcal{K} = \mathcal{K}_1 \times \mathcal{K}_2 \times \cdots \times \mathcal{K}_m. \tag{9.64}$$

Under the above assumptions, we can formulate the problem of finding the Bayes estimate of R_0^{**}, optimal in the sense of minimum of prior risk (the second asterisk appears due to the repeated optimality over the domain $\mathcal{K}$), i.e., the problem is to find the estimate of R_0^{**}

guaranteeing the minimum of a prior risk

$$G\left(\hat{R}_0\right) = \int_k L\left(\hat{R}_0, R_0^*\left(p(K_X), q(K_X)\right) h(K_X)\right) dK_X \tag{9.65}$$

for the given prior density $h(K_X)$ and a loss function ℓ. In (9.64) one uses a mean square error loss function, then

$$R_0^{**} = \int_k R_0^*\left(p(K_X), q(K_X)\right) h(K_X) dK_X. \tag{9.66}$$

Since we have to carry out multiple integrations, the use of (9.66) in practical calculations is almost impossible. Simplification may be achieved, if we pass, starting from $h(K_X)$ and transformations of $p(K_X)$ and $q(K_X)$, to the prior density for m_Z and σ_Z.This problem may be solved approximately in the following way.

Due to the small length of the intervals K_i $(i = 1, 2, \ldots, m)$, we represent $p(K_X)$ and $q(K_X)$ with the help of linear portions of the Taylor series

$$m_Z = p(K_X) \cong p\left(K_X^{(0)}\right) + \sum_{i=1}^{m} p_i'\left(K_X^{(0)}\right)\left(K_i - K_i^{(0)}\right);$$

and

$$\sigma_Z = q(K_X) \cong q\left(K_X^{(0)}\right) + \sum_{i=1}^{m} q_i'\left(K_X^{(0)}\right)\left(K_i - K_i^{(0)}\right).$$

Thereafter, we find the mean values $m_Z^{(0)}$, $\sigma_Z^{(0)}$ and variances s_m^2, s_σ^2 of the parameters m_Z and σ_Z, respectively:

$$m_Z^{(0)} = p\left(K_X^{(0)}\right), \quad \sigma_Z^{(0)} = q\left(K_X^{(0)}\right), \tag{9.67}$$

and

$$s_m^2 = \sum_{i=1}^{m} p_i'\left(K_X^{(0)}\right)\sigma_{K_i}^2, \quad s_\sigma^2 = \sum_{i=1}^{m} q_i'\left(K_X^{(0)}\right)\sigma_{K_i}^2, \tag{9.68}$$

where

$$K_i^{(0)} = \int_{K_i} K_i h_i(K_i) dK_i \ \text{ and } \ \sigma_{K_i}^2 = \int K_i^2 h_i(K_i) dK_i - K_i^{(0)2}.$$

Next we approximate the prior densities $h_m(m_Z)$ and $h_\sigma(\sigma_Z)$ of the parameters m_Z and σ_Z, respectively, by some two-parametric family. For a large dimension of K_z, taking into account the statement of a central limit theorem, we may use a normal approximation for $h_m(m_Z)$ and $h_\sigma(\sigma_Z)$. Such an approach enables us to use instead of m-dimensional integral (9.66) a two-dimensional integral for obtaining R_0^{**}:

$$R_0^{**} = \int_{-\infty}^{\infty}\int_0^{\infty} R_0^*(m_Z, \sigma_Z) h_m(m_Z) h_\sigma(\sigma_Z) dm_Z d\sigma_Z \tag{9.69}$$

Finally, instead of integral (9.69), we can use its estimate obtained after the approximation of $R_0^*(m_Z, \sigma_Z)$ under the integral sign by the portion of the Taylor series up to the second order terms, inclusively:

$$R_0^{**} \cong R_0^*\left(m_Z^{(0)}, \sigma_Z^{(0)}\right) + a_2 s_m^2 + b_2 s_\sigma^2,$$

where

$$a_2 = \frac{\partial^2 R_0^*\left(m_Z^{(0)}, \sigma_Z^{(0)}\right)}{\partial m_Z^{(0)2}} \quad \text{and} \quad b_2 = \frac{\partial^2 R_0^*\left(m_Z^{(0)}, \sigma_Z^{(0)}\right)}{\partial \sigma_Z^{(0)2}}.$$

9.4.5 *A numerical example*

For the numerical example we choose an element important for the working capacity of different mechanical and hydraulic transmitters: a spiral cylindrical ring. Assume that a central static force T (expanding or contracting) acts on the ring. The cross section of the ring works on torsion, where the maximal tangent tension is computed by the formula

$$T_{\max} = \frac{M_k}{W_k},$$

where M_k is a torsion moment, W_k is a moment of resistance of the ring to a torsion. For M_k in [23] is proposed the following formula:

$$M_k = \frac{kTD}{2},$$

in which D is a mean diameter of the ring, k is a coefficient depending on the curvature of the ring loops and form of the cross-section. From this point on we will assume that the ring is made of a round wire with the index $c = D/d$ (d is the wire diameter) which is greater than 4. In this case, for the correction coefficient we recommend [23] the following dependence:

$$k = \frac{4c-1}{4c+1} + \frac{0.615}{c}.$$

Taking into account the above arguments, we rewrite the working capacity condition in the form

$$\phi(T, \tau_T, D, d) = \tau_T - \tau_{\max}(T, d, D) > 0, \tag{9.70}$$

where τ_T is a fluctuation limit of the material, and $\tau_{\max}$ is computed by the formula

$$\tau_{\max} = \frac{8}{\pi} T\left(\frac{4D-d}{4D+d} \cdot \frac{D}{d^3} + 0.615 \cdot \frac{1}{d^2}\right).$$

As seen from the represented working capacity model, the vector of initial variables $\mathbf{X}$ is composed of the following random variables: T, τ_T, D, d.

Table 9.1 Numerical Characteristics for the TTF Calculation

X_i	$T,\ H$	$\tau_T,\ H/m^2$	$D,\ m$	$d,\ m$
m_i	$0.5\cdot 10^3$	$0.95\cdot 10^9$	$4\cdot 10^{-2}$	$4\cdot 10^{-3}$
σ_i	10	$0.95\cdot 10^7$	10^{-3}	$0.667\cdot 10^{-4}$

For the sake of simplicity of calculations, we pass the dimensionless analog of the working capacity condition (9.70). To this end, we divide all terms of the inequality (9.70) by the number $A = E\left[\tau_T\right]$. This gives the following relation for the status variable:

$$Z = \frac{\tau_T}{A} - \frac{\tau_{\max}\left(T, d, D\right)}{A}.$$

All further calculations will be carried out in accordance with 9.4.1 and 9.4.2. As a ring material the steel 50XBA has been chosen. The numerical characteristics for the TTF calculation (the set K_X are given in Table 9.1). With the help of these data and formulas (9.24) and (9.25) we obtain $\rho_{ij} = 0$, $m_Z = 1.488\cdot 10^{-1}$ and $\sigma_Z = 0.5109\cdot 10^{-1}$. If the ring TTF is computed by only a theoretical model, the TTF value equals $R = 0.9982$.

Let us now find the Bayes estimate taking into account the model error. Suppose we know a priori that the additive model error leads us to overstate the carrying capability of the ring. This corresponds to the calculation case with a negative additive error. The distribution density has the form (9.14) in which the parameter θ has the sense of a mean value of the error. Let us find the segment of a prior uncertainty for θ. Assuming that under the static loading one uses the safety coefficient $\eta = 1.3$ [23], we determine the limit value of the additive error $\varepsilon_p = -(\eta - 1)/\eta = -0.23$. With the help of recommendations given in 9.4.1, we find the limit value of the mean error (with $p = 0.99$):

$$\theta_\pi = -\frac{\varepsilon_p}{\ln(1-p)} \approx -0.05.$$

Taking into account a hypothetical experience, we choose as an interval of a prior uncertainty $E_\theta = [-0.05; -0.01]$ and will assume that θ has a normal distribution in E_θ. This distribution corresponds to the situation when a designer supposes that the mean model error lies in the limits from -5% to -1%, and cannot give a preference to some value from this interval. Having chosen a mean square error loss function, we define a pointwise TTF estimate by the formula (9.49) with $\theta_1 = \theta$ and $\theta_2 = 0$. This yields $R_0^* = 0.9778$.

Such an essential decreasing of the TTF estimate in comparison with a theoretical one may be explained by the fact that the assumption of a theoretical working capacity model always overstates the real carrying capability. In Fig. 9.3 we represent the dependence of a prior

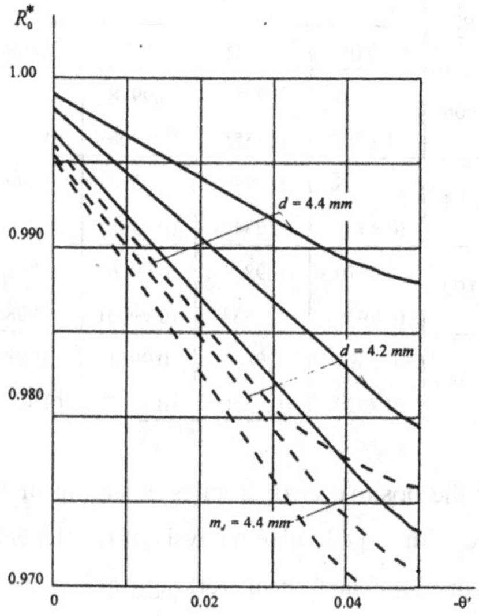

Fig. 9.3 The Estimate of TTF as Function of the Limiting Value of the Mean Error: Solid (Dashed) Line Without (With) Error in the Numerical Characteristics

TTF estimate on the left limit θ' of the uncertainty interval for θ as $\theta'' = 0$ and different values of a mean of the wire diameter d. As seen from Figure 9.3, while the absolute value of θ' increases, a TTF estimate decreases. At the same time, by increasing the diameter of the wire we may ensure the desired TTF value. In the same figure we denote by dotted lines TTF estimates which touch upon uncertainty of the initial data. Carrying out the calculation, we assume that the mean value of the loading m_T and its scattering σ_T have a symmetric 10% uncertainty interval. It may be observed that a TTF estimate decreases because of its uncertainty.

For the values of numerical characteristics of the theoretical status variable $m_Z = 0.1448$ and $\sigma_Z = 0.05109$, one has carried out a lot of numerical calculations of prior TTF estimates for different intervals of a prior uncertainty $\Theta_1 = [\theta_1', \theta_1'']$ and $\Theta_2 = [\theta_2', \theta_2'']$. In Table 9.2 we present the results of calculations of TTF estimates R_0^* and $\underline{R}_{0\gamma}^*$, corresponding to the case $\theta_1'' = \theta_2' = 0$ for different values θ_1' and θ_2'' (values of $\underline{R}_{0\gamma}^*$ are given in the round brackets). As can be seen from the table, enlarging of the prior uncertainty interval for the negative error implies decreasing of the Bayes TTF estimate. At the same time, enlarging of the

Table 9.2 A prior estimate for TTF with $\theta_1'' = \theta_2' = 0$.

θ_2''	θ_1'			
	−0.06	−0.04	−0.02	0.00
0.06	0.9746 (0.8948)	0.9904 (0.9555)	0.9978 (0.9908)	0.9993 (0.9987)
0.04	0.9715 (0.8948)	0.9889 (0.9544)	0.9974 (0.9904)	0.9991 (0.9986)
0.02	0.9670 (0.8930)	0.9867 (0.9533)	0.9966 (0.9900)	0.9988 (0.9984)
0.00	0.9599 (0.8920)	0.9826 (0.9526)	0.9951 (0.9867)	0.9982 (0.9982)

uncertainty interval for the positive error implies enlarging of the Bayes TTF estimate. These conclusions agree with a qualitative analysis of the dependence of the TTF on the value and sign of the error of the theoretical working capacity model.

Chapter 10

Statistical Reliability Analysis Posterior Bayes Estimates

10.1 The likelihood function for independent trials

This chapter is a continuation of Chapter 9, generalizing the results in the case of a posterior estimation when experimental data about the parameters of the tested system are known. When we project and build technical devices, it is customary that two types of testing are carried out: functional and exploratory ones. The purpose of the researches of the first type is to establish factual levels of the functional capability of the system with the help of tests in laboratories or on test benches. With the help of the second type of tests, one verifies a model's working capacity under the exploitation conditions or under the conditions which are similar to them. In the problem considered below, we unite both such results in order to define more exactly the errors of the working capacity model and the time to failure probability. The solution of this problem follows the general scheme of the Bayes statistical estimation including the definition of a likelihood function, construction of a posterior distribution, and the obtaining of a corresponding estimate starting with a chosen loss function. At the end of this chapter we shall give some examples of using the proposed procedures of a Bayes posterior estimation for the solution of some applied problems.

10.1.1 *A likelihood function from the results of research tests*

The essence of research tests is that each test is carried out until a failure occurs; as a result, we find a real level of an object's functional capability. If one carries out tests under loading which increases constantly, then a loading value causing a failure is chosen as a real value of a functional capability.

Let us return to the example considered in § 9.1. We are reminded that the purpose of research tests is to obtain empirical information, which helps us to correct Euler's formula (9.3). Suppose that the first element put to testing has an elasticity module E_1, length ℓ_1, and moment of inertia J_1. The loading which implies a failure will be denoted by T_1^*. The value T is a factual level of a carrying capability for the first test. At the same time, a theoretical value of a carrying capability is defined by the formula (9.3) and equals

$$T_{cr1} = \frac{\pi^2 E_1 J_1}{\mu^2 \ell_1^2}.$$

Clearly, the difference $T_1^* - T_{cr1}$ determines the error of the Euler formula for the first test. If we use a relative additive error e and generalized working capacity model of the form (9.5), then the fact of the appearance of a failure during the first test is written formally in the following way:

$$\frac{T_{cr1}}{A} - \frac{T_1^*}{A} + \varepsilon = 0,$$

where $A = E\left[T_{cr}\right]$, and an experimental value of the relative additive error ε in the first test is determined uniquely by this expression, i.e., $\varepsilon_1 = -\left(T_{cr1} - T_1^*\right)/A$. Analogously, we can determine the value ε_j for each research test.

In a common case for the generalized working capacity model of the form $\phi(\mathbf{X}) + \varepsilon > 0$, the value of the additive error is determined by the expression

$$\varepsilon_j = -\phi\left(\mathbf{x}_j\right), \tag{10.1}$$

where x_j is a realization of the vector of initial variables which is fixed in the j-th test. If we obtain x_j by the scheme of independent tests, and a random variable of the additive error ε obeys a probability distribution with a density $f_\varepsilon(\varepsilon;\theta)$, then the likelihood function (in accordance with [123]) has the form

$$\ell_i(\theta \mid \underset{\sim}{\varepsilon}) = \prod_{j=1}^{n_i} f\left(\varepsilon_j;\theta\right), \tag{10.2}$$

where $\underset{\sim}{\varepsilon}$ is the set of all values ε_j $(j = 1, 2, \ldots, n_i)$. Let us write the resulting expressions of two calculating cases introduced in § 9.3.

The case of a generalized exponential error:

$$\ell_i(\theta_1, \theta_2 \mid \underset{\sim}{\varepsilon}) = \frac{1}{\left(\theta_2 - \theta_1\right)^{n_i}} \exp\left[-\left(\frac{\omega_1}{\theta_1} + \frac{\omega_2}{\theta_2}\right)\right]. \tag{10.3}$$

Here the statistics ω_1 and ω_2 are computed by the formulas

$$\omega_1 = \sum_{i=1}^{k_i} \xi_i, \quad \omega_2 = \sum_{i=1}^{\ell_i} \zeta_i,$$

and the sets $(\xi_1, \xi_2, \ldots, \xi_{k_i})$ and $(\zeta_1, \zeta_2, \ldots, \zeta_{\ell_i})$ are generated respectively by negative and positive elements of the sample $\underset{\sim}{\varepsilon}$, where $k_i + \ell_i = n_i$.

Table 10.1 Bayes Estimators for TTF.

Empirical Information	Result of j-th Test		
	A_1	A_2	A_3
Qualitative Information	$W_j > 0$	$W_j = 0$	$W_j < 0$
Quantitative Information Based on the Theoretical Model	$z'_j = \varphi(x_j)$	$z^*_j = \varphi(x_j)$	$z''_j = \varphi(x_j)$
Quantitative Information for the Additive Error	$\varepsilon_j > -z'_j$	$\varepsilon_j = -z^*_j$	$\varepsilon_j < -z''_j$

The case of a Gaussian error without a systematic bias:

$$\ell_i(\sigma_\varepsilon \mid \underset{\sim}{\varepsilon}) = \frac{1}{(2\pi)^{n_i/2}\sigma_\varepsilon^{n_i}} \exp\left(-\frac{s^2}{2\sigma_\varepsilon^2}\right), \tag{10.4}$$

where

$$s^2 = \sum_{j=1}^{n_i} \varepsilon_j^2.$$

10.1.2 *A likelihood function from the results of functional tests*

A distinctive peculiarity of functional tests is that they are carried out under conditions coinciding with the exploitation conditions or ones similar to them. Because of this circumstance, we cannot, as a rule, fix a failure fact. Therefore, during each test only one of the following three events may be observed: A_1 is a working capacity of the device, A_2 is a failure, A_3 and is a nonworking state of the device. Note that events A_3 and A_2 do not coincide. The failure is observed only when the loading takes on a value equal to a functional capability (in this case the generalized status variable W takes on value zero). At the same time, a nonworking state corresponds to the situation under which the loading is higher than a functional capability; a generalized status variable will be negative in this case.

Assume that in the j-th test some realization of the vector of initial variables x_j ($j = 1, 2, \ldots, n$) is fixed. Each element from x_j can be measured in the tests or its value is assumed to be equal to the calculating one. It enables us (in accordance with a chosen working capacity model) to find the value of Z. For empirical value of a theoretical status variable for each of the three possible outcomes of the test we will denote A_1 by z'_j ($j = 1, 2, \ldots, r$), A_2 by z^*_j ($j = 1, 2, \ldots, d$) and A_3 by z''_j ($j = 1, 2, \ldots, s$). This data gives us quantitative information about the value of an additive error ε for each test. Suppose that during the j-th test a working capacity (event A_1) is observed, i.e., a generalized state variable $W_j > 0$. Since $W = Z + \varepsilon$, from the condition $W_j > 0$ we have $\varepsilon_j > -z'_j$. A complete description of all test outcomes is given in Table 10.1. The results of the functional tests will be represented in the form of the set $\underset{\sim}{z}$, including $\underset{\sim}{z}' = (z_1', z_2', \ldots, z_r')$, $\underset{\sim}{z}^* = (z_1^*, z_2^*, \ldots, z_d^*)$, and $\underset{\sim}{z}'' = (z_1'', z_2'', \ldots, z_S'')$. If one considers these tests as experimental findings of the additive error ε, then the vector $\underset{\sim}{z}$ may be interpreted as censored from the left and right sample of a random variable ε. When a distribution density $f_\varepsilon(\varepsilon;\theta)$ is given, we represent the likelihood function for the sample in accordance with [123] in the following way:

$$\ell_\Phi(\theta \mid \underset{\sim}{\varepsilon z}) = \prod_{j=1}^{r} \int_{-z_j'}^{\infty} f_\varepsilon(\varepsilon;\theta)d\varepsilon \prod_{j=1}^{d} f_\varepsilon(-z_j^*;\theta) \prod_{j=1}^{s} \int_{-\infty}^{-z_j''} f_\varepsilon(\varepsilon;\theta)d\varepsilon,$$

or

$$\ell_\Phi(\theta \mid \underset{\sim}{\varepsilon z}) = \prod_{j=1}^{r} \int_{-z_j'}^{\infty} [1 - F_\varepsilon(-z_j';\theta)] \prod_{j=1}^{d} f_\varepsilon(-z_j^*;\theta) \prod_{j=1}^{s} F_\varepsilon(-z_j'';\theta), \tag{10.5}$$

where $F_\varepsilon(\varepsilon;\theta)$ is the cumulative distribution function, corresponding to $f_\varepsilon(\varepsilon;\theta)$.

A *likelihood function for calculating the case of the generalized exponential error.* The expression for the p.d.f. $f_\varepsilon(\varepsilon;\theta)$ was written earlier in the form (9.13). Then the corresponding distribution function may be written in the following way:

$$F_\varepsilon(\varepsilon;\theta_1,\theta_2) = \begin{cases} -\dfrac{\theta_1}{\theta_2-\theta_1}\exp\left(-\dfrac{\varepsilon}{\theta_1}\right), & \varepsilon < 0, \\ 1 - \dfrac{\theta_2}{\theta_2-\theta_1}\exp\left(-\dfrac{\varepsilon}{\theta_2}\right), & \varepsilon \geqslant 0. \end{cases} \tag{10.6}$$

Represent each of the vectors, $\underset{\sim}{z}'$, $\underset{\sim}{z}^*$, $\underset{\sim}{z}''$ as a union of two vectors consisting of negative and nonnegative components: $\underset{\sim}{z}' = \{\xi', \zeta'\}$, $\underset{\sim}{z}^* = \{\xi^*, \zeta^*\}$, $\underset{\sim}{z}'' = \{\xi'', \zeta''\}$. Dimensions of components of new vectors we denote respectively by r_- and r_+ for $\underset{\sim}{\xi}'$ and $\underset{\sim}{\zeta}'$, d_- and d_+ for $\underset{\sim}{\xi}^*$ and $\underset{\sim}{\zeta}^*$, s_- and s_+ for $\underset{\sim}{\xi}''$ and $\underset{\sim}{\zeta}''$. Clearly, the sample $\underset{\sim}{\xi} = (\underset{\sim}{\xi}', \underset{\sim}{\xi}^*, \underset{\sim}{\xi}'')$ has the dimension $m_- = r_- + d_- + s_-$, and the sample $\underset{\sim}{\zeta} = (\underset{\sim}{\zeta}', \underset{\sim}{\zeta}^*, \underset{\sim}{\zeta}'')$ the dimension $m_+ = r_+ + d_+ + s_+$. The likelihood function (10.5) transforms to:

$$\ell_\Phi(\theta_1,\theta_2 \mid \underset{\sim}{z}) = Q(\theta_1,\theta_2;d,r_-,s_+)P(\theta_1,\theta_2;\omega_1,\omega_2)R_+(\theta_1,\theta_2;\underset{\sim}{\zeta}')S_-(\theta_1,\theta_2;\underset{\sim}{\xi}'') \tag{10.7}$$

$$Q(\theta_1,\theta_2;d,r_-,s_+) = \frac{|\theta_1|^{s_+}\theta_2^{r_-}}{(\theta_2-\theta_1)^{d+r_-+s_+}}, \tag{10.8}$$

$$P(\theta_1,\theta_2;\omega_1,\omega_2) = \exp\left(\frac{\omega_1}{\theta_1} + \frac{\omega_2}{\theta_2}\right) \tag{10.9}$$

$$\omega_1 = \sum_{j=1}^{d_+} \zeta_j^* + \sum_{j=1}^{s_+} \zeta_j'', \quad \omega_2 = \sum_{j=1}^{d_-} \xi_j^* + \sum_{j=1}^{r_-} \xi_j',$$

$$R_+\left(\theta_1,\theta_2;\zeta'\right) = \prod_{j=1}^{r_+}\left[1+\frac{\theta_1}{\theta_2-\theta_1}\exp\left(\frac{\zeta_j'}{\theta_1}\right)\right], \tag{10.10}$$

and

$$S_-\left(\theta_1,\theta_2;\underset{\sim}{\xi}''\right) = \prod_{j=1}^{s}\left[1-\frac{\theta_2}{\theta_2-\theta_1}\exp\left(\frac{\xi_j''}{\theta_2}\right)\right]. \tag{10.11}$$

Note one interesting peculiarity of the obtained likelihood function. To this end, we consider a particular case of a generalized exponential error for which $02 = 0$, thus $e < 0$. The distribution function (10.6) in this case has the form

$$F_\varepsilon(\varepsilon;\theta_1,0) = \begin{cases} \exp\left(-\dfrac{\varepsilon}{\theta_1}\right), & \varepsilon < 0, \\ 1, & \varepsilon \geqslant 0. \end{cases} \tag{10.12}$$

If the assumption $\varepsilon < 0$ is true, then the values z_j' and z_j^* observed during the test must be always nonnegative. Since $W = Z+\varepsilon$ and $W > 0$, as $\varepsilon \leqslant 0$, we obtain $z_j' > 0$. Analogously, as $W = 0$ and $\varepsilon \leqslant 0$, we obtain $z_j^* \geqslant 0$. For the nonworking state ($W = 0$) the values z_j'' may be either negative or positive. But for the negative values z_j'', in accordance with (10.12), we have, $F_\varepsilon(-z_j'';\theta_1,0) = 1$, i.e., negative values z_j'' for the likelihood function will not be noninformative. The conclusion we have made has an evident explanation. If $\varepsilon \leqslant 0$, i.e., a theoretical model overstates the real functional capability, then for $Z < 0$ always $W < 0$. Thus, even if we don't carry out tests, we can write the great number of negative values z_j'' and ascertain that for all these values in the tests the nonworking states of the system will be realized. In other words, without tests we would find their outcomes and use them in the likelihood function. However, this has not occurred, since under the condition $F_\varepsilon(-z_j'';\theta_1,0) = 1$ for all $z_j'' < 0$, the likelihood function doesn't react on the negative values z. This wonderful property of the considered Bayes procedure emphasizes its validity.

A likelihood function for the Gaussian error without a systematic bias. Here we assume that a theoretical status variable may take on positive or negative values. The resulting expression for the likelihood function has the form

$$\ell_\Phi(\sigma_\varepsilon \mid \underset{\sim}{\varepsilon z}) = \frac{1}{(2\pi)^{d/2}}\cdot\frac{1}{\sigma_\varepsilon^d}\exp\left(-\frac{\omega^{*2}}{2\sigma_\varepsilon^2}\right)\prod_{j=1}^{s}\left[1-\Phi\left(\frac{z_j''}{\sigma_\varepsilon}\right)\right]\prod_{j=1}^{r}\Phi\left(\frac{z_j'}{\sigma_\varepsilon}\right), \tag{10.13}$$

where $\omega^{*2} = \sum_{j=1}^{d} z_j^{*2}$.

10.2 The posterior distribution of the error parameters of a theoretical working capacity model

In the general case the posterior distribution of the vector θ is determined with the help of the Bayes theorem. In this section we investigate in detail different questions in obtaining the interesting posterior distributions from a practical point-of-view. We consider separately densities $\hbar_i(\theta \mid \underset{\sim}{\varepsilon})$ and $\hbar_\Phi(\theta \mid \underset{\sim}{z})$ which characterize, respectively, research and theoretical tests, and also the density of the distribution $\hbar(\theta \mid \underset{\sim}{\varepsilon}, \underset{\sim}{z})$ corresponding to the set of tests of both types. In addition to this, we investigate the possibility of using improper prior Jeffrey's distributions. The discrete form of representation of prior and posterior distributions will be considered separately.

A **posterior distribution of the parameters of error ε for research tests.** In accordance with the Bayes theorem,

$$\hbar_i(\theta \mid \underset{\sim}{\varepsilon}) \sim h_i(\theta)\ell_i(\theta \mid \underset{\sim}{\varepsilon}). \tag{10.14}$$

For calculating case of a generalized exponential error ε with a likelihood function (10.3), a posterior density in accordance with (10.14) is written in the following way:

$$\hbar_i(\theta_1, \theta_2 \mid \underset{\sim}{\varepsilon}) = \frac{1}{\beta_i} \cdot \frac{h_1(\theta_1)h_2(\theta_2)}{(\theta_2 - \theta_1)^{n_i}} \exp\left[-\left(\frac{\omega_1}{\theta_1} + \frac{\omega_2}{\theta_2}\right)\right], \quad \theta_1 \in \Theta_1, \quad \theta_2 \in \Theta_2, \tag{10.15}$$

where the normalizing factor β_i is determined by the integral

$$\beta_i = \frac{h_1(\theta_1)h_2(\theta_2)}{(\theta_2 - \theta_1)^{n_i}} \exp\left[-\left(\frac{\omega_1}{\theta_1} + \frac{\omega_2}{\theta_2}\right)\right] d\theta_1 d\theta_2. \tag{10.16}$$

For evaluation of (10.18), we need to apply numerical methods even in the case of uniform prior $h_1(\theta_1)$ and $h_2(\theta_2)$.

Consider a possibility of using improper prior $h_1(\theta_1)$ and $h_2(\theta_2)$ for obtaining $\hbar_i(\theta_1, \theta_2 \mid \underset{\sim}{\varepsilon})$. Taking into account Jeffrey's theory [114], we conclude the following prior densities correspond to the absence of information about the parameters θ_1 and θ_2:

$$h_1(\theta_1) \sim \frac{1}{\theta_1}, \quad \theta_1 \in (-\infty, 0], \quad h_2(\theta_2) \sim \frac{1}{\theta_2}, \quad \theta_2 \in [0, \infty). \tag{10.17}$$

Substituting (10.17) into (10.15), we get

$$\hbar_i(\theta_1, \theta_2 \mid \underset{\sim}{\varepsilon}) \sim \frac{1}{\theta_1\theta_2(\theta_2 - \theta_1)^{n_i}} \exp\left[-\left(\frac{\omega_1}{\theta_1} + \frac{\omega_2}{\theta_2}\right)\right],$$
$$-\infty < \theta_1 \leqslant 0, \quad 0 \leqslant \theta_2 < \infty. \tag{10.18}$$

It is easy to verify that

$$\beta_i = \int_{-\infty}^{0}\int_{0}^{\infty} \frac{1}{\theta_1\theta_2(\theta_2 - \theta_1)^{n_i}} \exp\left[-\left(\frac{\omega_1}{\theta_1} + \frac{\omega_2}{\theta_2}\right)\right] d\theta_2 d\theta_1 < \infty$$

Consequently, in spite of the fact that prior distribution densities are improper, the posterior density (10.18) is proper and may be used as a basis for obtaining the conclusion about a TTF and error value.

For calculating the case of a Gaussian non biased additive error, the posterior density has the form

$$\hbar_i(\sigma_\varepsilon \mid \underset{\sim}{\varepsilon}) = \frac{1}{\beta_i} \cdot \frac{h(\sigma_\varepsilon)}{\sigma_\varepsilon^{n_i}} \exp\left(-\frac{s^2}{2\sigma_\varepsilon^2}\right), \quad \sigma_\varepsilon \in E_\sigma \subset [0,\infty), \tag{10.19}$$

where

$$\beta_i = \frac{h(\sigma_\varepsilon)}{\sigma_\varepsilon^{n_i}} \exp\left(-\frac{s^2}{2\sigma_\varepsilon^2}\right) d\tau_\varepsilon.$$

The use of improper prior density $h(\sigma_\varepsilon) \sim \sigma_\varepsilon^{-1}$ leads to the proper posterior density for which

$$\hbar_i(\sigma_\varepsilon \mid \underset{\sim}{\varepsilon}) = \frac{1}{\sigma_\varepsilon^{n_i+1}} \exp\left(-\frac{s^2}{2\sigma_\varepsilon^2}\right), \quad \sigma_\varepsilon \in [0,\infty). \tag{10.20}$$

As seen from the relations obtained above, posterior densities of the parameters of the additive error of the working capacity model have the same structure, besides, for evaluation of the normalizing factor we need to use methods of numerical integration.

10.2.1 *The posterior distribution of the parameters of the error ε for functional tests*

If the prior density $h(\theta)$ is given and the likelihood function $\ell_\Phi(\theta \mid \underset{\sim}{\varepsilon z})$ is known, for the posterior density, corresponding to the results of functional tests, we write, applying the Bayes theorem, we write, applying the Bayes theorem,

$$\hbar_\Phi(\theta \mid \underset{\sim}{\varepsilon z}) \sim h(\theta)\ell_\Phi(\theta \mid \underset{\sim}{\varepsilon z}), \quad \theta \in \Theta. \tag{10.21}$$

All further arguments connected with obtaining concrete expressions for the posterior density are based on item-by-item examination of all possible combinations of $h(\theta)$ and $\ell_\Phi(\theta \mid \underset{\sim}{z})$ in the right hand part of the expression (10.21). In particular, for calculating the case of the generalized exponential error with a likelihood function (10.11), we will have

$$\hbar_\Phi(\theta_1,\theta_2 \mid \underset{\sim}{z}) \sim h_1(\theta_1)h_2(\theta_2)Q(\theta_1,\theta_2;d,r_-,s_+)P(\theta_1,\theta_2;\omega_1,\omega_2)$$
$$\times R_+(\theta_1,\theta_2;\zeta')S_-(\theta_1,\theta_2;\xi''), \quad \theta_1 \in \Theta_1, \quad \theta_2 \in \Theta_2. \tag{10.22}$$

Moreover, for the improper prior density $h(\theta_1,\theta_2) \sim -\theta_1^{-1}\theta_2^{-1}$ this expression is changed to

$$\hbar_\Phi(\theta_1,\theta_2 \mid \underset{\sim}{z}) \sim -\theta_1^{-1}\theta_2^{-1}Q(\theta_1,\theta_2;d,r_-,s_+)P(\theta_1,\theta_2;\omega_1,\omega_2)$$
$$\times R_+(\theta_1,\theta_2;\underset{\sim}{\xi}'S_-(\theta_1,\theta_2;\xi''), \quad \theta_1 \in (-\infty,0], \quad \theta_2 \in [0,\infty). \tag{10.23}$$

We shall investigate the possibility of using (10.23) in practical calculations. The posterior density (10.23) is proper, if

$$\int_{-\infty}^{0}\int_{0}^{\infty}\frac{1}{|\theta_1|\theta_2}\ell_\Phi(\theta_1,\theta_2 \mid \underset{\sim}{\varepsilon z})\,d\theta_2\,d\theta_1<\infty. \tag{10.24}$$

Analyzing expressions (10.8)–(10.11) we conclude that condition (10.24) is fulfilled if and only if at least one of the numbers d, r_-, s_+ doesn't equal zero. Under the condition $d=r_-=s_+=0$, it is impossible to use the posterior density (10.23) in order to obtain an informative conclusion about a TTF. For calculating the case of the Gaussian error ε, we have

$$\hbar_\Phi(\sigma_\varepsilon \mid \underset{\sim}{z}) \sim \frac{h(\sigma_\varepsilon)}{\sigma_\varepsilon^d}\exp\left(-\frac{\omega^{*2}}{2\sigma_\varepsilon^2}\right)\prod_{j=1}^{s}\left[1-\Phi\left(\frac{z_j''}{\sigma_\varepsilon}\right)\right]\prod_{j=1}^{r}\Phi\left(\frac{z_j'}{\sigma_\varepsilon}\right),$$
$$\sigma_\varepsilon\in E_\sigma\subset[0,\infty). \tag{10.25}$$

For the improper prior $h(\sigma_\varepsilon)\sim\sigma_\varepsilon^{-1}$, $0\leqslant\sigma_\varepsilon<\infty$, relation (10.25) takes the form

$$\hbar_\Phi(\sigma_\varepsilon \mid z) \sim \frac{1}{\sigma_\varepsilon^{d+1}}\exp\left(-\frac{\omega^{*2}}{2\sigma_\varepsilon^2}\right)\prod_{j=1}^{s}\left[1-\Phi\left(\frac{z_j''}{\sigma_\varepsilon}\right)\right]\prod_{j=1}^{r}\Phi\left(\frac{z_j'}{\sigma_\varepsilon}\right). \tag{10.26}$$

10.2.2 *The posterior distribution of the parameters of the error ε by the set of results of research and functional tests*

If a researcher has a possibility of carrying out research tests for the construction of the posterior density characterizing the form of information after the termination of the last test, one can use a consecutive Bayes procedure. The essence of this procedure is: at the first stage, including research tests, in full accordance with recommendations given in 10.2.1, we determine a posterior density of the distribution

$$\hbar_i(\theta \mid \underset{\sim}{\varepsilon}) \sim h(\theta)\ell_i(\theta \mid \underset{\sim}{\varepsilon}). \tag{10.27}$$

If functional tests are carried out after the research tests, for the determination $\hbar_\Phi(\theta \mid \underset{\sim}{z})$ it is more reasonable to use not $h(\theta)$ but $\hbar_i(\theta \mid \underset{\sim}{\varepsilon})$.
Then

$$\hbar_\Phi(\theta \mid \underset{\sim}{z}) \sim \hbar_i(\theta \mid \underset{\sim}{\varepsilon})\ell_\Phi(\theta \mid \underset{\sim}{z}). \tag{10.28}$$

The posterior density $\hbar_\Phi(\theta \mid \underset{\sim}{z})$ should be interpreted as resulting for a whole two-stage sequence of tests. We will take into account this fact, denoting by $\hbar(\theta \mid \underset{\sim}{\varepsilon},\underset{\sim}{z})$ the resulting posterior density of the parameter θ.

Substituting (10.27) into (10.28) we write the final expression

$$\hbar(\theta \mid \underset{\sim}{\varepsilon}, \underset{\sim}{z}) \sim h(\theta)\ell_i(\theta \mid \underset{\sim}{\varepsilon})\ell_\Phi(\theta \mid \underset{\sim}{z}). \tag{10.29}$$

We will call the product $\ell(\theta \mid \underset{\sim}{\varepsilon}, \underset{\sim}{z}) = \ell_i(\theta \mid \underset{\sim}{\varepsilon})\ell_\Phi(\theta \mid \underset{\sim}{z})$ a cumulative likelihood function. Using (10.2) and (10.5) for $\ell(\theta \mid \underset{\sim}{\varepsilon}, \underset{\sim}{z})$ we obtain

$$\ell(\theta \mid \underset{\sim}{\varepsilon}, \underset{\sim}{z}) \tag{10.30}$$

$$= \prod_{j=1}^{r} [1 - F_\varepsilon(-z_j'; \theta)] \prod_{j=1}^{d} f_\varepsilon(-z_j^*; \theta) \prod_{j=1}^{n_i} f_\varepsilon(\varepsilon_j; \theta) \prod_{j=1}^{s} F_\varepsilon(-z_j''; \theta),$$

$$\theta \in \Theta. \tag{10.31}$$

Having remembered expression (10.1) for the element of the sample of research tests we have $\varepsilon_j = -\phi(x_j)$, $j = 1, \ldots, n_i$. Table 10.1 shows $z_j^* = -\phi(x_j)$. Therefore, ε_j and $-z_j^*$ have the same values of the theoretical status variable Z at the failure moment appearance, i.e., when the acting loading becomes equal to a functional capability. Taking into account this circumstance, we may draw the important practical conclusion: if the results of research tests are put together with the results of functional tests in which the failure has occurred, then a cumulative likelihood function $\ell(\theta \mid \underset{\sim}{\varepsilon}, \underset{\sim}{z})$ coincides with the functional $\ell_\Phi(\theta \mid \underset{\sim}{z})$. This conclusion lets us use the results of 10.2.2 for the determination of the posterior density $\hbar(\theta \mid \underset{\sim}{\varepsilon}, \underset{\sim}{z})$. To this end, one should include in the sample $\underset{\sim}{z}^*$ the elements of the sample $\underset{\sim}{\varepsilon}$ taken with the opposite sign. That is why later we will assume $\underset{\sim}{z}^* = (z_1^*, z_2^*, \ldots, z_d^*, -\varepsilon_1, -\varepsilon_2, \ldots, -\varepsilon_{n_i})$. We can also use a similar method in the case when under the research tests it is assumed, for some reason, that non attainment of a limit state takes place.

In conclusion, we note that the posterior distribution density is an exhaustive characteristic of the working capacity model error. However, due to the practices existing now, to make a conclusion about the properties of the device with the help of numerical criteria, it is not sufficient for estimating the TTF of the system and the value of the error of the theoretical working capacity model to have knowledge of a posterior density. In 10.3 we will find corresponding numerical estimates with the help of the posterior densities obtained above. The more visual method of analysis of the system properties may be obtained from a discrete representation of prior distribution considered below.

10.2.3 *The discrete posterior TTF distribution*

Using discrete prior distributions of the parameters of the error ε, we will find corresponding posterior distributions of the TTF. Let us restrict ourselves to the case of the generalized exponential error ε, obeying the probability distribution with the density (9.13). Suppose θ_1 and θ_2 have prior distributions respectively, (p_{1i}, θ_{1i}), $i = 1, 2, \ldots, m$, and (p_{2k}, θ_{2k}), $k = 1, 2, \ldots, \ell$, where $p_{1i} = P\{\theta_1 = \theta_{1i}\}$, $p_{2k} = P\{\theta_2 = \theta_{2k}\}$. With the help of these distributions and the relation (9.19) we can find a prior distribution for the TTF (P_{Rj}, R_j), $j = 1, 2, \ldots, mk$, where $R_j = R(\theta_{1i}, \theta_{1k})$, $p_{Rj} = p_{1i}p_{1k}$. The correspondence between the index j and a pair of indices (i,k) is given by the elation $R_{j-1} \leqslant R_j$, i.e., in order to write the distribution series for all the TTF R we have to carry out calculations of $R_{ik} = R(\theta_{1i}, \theta_{2k})$ for all possible pairs (i,k), and write the obtained values in ascending order, and renumber them from 1 to mk. Thereafter, each value R_j is associated with the corresponding probability $p_{1i}\, p_{2k}$. Here and further on we shall assume that among the values of R_j there are no repeated values.

Using the likelihood function (10.11) and applying the Bayes theorem, wefind in the discrete representation the posterior probabilities $\widetilde{p}_{Rj} = P\{R = R_j \mid \underset{\sim}{z}\}$:

$$\widetilde{p}_{R_j} = \frac{p_{R_j} \ell_\Phi(\theta_{1i}, \theta_{2i}, \theta_{2k} \mid \underset{\sim}{z})}{\sum\limits_{i=1}^{m} \sum\limits_{k=1}^{\ell} p_{\ell i} p_{2k} \ell_\Phi(\theta_{1i}, \theta_{2i}, \theta_{2k} \mid \underset{\sim}{z})}, \quad j = 1, 2, \ldots, mk, \tag{10.32}$$

where the correspondence between j and a pair of indices (i, k) is found with the help of the already mentioned procedure. The distribution series $(\widetilde{p}_{Rj}, R_j)$, $j = 1, 2, \ldots, mk$ is an exhaustive characteristic of the TTF and is more visual in comparison to a continuous posterior density. Besides, it is free of known arbitrariness and is connected with the choice of a loss function.

A *numerical example.*The automatic control system is described by the differential equation

$$\frac{dY}{dt} + Y_2 = (\lambda + 1)^2, \quad Y(0) = 0, \tag{10.33}$$

where λ is a random variable obeying the normal distribution with the mean value O and variance 0.01. The system is assumed to survive, if at the moment $t = 1$ the variable Y is greater than the value $y_0 = 0.42$.

The theoretical model of the system (10.33) consists of an additive error ε, which can be described by the generalized exponential distribution (9.13), where, the parameters θ_1 and θ_2 belong to the intervals $\Theta_1 = [0.08; 0]$, $\Theta_2 = [0; 0.06]$. The prior distributions for θ_1 and θ_2 are given in Fig. 10.1 and Fig. 10.2 by the dotted lines. As a TTF of the system the probability $R = P\{Z + \varepsilon > 0\}$ has been chosen, where $Z = Y(1) - y_0$. Using the interpolation method [42], we obtain $E[Y(1)] = 0.7622$, $D[Y(1)] = 0.01381$, whence $m_Z = 0.3422$, $\sigma_Z = 0.1175$.

The following values of the theoretical status variable have been fixed during the seven tests $\underset{\sim}{z}^* = (0.2663; 0.4309; 0.3567; 0.5783; 0.2619; 0.3385; 0.4851)$, $\underset{\sim}{z}^* = \phi$, $\underset{\sim}{z}'' = \phi$. Figs. 10.1–10.2 represent the posterior distributions of the parameters of the error θ_1 and θ_2, and TTF R. As seen from the figures, the experiment results correctly identify the prior distributions (they are represented by the dotted lines).

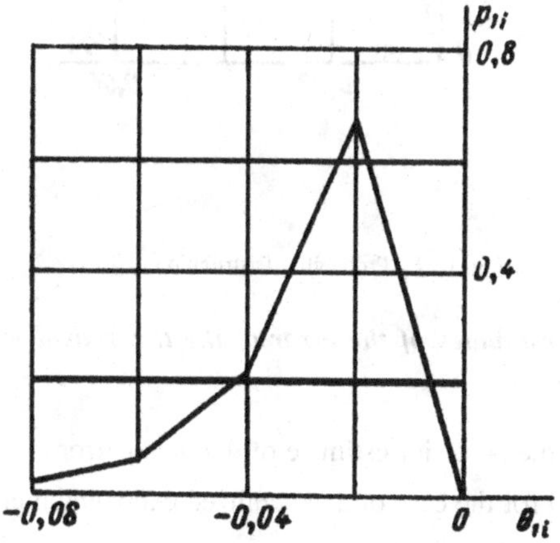

Fig. 10.1 Probability Distributions of the Parameters θ_1 and θ_2.

10.3 Bayes posterior estimates

The procedure of the posterior TTF estimation coincides with the procedure of a prior Bayes estimation given in § 9.4. The difference is that instead of the prior density $h(\theta)$ we must use the posterior one, $\hbar(\theta \mid \underset{\sim}{z})$ obtained by the results of a joint experiment, including research and functional tests. In this chapter we adhere to the following scheme. At first, we consider obtaining the estimates of the parametric additive error ε, and thereafter we find the corresponding TTF estimates.

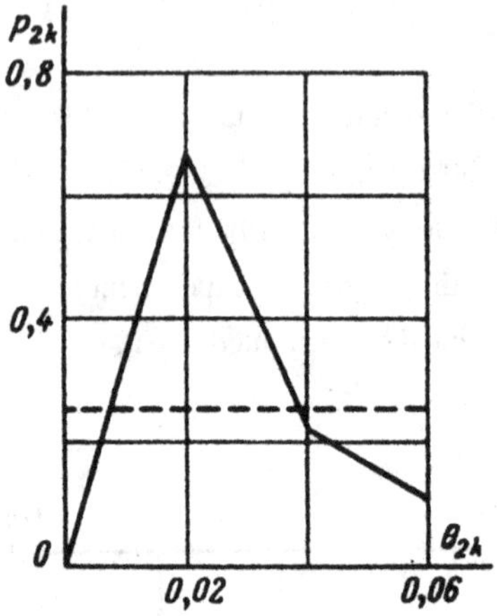

Fig. 10.2 Probability Distribution of TTF.

10.3.1 *The posterior estimates of the error of the theoretical working capacity model*

The problem is to Bud the posterior estimate of the mean error $\varepsilon = E_{[\varepsilon]}$ of the theoretical working capacity model for the case of a generalized exponential error and an estimate of σ_ε for the Gaussian error without a bias.

Calculating the case of a generalized exponential error. Obtain the dependence $\varepsilon_0 = \varepsilon_0(\theta_1, \theta_2)$. With the help of (9.13) we easily find

$$\varepsilon_0 = E[\varepsilon] = \int_{-\infty}^{\infty} \varepsilon f_\varepsilon(\varepsilon; \theta_1, \theta_2) d\varepsilon = \theta_1 + \theta_2. \tag{10.34}$$

Because of the linear dependence (10.34) we find first the estimates of the parameters θ_1 and $\widehat{\theta}_1^*$ in the form $\widehat{\theta}_1^*$ and, an thereafter, summing them, we determine the estimate. The estimates $\widehat{\theta}_1^*$ and $\widehat{\theta}_1^*$ will be determined as corresponding posterior mean values by the formulas

$$\widehat{\theta}_1^* = \iint_{\Theta_1 \times \Theta_2} \theta_1 \hbar(\theta_1, \theta_2 \mid \underset{\sim}{\varepsilon z}) d\theta_1 d\theta_2, \tag{10.35}$$

and

$$\widehat{\theta}_2^* = \iint_{\Theta_1 \times \Theta_2} \theta_2 \hbar(\theta_1, \theta_2 \mid \underset{\sim}{\varepsilon z}) d\theta_1 d\theta_2, \tag{10.36}$$

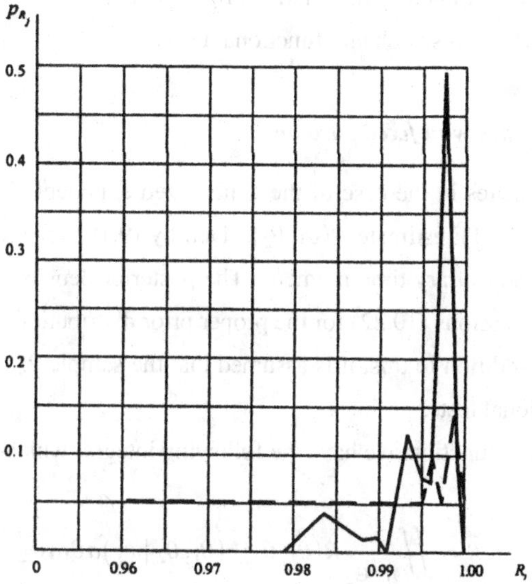

Fig. 10.3 Trend of the Operational Capacity during the Experiment.

where $\hbar(\theta_1, \theta_2 \mid \underset{\sim}{z})$ is determined by the relation (10.22) under the assumption that the sample $\underset{\sim}{z}$ contains the results of research and functional tests. Simplification of the integrals (10.35) and (10.36) does not seem possible, and, in order to carry out practical calculations we need to apply methods of numerical integration for the double integrals. There is a possibility of determination of exactness of the $\widehat{\varepsilon}_0^* = \widehat{\theta}_1^* + \widehat{\theta}_2^*$ in the form of posterior mean squared value $\sigma_{\widehat{\varepsilon}_0^*} = \{D[\varepsilon]\}^{1/2}$ with the help of the following formula

$$\sigma^2_{\widehat{\varepsilon}_0^*} = D[\theta_1] + D[\theta_2] + 2K[\theta_1, \theta_2], \tag{10.37}$$

where

$$S[\theta_i] = \iint_{\Theta_1\times\Theta_2} \theta_i^2 \hbar(\theta_1, \theta_2 \mid \underset{\sim}{\varepsilon z}) d\theta_1 d\theta_2 - \hat{\theta}_i^{*2}, \quad i = 1, 2,$$

$$K[\theta_1, \theta_2] = \iint_{\Theta_1\times\Theta_2} \theta_1\theta_2 \hbar(\theta_1, \theta_2 \mid \underset{\sim}{\varepsilon z}) d\theta_1 d\theta_2 - \hat{\theta}_1^* \hat{\theta}_2^*.$$

Calculating the case of a Gaussian error of a working capacity model is reduced to the analogous (but one-dimensional) integrals. With the help of these integrals we determine the estimate 6 and its error in the form of the posterior variance $D[\sigma_\varepsilon]$:

$$\hat{\sigma}_\varepsilon^* = \int_0^\infty \sigma_\varepsilon \hbar(\sigma_\varepsilon \mid \underset{\sim}{\varepsilon z}) d\sigma_\varepsilon, \tag{10.38}$$

and

$$D[\sigma_\varepsilon] = \int_0^\infty \sigma_\varepsilon^2 \hbar(\sigma_\varepsilon \mid \underset{\sim}{\varepsilon z}) d\sigma_\varepsilon - \hat{\sigma}_\varepsilon^{*2}, \tag{10.39}$$

where $\hbar(\sigma_\varepsilon \mid \underset{\sim}{\varepsilon z})$ is determined by the relation (10.25) under the assumption that the sample $\underset{\sim}{\varepsilon z}$ contains the results of research and functional tests.

10.3.2 *TTF Estimates with fixed parameters*

To obtain TTF estimates in the case of the generalized exponential error ε, we will start from the conditional TTF estimate $R(\theta_1, \theta_2)$ given by (9.19) for the fixed time moment, and by (9.35) for an arbitrary time moment. The posterior density $\hbar(\theta_1, \theta_2 \mid \underset{\sim}{\varepsilon z})$ is determined either by expressions (10.22) for the proper prior distributions, or by (10.23) for the improper ones. In addition to this, it is assumed that the sample $\underset{\sim}{\varepsilon z}$ contains the results of research and functional tests.

For the quadratic loss function, we have the following integral which enables us to find the TTF estimate R^*:

$$\widehat{R} = \iint_{\Theta_1 \times \Theta_2} R(\theta_1, \theta_2) \hbar(\theta_1, \theta_2 \mid \underset{\sim}{\varepsilon z}) d\theta_1 d\theta_2 \tag{10.40}$$

If one uses the loss function of the form (9.46) for obtaining the estimate R^*, it yields the optimization problem, analogous to (9.53):

$$\widehat{R}^* = \arg \min_{x \in [0,1]} \iint_{\Theta_1 \times \Theta_2} F(\theta_1, \theta_2; x) d\theta_1 d\theta_2. \tag{10.41}$$

Where

$$F(\theta_1, \theta_2; x) = \begin{cases} K_1 \left[x - R(\theta_1, \theta_2)\right]^2 \hbar(\theta_1, \theta_2 \mid \underset{\sim}{z}), & x \leqslant R(\theta_1, \theta_2), \\ \left[K_1 \left(x - R(\theta_1, \theta_2)\right)^2 + K_2 \left(x - R(\theta_1, \theta_2)\right)\right] \hbar(\theta_1, \theta_2 \mid \underset{\sim}{z}), & x > R(\theta_1, \theta_2). \end{cases}$$

The Bayes lower confidence limit $\underline{R}_\gamma^*$ will be determined analogously to the approach proposed in 9.4.2 as

$$\underline{R}_\gamma^* = R(\theta_1, \theta_2), \tag{10.42}$$

where $\underline{\theta}_1$ and $\underline{\theta}_2$ are found from the transcendental equations

$$\int_{\underline{\theta}_1}^{\theta_1''} \int_{\theta_2'}^{\theta_2''} \hbar(\theta_1, \theta_2 \mid \underset{\sim}{\varepsilon z}) d\theta_1 d\theta_2 - \gamma^{1/2} = 0, \tag{10.43}$$

and

$$\int_{\theta_1'}^{\theta_1''} \int_{\underline{\theta}_2}^{\theta_2''} \hbar(\theta_1, \theta_2 \mid \underset{\sim}{\varepsilon z}) d\theta_1 d\theta_2 - \gamma^{1/2} = 0.$$

We use a similar calculation approach in the case of Gaussian error. The pointwise estimate $\widehat{R}^*$ is determined with the help of the one-dimensional integral

$$\hat{R}^* = \int_{\sigma_\varepsilon'}^{\sigma_\varepsilon''} R(\sigma_\varepsilon) \hbar(\sigma_\varepsilon \mid \underset{\sim}{\varepsilon z}) d\sigma_\varepsilon \tag{10.44}$$

for the quadratic loss function, or with the help of the following minimization problem that we have to solve:

$$\hat{R}^* = \arg\min_{x\in[0,1]} \int_{\sigma'_\varepsilon}^{\sigma''_\varepsilon} F(\sigma_\varepsilon;x)\, d\sigma_\varepsilon, \tag{10.45}$$

where

$$F(\sigma_\varepsilon;x) = \begin{cases} K_1\,(x-R(\sigma_\varepsilon))^2\,\hbar(\sigma^\varepsilon \mid \underset{\sim}{z}) & x \leqslant R(\sigma_\varepsilon), \\ \left[K_1\,(x-R(\sigma_\varepsilon))^2 + K_2\,(x-R(\sigma_\varepsilon))\right]\hbar(\sigma_\varepsilon \mid \underset{\sim}{z}), & x > R(\sigma_\varepsilon). \end{cases} \tag{10.46}$$

In the relations (10.44)–(10.46), $R(\sigma_\varepsilon)$ is determined by the formula (9.23) for the TTF at the fixed time moment t_0, or by the formula (9.40) for the TTF during the time τ. For the posterior density $\hbar(\sigma_\varepsilon \mid \underset{\sim}{z})$ one should use the expression (10.25), assuming that the sample $\underset{\sim}{z}$ contains the results of research and functional tests. When the confidence level γ is given, we obtain the Bayes lower confidence limit of the TTF $\underline{R}^*_\gamma$ by the usual approach. In accordance with it,

$$\underline{\hat{R}}^* = R(\underline{\sigma}_\varepsilon). \tag{10.47}$$

In order to find $\underline{\sigma}_\varepsilon$ we need to solve the equation

$$\int_{\underline{\sigma}_\varepsilon}^{\sigma''_\varepsilon} \hbar(\sigma_\varepsilon \mid \varepsilon\underset{\sim}{z})\,d\sigma_\varepsilon - \gamma = 0. \tag{10.48}$$

10.3.3 *Investigation of certainty of the Bayes estimates*

We carry out numerous calculations of TTF estimates for the samples of different volumes and a broad range of a priori data with the help of the method proposed above on the basis of Example 9.4.5 in order to obtain information about the quality of this method.

Investigation of posterior Bayes TTF estimates has been carried out with the help of samples of values of the theoretical status variable Z which have been modeled by the special algorithm. The essence of this follows: for each j-th testing two numbers are generated. They obey a normal law with the parameters m_Z, σ_Z and ε_j which follows the probability distribution with the density $f_\varepsilon\left(\varepsilon;\, \theta_1^{(0)},\, \theta_2^{(0)}\right)$, given by the expression (9.13). The quantities $\theta_1^{(0)}$ and $\theta_2^{(0)}$ have the meaning of real values of the parameters θ_1 and θ_2, which are determined by the uncertainty intervals Θ_1 and Θ_2. The chosen values of m_Z, σ_Z, $\theta_1^{(0)}$ and $\theta_2^{(0)}$ determine uniquely the real TTF value R. For each j-th random probe we determine the value of the error ε of settling the generalized status variable $\omega_j = z_j + \varepsilon_j$. Having chosen some error value δ of settling the generalized types of outcomes we find: a working capacity, if $\omega_j > \delta$; a failure, if $|\omega_j| < \delta$; a nonworking state, if $\omega_j < -\delta$. In accordance

Table 10.2 Bayes Estimators for TTF.

θ_1'	θ_2''	$n=10$	$n=50$	$n=100$
−0.06	0.06	0.9746	0.9755	0.9684
−0.06	0.04	0.9715	0.9710	0.9675
−0.06	0.02	0.9670	0.9693	0.9864
−0.06	0.00	0.9599	0.9672	0.9650
−0.04	0.06	0.9904	0.9821	0.9769
−0.04	0.04	0.9889	0.9803	0.9753
−0.04	0.02	0.9867	0.9776	0.9729
−0.04	0.00	0.9826	0.9736	0.9695
−0.02	0.06	0.9978	0.9950	0.9904
−0.02	0.04	0.9974	0.9944	0.9936
−0.02	0.02	0.9966	0.9936	0.9874

Table 10.3 Posterior Estimators for TTF.

θ_1'	θ_2''	$n=20$	$n=40$	$n=60$	$n=80$
−0.06	0.06	0.9860	0.9719	0.9787	0.9640
−0.06	0.04	0.9849	0.9704	0.9780	0.9625
−0.04	0.06	0.9923	0.9827	0.9825	0.9772
−0.04	0.04	0.9912	0.9809	0.9836	0.9752

with the type of outcomes of the j-th trial, the corresponding values z_j are included in $\underset{\sim}{\varepsilon z}'$ for the first outcome, $\underset{\sim}{\varepsilon z}^*$ for the second one and $\underset{\sim}{\varepsilon z}''$ for the third outcome.

In Table 10.2 we represent the Bayes pointwise TTF estimates, obtained for different intervals of a prior uncertainty $\Theta_1 = \left[\theta_1', \theta_1''\right]$ and $\Theta_2 = \left[\theta_2', \theta_2''\right]$ for the sample sizes $n = 0, 50, 100$. In order to learn the behavior of the posterior Bayes TTF estimation, we give in Table 10.3 the TTF estimates for the larger number of samples. During the modeling we have chosen $m_Z = 0.1488$, $\sigma_Z = 0.05109$, $\theta_1^{(0)} = -0.04$, $\theta_2^{(0)} = 0.02$ which corresponds to the TTF value $R = 0.9639$. By inspecting the analysis given in Table 10.2 and Table 10.3, we conclude that with increasing the sample sizes the Bayes pointwise estimate approaches the real TTF value. This pattern is common. It appears more frequently in calculating variants where the uncertainty interval has been chosen more successfully. As seen from Table 10.3, the pattern of approaching the posterior TTF estimate to its real value is nonmonotonic. This is explained by the randomness of the modeled samples.

10.3.4 *Bayes TTF estimates for undefined parameters*

Below we represent the development of the previous results for the case where the initial data is given with the errors and during the testing this data is corrected in accordance with the testing outcomes. The essence of this problem is that the correction of initial data is performed only by the results of functional tests. For the research test we artificially give the loadings which made the system achieve the limit state, and, consequently it implies a failure. Thereby the observed test loading value cannot be considered as an element of a sample of real loading.

Consider a situation when a TTF is estimated at the fixed time moment. Suppose, in accordance with 10.3.2, that we have found the Bayes estimate $\widehat{R}_0^*$ using the results of research and functional tests. The obtained estimate depends on the mean value m_Z and on the mean squared value σ_Z, i.e., $\widehat{R}_0^* = \widehat{R}_0^*(m_Z, \sigma_Z)$. This is valid, since the conditional TTF estimate $R(\theta_1, \theta_2)$ is parameterized with the help of m_Z and σ_Z. In view of the uncertainty of the initial data, the parameters m_Z and σ_Z appear to be also uncertain. Besides, this uncertainty is expressed with the help of prior densities $h_m(m_Z)$ and $\hbar_\sigma(\sigma_Z)$. One possible way of obtaining $h_m(m_Z)$ and $\hbar_\sigma(\sigma_Z)$ has been given in 9.4.4.

The problem of estimating TTF for the case when uncertain characteristics, connected with the error of initial data, are corrected by the results of functional tests will be solved by the following scheme:

1) Starting from prior densities $h_m(m_Z)$ and $\hbar_\sigma(\sigma_Z)$ and qualitative results of functional tests $\underset{\sim}{\varepsilon}_Z = (z_1, z_2, \ldots, z_n)$ we find the corresponding posterior density $\hbar_{m\sigma}(m_Z, \sigma_Z \mid \underset{\sim}{z})$ with the help of the Bayes theorem;
2) Having chosen some loss function we find the Bayes estimate $\widehat{R}_0^{**}$ of the function $\hat{R}_0^*(m_Z, \sigma_Z)$ by minimization of the corresponding posterior risk.

To determine the posterior density $\hbar_{m\sigma}(m_Z, \sigma_Z \mid \underset{\sim}{z})$ we use the known
Bayes solution [202], based on prior densities conjugated with the Gaussian likelihood kernel. Instead of the parameters m_Z and σ_Z we will use the parameters m_Z and $c_Z = \sigma_Z^{-2}$, following the procedure given in [202]. As a prior density for m_Z and c_Z we use a gamma-normal probability density

$$h(m_Z, c_Z) = h_c(c_Z)\, h_m(m_Z \mid c_Z) \tag{10.49}$$

where

$$h_c(c_Z) = h_c(c_Z; s'^2, \nu') = \left(\frac{\nu' s'^2}{2}\right)^{\nu/2} \frac{c_Z^{\nu'/2-1}}{\Gamma\left(\frac{\nu'}{2}\right)} \exp\left(-\frac{1}{2}\nu' s'^2 c_Z\right), \quad c_Z > 0, \; \nu' > 0, \tag{10.50}$$

and

$$h_m(m_Z \mid c_Z) = h_m\left(m_Z; m', \frac{1}{c_Z n'}\right) = \frac{(c_Z n')^{1/2}}{\sqrt{2\pi}} \exp\left[-\frac{1}{2} c_Z n' (m_Z - m')^2\right]. \tag{10.51}$$

The parameters of the joint density (10.49) are determined with the help of the earlier obtained numerical results (see expressions (9.67) and (9.68) by equating the theoretical moments of the distributions (10.50) and (10.51) to the corresponding calculating values:

$$m' = m_Z^{(0)}, \quad n' = \frac{\left[\sigma_Z^{(0)}\right]^2}{s_m^2}, \tag{10.52}$$

and

$$s'^2 = \left[\sigma_Z^{(0)}\right], \quad \nu' = \frac{\left[\sigma_Z^{(0)}\right]^2}{2 s_\sigma^2}. \tag{10.53}$$

In the given case the sufficient statistic is generated by the following quantities [202]: The posterior density of the parameters m_Z and $\sigma_Z$has the same form as in (10.49), but instead of n', m', ν' and $\nu' s'^2$ we correspondingly use

$$n'' = n' + n, \quad m'' = \frac{n'm' + n\hat{m}}{n' + n}, \quad \nu'' = \nu' + n, \tag{10.54}$$

and

$$\nu'' s''^2 = \nu' s'^2 + n' m'^2 + n\hat{D} + n\hat{m}^2 - n'' m''^2. \tag{10.55}$$

With the help of these expressions we can find, in particular, the posterior mean values $\hat{m}_Z^{(0)}$ and $\widehat{\sigma}_Z^{(0)}$ and variances $\widehat{s}_m^2$ and $\widehat{s}_\sigma^2$ of the parameters m_Z and, σ_Z respectively, which correct the prior estimates (9.67) and (9.68) according to the experiment's results:

$$\hat{m}_Z^{(0)} = \frac{n' m_Z^{(0)} + n\hat{m}}{n' + n}, \quad \hat{\sigma}_Z^{(0)} = s'', \tag{10.56}$$

and

$$\hat{s}_m^2 = \frac{\hat{\sigma}_Z^{(0)2} + n\widehat{m}}{n' + n}, \quad \hat{s}_\sigma^2 = \frac{s''^2}{2\nu''}. \tag{10.57}$$

So, with the help of this approach, using the conjugated prior densities, we have obtained the joint distribution density $\hbar_{m\sigma}\left(m_Z,\sigma_Z \mid \underset{\sim}{\varepsilon}_Z\right)$ which is written with the help of formulas (10.49)–(10.51), where, instead of each parameter with one prime, it is necessary to substitute the parameters denoted by the same symbols but having two primes. The last ones are computed by the formulas (10.52)–(10.57) with the help of prior data and experiment results.

The second part of the problem, connected with obtaining the final Bayes TTF estimate R_0^{**} which takes into account new experimental information for the correction of the initial information about the numerical characteristics of initial variables is solved almost analogously to 9.4.4. The simplest way of obtaining $R*$ is by substituting into R the posterior pointwise estimates given by formulas (10.56), i.e,

$$\hat{R}_0^{**} \cong \hat{R}_0^{*}\left(\hat{m}_Z^{(0)}, \hat{\sigma}_Z^{(0)}\right). \tag{10.58}$$

The exact solution may be found in the form

$$\hat{R}_0^{**} = \int_{-\infty}^{\infty}\int_0^{\infty} \hat{R}_0^{*}(m_Z,\sigma_Z)\hbar_{m\sigma}\left(m_Z,\sigma_Z \mid \underset{\sim}{\varepsilon}_Z\right) d\sigma_Z\, dm_Z. \tag{10.59}$$

In order to avoid the necessity of a double numerical integration, we represent $\widehat{R}_0^{*}(m_Z,\sigma_Z)$ in the integrand of (10.59) in the form of a Taylor series with respect to $\widehat{m}_Z^{(0)}$ and $\widehat{\sigma}_Z^{(0)}$. Leaving only the terms up to the second order of smallness, that is,

$$\hat{R}_0^{**} \cong \hat{R}_0^{*}\left(\hat{m}_Z^{(0)}, \hat{\sigma}_Z^{(0)}\right) + a_2^{*}\hat{s}_m^2 + b_2^{*}\hat{s}_\sigma^2, \tag{10.60}$$

where

$$\partial_2^{*} = \frac{\partial^2 \hat{R}_0^{*}\left(\hat{m}_Z^{(0)}, \hat{\sigma}_Z^{(0)}\right)}{\partial \hat{m}_Z^{(0)2}} \quad \text{and} \quad \frac{\partial^2 \hat{R}_0^{*}\left(\hat{m}_Z^{(0)}, \hat{\sigma}_Z^{(0)}\right)}{\partial \hat{\sigma}_Z^{(0)2}}.$$

10.4 A procedure for controlling the operational capacity of a system

In this section we present and solve one applied problem with the operational capacity control of the object by the results of measurement of the key parameter. The main part of the diagnostic procedures used in this area is based on the binary representation of the control results [134], when each testing is fixed the fact of the key parameters being in the admissible domain or not being in this domain. In the first case, the system is regarded as having survived, in the second one as non-survival. We cannot say that such an approach is flexible enough in spite of the fact that it is simple and operative. This is explained by the reason that the testing results giving the values of the key parameter which are situated dangerously near to the admissible domain but assumed to be as successful as the results of testing in which the values of the key parameter are situated far away from the boundary. Besides, the control of attainment of the desired reliability level cannot be done often (for example, for the case of a small number of successful tests). Below we have formulated and solved for one case of calculating the problem of the working capacity. This problem enables us to make a conclusion about the attainment of the given reliability level. The contents of this section are based on the results of the previous one and essentially use the notion of the coefficient of the working capacity inventory.

10.4.1 *Setting of the problem*

Let Y be a unique key parameter, U its admissible value. We will assume that Y and $\underline{U}$ are random variables obeying the Gaussian probability distribution with the parameters m_Y, σ_Y and m_U and σ_U, respectively. The values of these parameters are estimated beforehand, when we carry out the project testing of the system. Therefore, before we begin testing for some prior estimates, $m_Y^{(0)}$, $\sigma_Y^{(0)}$ and $m_U^{(0)}$, $\sigma_U^{(0)}$ are known. Since these estimates in a common case are very rough, we will assume also that given corresponding intervals of prior uncertainty: for the mean values, $[m'_Y, m''_Y]$ and $[m'_U, m''_U]$, for the variation coefficients u_Y and v_U of the random variables Y and U, correspondingly $[v'_Y, v'_Y]$ and $[v, v]$. Each interval will be represented with the help of the quantity Δ equal to a half of the length of this interval, i.e., we will assume that we know the values

$$\Delta_Y = \frac{m''_Y - m'_Y}{2}, \quad \Delta_U = \frac{m''_U - m'_U}{2}.$$

$$\Delta_1 = \frac{v''_Y - v'_Y}{2}, \quad \Delta_2 = \frac{v''_U - v'_U}{2}.$$

Hence, before testing we know that $\left\{m_Y^{(0)}, \Delta_Y\right\}$, $\left\{v_Y^{(0)}, \Delta_1\right\}$, $\left\{m_U^{(0)}, \Delta_U\right\}$, $\left\{v_U^{(0)}, \Delta_2\right\}$, where $v_Y^{(0)} = \sigma_Y^{(0)}/m_Y^{(0)}$, $v_U^{(0)} = \sigma_U^{(0)}/m_U^{(0)}$.

During the experimental data processing we carry out n independent tests with a modification, fixing the values of key parameters Y and admissible value U. For each j-th stage of testing during which j tests have been carried out, the testing results generate a sample $\underset{\sim}{y}^{(j)} = (y_1, y_2, \ldots, y_j)$ and $\underset{\sim}{u}^{(j)} = (u_1, u_2, \ldots, u_j)$ so that all the results of n tests are written in the form $\{y, u\}$, where $\underset{\sim}{y} = \underset{\sim}{y}^{(n)}$, $\underset{\sim}{u} = \underset{\sim}{u}^{(n)}$.

We will assume that given the desired probability R_{req} of fulfillment of the working capacity condition, $Y > U$. The problem is to construct the control procedure for the fulfillment of the condition

$$\hat{R}_j = \hat{R}_j\left(\underset{\sim}{\varepsilon y}^{(j)}, \underset{\sim}{\varepsilon u}^{(j)}\right) \geqslant R_{\text{req}} \tag{10.61}$$

for each j-th stage of testing and obtaining of the conclusion about the fulfillment of the requirement about the reliability of all n tests.

10.4.2 *A problem solution in the general case*

To find a more laconic writing of the control procedure, we introduce the so called working capacity inventory coefficient $g = m_Y/m_U$. The probability of fulfillment of the condition $Y > U$ under the given values of v_Y and v_U is written as

$$R = P\{Y - U > 0\} = \Phi\left(\frac{g-1}{\sqrt{g^2 v_Y^2 + v_U^2}}\right),$$

which allows us to find from the condition

$$\Phi\left(\frac{g-1}{\sqrt{g^2 v_Y^2 + v_U^2}}\right) - R_{\text{req}}$$

the least value of the coefficient g guaranteeing the fulfillment of the reliability requirement:

$$g_{\text{req}} = g_{\text{req}}(v_U, v_U) = \frac{1 - \left[1 - \left(1 - v_U^2\right)\left(1 - z_{\text{req}} v_Y^2\right)\right]^{1/2}}{1 - z_{\text{req}} v_Y^2}, \tag{10.62}$$

where z_{req} is the quantile of the normal distribution of the probability of R_{req}. The idea of construction of the control procedure consists of obtaining the posterior Bayes lower γ-confidential $\underline{g}_\gamma = \underline{g}_\gamma(\underset{\sim}{\varepsilon u}, \underset{\sim}{\varepsilon y})$ and comparing this limit with g_{req}. To ensure the possibility of such a construction we give the following arguments. Choose as RJ in the condition (10.61) the Bayes lower confidence limit E and assume that the variation coefficients VU and VY are known. In view of the monotonicity of the function

$$R(g, v_U, v_Y) = \Phi\left(\frac{g-1}{\sqrt{g^2 u_Y^2 + v_U^2}}\right) \tag{10.63}$$

with respect to the variable g the following relation holds:

$$P\left\{\underline{R}_\gamma^* \geqslant R_{\text{req}}\right\} = P\left\{R\left(\underline{g}_\gamma; v_U, v_Y\right) \geqslant R\left(g_{\text{req}}, v_U, v_Y\right)\right\}. \tag{10.64}$$

Since only the posterior probabilities are considered, one should use instead of the values v_U and v_Y their posterior estimates $\hat{v}_U$ and $\hat{v}_Y$. Hence, it follows that the condition of reliability (10.61) is fulfilled, if the following inequality for the estimation of the inventory coefficient of the operational capacity of the system:

$$\underline{g}_\gamma(\underset{\sim}{\varepsilon}y, \underset{\sim}{\varepsilon}u) \geqslant g_{\text{req}}(\hat{v}_U, \hat{v}_Y), \tag{10.65}$$

where $g_{\text{req}}(v_U, u_Y)$ is determined by formula (10.62), and the problem is to obtain the Bayes lower confidence level $\underline{g}_\gamma$ for the inventory coefficient.

For obtaining $\underline{g}_\gamma$ we find the posterior density $\hbar(m_Y, m_U \mid \underset{\sim}{\varepsilon}u, \underset{\sim}{\varepsilon}y)$ and apply thereafter the Bayes estimation procedure for the function of two random variables m_Y and m_U of the form $g = m_Y/m_U$. Under the assumption, Y and U obey the Gaussian distribution. Therefore, the kernel of the likelihood function $\ell_0(m_Y, m_U \mid \underset{\sim}{\varepsilon}u, \underset{\sim}{\varepsilon}y)$ with given σ_Y and σ_U is written as

$$\ell_0(m_Y, m_U \mid \underset{\sim}{\varepsilon}u, \underset{\sim}{\varepsilon}y) = \exp\left[-\frac{n}{2\sigma_U^2}\left(m_U^2 - 2\bar{u}m_U\right) - \frac{n}{2\sigma_Y^2}\left(m_Y^2 - 2\bar{u}m_Y\right)\right],$$

where $\bar{u}$ and $\bar{y}$ are correspondingly the sample means for U and Y. Assuming that in the intervals of a prior uncertainty m_Y and m_U obey the normal law, we obtain the following relation for the posterior density of the parameters m_Y and m_U

$$\hbar(m_Y, m_U \mid \underset{\sim}{\varepsilon}u, \underset{\sim}{\varepsilon}y) \sim a_0(m_Y, m_U) = \exp\left[-\frac{n}{2\sigma_U^2}\left(m_U^2 - 2\bar{u}m_U\right) - \frac{n}{2\sigma_Y^2}\left(m_Y^2 - 2\bar{y}m_Y\right)\right],$$

$$m'_U \leqslant m_U \leqslant m''_U, \quad m'_Y \leqslant m_Y \leqslant m''_Y. \tag{10.66}$$

Following the concept of the Bayes confidence estimation, we determine the value $\underline{g}_\gamma$ with the help of the following equation:

$$\iint_{\Omega(\underline{g}_\gamma)} a_0(m_Y, m_U)\, dm_Y dm_U = \gamma \int_{m'_U}^{m''_U} dm_U \int_{m'_Y}^{m''_Y} a_0(m_Y, m_U)\, dm_Y \tag{10.67}$$

where the domain $\Omega(\underline{g}_\gamma)$ containing the unknown limit $\underline{g}_\gamma$ represents by itself the intersection of the domains $\omega_1(\underline{g}_\gamma) = \{(m_Y, m_U) : m_Y \geqslant \underline{g}_\gamma m_U\}$ and $\omega_2 = [m'_U \leqslant m_U \leqslant m''_U,\ m'_Y \leqslant m_Y \leqslant m''_Y]$ the values of the variances σ_Y^2 and σ_U^2 are replaced by the corresponding posterior estimates.

The control procedure given below has an algorithmic nature and cannot be reduced to simpler calculations. The essential simplification may be achieved only for calculating the case with a constant admissible value.

10.4.3 *Calculating the case of a nonrandom admissible value*

Assume that Y obeys the normal law with the parameters m_Y and σ_Y, and the admissible value U always takes on a nonrandom value u. The probability that the condition of the operational capacity of the system holds, that is,

$$R = P\left\{\frac{Y}{u} > 1\right\} = \Phi\left(\frac{g-1}{\sigma_Y/u}\right). \tag{10.68}$$

The value of the inventory coefficient of the operational capacity of the system guaranteeing the fulfilment of the requirement about the reliability R_{req} is determined in accordance with (10.68) by the formula

$$g_{\text{req}} = z_{\text{req}}\frac{\sigma Y}{u} + 1, \tag{10.69}$$

where Z_{req} is the quantile of the normal distribution of the probability R_{req}. From this point we will follow the scheme of 10.4.3: using the results of testing $\underset{\sim}{\varepsilon_Y}$ we estimate the lower confidence limit $\underline{g}_\gamma$ for the coefficient $g = m_Y/u$ and control the reliability behavior of the system with the help of the condition $\underline{g}_\gamma \geqslant g_{\text{req}}$.

For the construction of the Bayes posterior estimate of $g = m_Y/u$, we use the known solution, based on the conjugated prior distributions [202]. As in 10.4.2 we will assume absolute error Δ_m and Δ_σ of the prior distribution of the parameters m_Y and σ_Y are given, i.e., we suppose that $[m'_Y, m''_Y]$ is the interval of a prior uncertainty for m_Y, where $m'_Y = m_Y^{(0)} - \Delta_m$, $m''_Y = m_Y^{(0)} + \Delta_m$, and for $\sigma_Y\,[\sigma'_Y, \sigma''_Y]$, where $\sigma''_Y = \sigma_Y^{(0)} + \Delta'_{\sigma Y} = \sigma_Y^{(0)}$. In accordance with [202], the prior distribution for m_Y and $c_Y = \sigma_Y^{-2}$ has the form

$$h(m_Y, c_Y) = h_c(c_Y)\,h_m(m_Y \mid c_Y), \tag{10.70}$$

where

$$h_c(c_Y) = h_c(c_Y; s'^2, \nu') = \left(\frac{\nu' s'^2}{2}\right)^{\nu'/2} \frac{c_Y^{\nu'/2-1}}{\Gamma\left(\frac{\nu'}{2}\right)} \exp\left(-\frac{1}{2}\nu' s'^2 c_Y\right), \quad c_Y > 0, \;\; \nu' > 0, \tag{10.71}$$

and

$$h_m(m_Y \mid c_Y) = \frac{(c_Y n')^{1/2}}{\sqrt{2\pi}} \exp\left[-\frac{1}{2}c_Y n' (m_Y - m')^2\right]. \tag{10.72}$$

The parameters of the densities (10.71) and (10.72) are determined by a priori known numerical characteristics $m_Y^{(0)}$, Δ_m, $\sigma_Y^{(0)}$, Δ_σ, analogously to the formulas (10.52) and (10.53):

$$m' = m_Y^{(0)}, \quad n' = \frac{g\sigma_Y^{(0)2}}{\Delta_m^2}, \tag{10.73}$$

$$s'^2 = \sigma_Y^{(0)2} \quad \text{and} \quad \nu' = \frac{9\sigma_Y^{(0)2}}{2\Delta_\sigma^2}. \tag{10.74}$$

For obtaining $\underline{g}_\gamma = \underline{m}_{Y\gamma}/u$ we need to know the posterior density $\bar{h}_m(m_Y/\hat{c}_Y)$, where $\hat{c}_Y$ is the posterior estimate of the parameter c_Y. In accordance with the theory of conjugated prior distributions, for the Gaussian case the desired posterior density is determined [202] by the expression (10.72), but with other parameters, i.e.

$$h_m(m_Y \mid \hat{c}_Y) = \left(\frac{\hat{c}_Y n''}{2\pi}\right)^{1/2} \exp\left[-\frac{1}{2}\hat{c}_Y n''(m_Y - m'')^2\right], \tag{10.75}$$

where

$$n'' = n' + n, \quad m'' = \frac{n'm'' + n\hat{m}}{n' + n}, \quad \hat{c}_Y = \left[\frac{v' + n}{v'}s'^2 + n'm'^2 + n\hat{D} + n\hat{m}^2 - n''m''\right]^{-1},$$

$$m' = \frac{1}{n}\sum_{i=1}^{n} y_i \quad \text{and} \quad \hat{D} = \frac{1}{n}\sum_{i=1}^{n}(y_i - \hat{m})^2.$$

In accordance with the concept of the Bayes confidence estimation, lower confidence limit $\underline{m}_Y$ with the confidence level γ is determined by equation

$$\int_{\underline{m}_Y}^{\infty} \tilde{\lambda}_m(m_Y \mid \hat{c}_Y)\,dm_Y = \gamma.$$

Having performed the necessary calculations, we finally obtain

$$\underline{g}_\gamma = \frac{m''}{u} - z_{1-\gamma}\cdot\frac{1}{u\hat{c}_Y n''}, \tag{10.76}$$

which allows us to control the attainment of the reliability level $R_{\text{req}}$with the help of the condition $\underline{g}_\gamma > g_{\text{req}}$.

Example 10.1 (A numerical example). Suppose that the required level of satisfaction of the operational capacity condition $R_{\text{req}} = 0.99$ while the admissible value of the parameter $u = 3.5$. A priori we are given $m_Y^{(0)} = 4.72$, $\Delta_m = 0.8$, $\sigma_Y^{(0)} = 0.4$, $\Delta_\sigma = 0.1$. The required value of the operational capacity inventory is $g_{\text{req}} = 1.266$. As seen from the example conditions, under the system elaborations the given TTF is ensured since $m_Y/u = 1.349 > g_{\text{req}}$.

During the experiment the first five tests, we demonstrate the following values of the key parameter $Y : y_1 = 4.85$, $y_2 = 4.90$, $y_3 = 5.08$, $y_4 = 3.60$, $y_5 = 3.85$. In Fig. 10.3 we depict the empirical curve of change of the estimate $\underline{g}_{0.9}$. As seen from the graph, after the fourth test the condition of fulfilment of the reliability requirement is broken. This implies some correction that results in the following values of three successive tests $y_6 = 5.26$, $y_7 = 4.94$, $y_8 = 5.08$. The curve $\underline{g}_{0.9}(j)$ has returned to the domain of required reliability.

As was mentioned in Chapter 9, a lot of engineering methods of calculation constructions and technical devices use essentially the notion of the safety coefficient without taking into account the random nature of the system parameters. The value of the safety coefficients are chosen, as a rule, from a wide range which are not connected in practice with the real

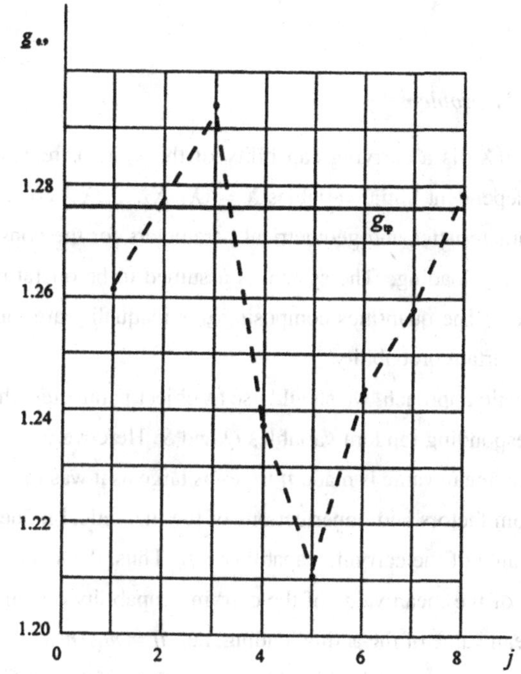

Fig. 10.4 Estimate for the Safety Coefficient as a Function of the Coefficient of Variation.

peculiarities of certain systems. If one applies the methods of a probability projection, i.e., chooses the system parameters in accordance with the required probability of its working capacity, then this shortcoming is eliminated, since the notion of a safety coefficient is not applied under the probability projection. As an example of this circumstance, we may choose the problems given in Chapters 8–10. However, due to the inertia of existing deterministic approaches to the projection (in particular, projection of the construction elements), safety coefficients will be used in practice for a long time. Therefore, the problem of development of the method of statistical estimation of the safety factors, applied for the calculations of certain objects, is very important. This method must, above all, take into account the required TTF level, probability characteristics of the parameters of the investigated system, and experimental data that let us verify the working capacity model of the system.

In this section we formulate and solve the problem of statistical estimation of the safety factors for the typical engineering method in the case of a Gaussian distribution of the status variable.

10.4.4 *Setting of the problem*

Suppose that $Q = \phi(\mathbf{X})$ is a carrying capability of the system, represented in the form of a function of independent initial variables $\mathbf{X} = (X_1, X_2, \ldots, X_n)$ containing in particular the mechanical characteristics and geometrical parameters for the construction elements. Denote by S the acting loading. The system is assumed to be operating if the condition $\phi(\mathbf{X}) \geqslant S$ is satisfied. The quantities composing this inequality are random, thus the inequality holds with certain probability.

Using the deterministic approach, we should use as object parameters the mean values m_Q and m_S of the corresponding random variables Q and S. Here we use the condition $m_Q = \eta m_S$, i.e., the loading mean value is made η times as large as it was in order to compensate for numerous random factors and imperfections of the theoretical model; $Q = \phi(\mathbf{X})$ leads to the calculating value of the carrying capability m_Q. Thus, the safety coefficient has the sense of a quotient of the mean value of the carrying capability obtained by a theoretical approach, to the mean value of the acting loading, i.e., $\eta = m_Q/m_S$.

Using the working capacity model with additive error considered in Chapter 9, we write the working capacity condition in the form

$$Q + m_Q\varepsilon - S > 0; \tag{10.77}$$

ε in this inequality has the sense of relative error of the theoretical dependence) $Q = \phi(\mathbf{X})$, and obeys the known distribution $f_\varepsilon(\varepsilon;\theta)$. The parameter θ is, generally speaking, unknown, but we are given the prior density $h(\theta)$ which concentrates by itself information about the error ε. It is assumed also that we know the distributions of probabilities of the random variables Q and S.

During the object design we can carry out such an experiment that may give us the factual level of carrying capability. Assume that in each of n independent tests the object is put in the condition of destruction, i.e., in such a condition when the applied loading will be equal to the factual (not calculating) carrying capability. In each j-th test we measure the values of destruction loading s_j^* and the values of all initial parameters included in the vector $\mathbf{x}_j$. This enables us to find the theoretical value of the carrying capability $q_j = \phi(\mathbf{x}_j)$. Since during the test a failure is observed, i.e., the condition $q_j + m_Q\varepsilon_j - s_j^* = 0$ holds, there is a possibility of determination of the factual value of the relative error ε_j:

$$\varepsilon_j = \frac{s_j^* - q_j}{m_Q}, \quad j = 1, 2, \ldots, n. \tag{10.78}$$

The problem is to find the posterior estimates of the safety coefficient η to account for the described set of the initial data and required value R_{req} of the probability of fulfillment of the condition (10.77).

10.4.5 *The case of Gaussian distributions*

Suppose that $Q \equiv N(m_Q, \sigma_Q)$, $S \equiv N(m_S, \sigma_S)$, and $\varepsilon \equiv N(m_\varepsilon, \sigma_\varepsilon)$, where we know the quotients $v_Q = \sigma_Q/m_Q$ and $v_S = \sigma_S/m_S$, which are called the variation coefficients of the theoretical carrying capability Q and loading S. The numerical characteristics m_ε and σ_ε are not given, but given the intervals of their prior uncertainty, correspondingly $[a,b]$ and $[c,d]$, where, $m_\varepsilon \equiv U(a,b)$, $\sigma_\varepsilon \equiv U(c,d)$.

For the Gaussian quantities Q, S and ε, the probability that the operational capacity condition (10.77) holds is written in the following way:

$$R = \Phi\left(\frac{m_Q - m_S + m_Q \cdot m_\varepsilon}{\sqrt{\sigma_Q^2 + \sigma_S^2 + m_Q^2\sigma_\varepsilon^2}}\right).$$

This probability is easily represented in the form of a function of the safety coefficient η, depending also on the parameters me m_ε, σ_ε, v_Q and v_S:

$$R(\eta) = \Phi\left(\frac{\eta(1 + m_\varepsilon) - 1}{\sqrt{v_Q^2\eta^2 + v_S^2 + \eta^2 m_Q^2 \sigma_\varepsilon^2}}\right). \tag{10.79}$$

Having equated $R(\eta) = R_{\text{req}}$ and using the expression (10.79), we obtain the equation for the safety coefficient, corresponding to the required TTF level

$$\eta(1 + m_\varepsilon) - 1 = z_{\text{req}}\left(v_Q^2\eta^2 + v_S^2 + \eta^2\sigma_\varepsilon^2\right)^{1/2},$$

where z_{req} is the quantile of the normal distribution of the probability of R_{req}. In the domain $\eta > 1$ this equation has a single root

$$\eta = \frac{(1 + m_\varepsilon)^2 + z_{\text{req}}\left[v_Q^2 + v_S^2 - z_{\text{req}}^2 v_Q^2 v_S^2 + \left(1 - z_{\text{req}}^2 v_S^2\right)\sigma_\varepsilon^2 + m_\varepsilon v_S^2\right]^{1/2}}{(1 + m_\varepsilon)^2 - z_{\text{req}}^2\left(v_Q^2 + \sigma_\varepsilon^2\right)}. \tag{10.80}$$

Since the variation coefficients v_Q and v_S are known, we will emphasize the dependence of the safety coefficient on the parameters of the model error, i.e., $\eta = \eta(m_\varepsilon, \sigma_\varepsilon)$.

The procedure of estimation of the coefficient η is followed further on by the standard scheme of Bayes estimation. Using the sample of the sample results $\underset{\sim}{\varepsilon} = (\varepsilon_1, \varepsilon_2, \ldots, \varepsilon_n)$

determined by the formula (10.78) and assumption $\varepsilon \equiv N(m_\varepsilon, \sigma_\varepsilon)$, we write the likelihood function

$$\ell(m_\varepsilon, \sigma_\varepsilon \mid \underset{\sim}{\varepsilon}) = \ell(m_\varepsilon, \sigma_\varepsilon; v_1, v_2) = \frac{1}{(2\pi)^{n/2}} \cdot \frac{1}{\sigma_\varepsilon^n} \exp\left[-\frac{n}{2\sigma_\varepsilon^2}\left(v_2 - 2m_\varepsilon v_1 + m_\varepsilon^2\right)\right],$$

and the testing statistics

$$v_k = \frac{1}{n}\sum_{j=1}^{n} \varepsilon_j^k \quad (k = 1, 2).$$

Since the parameters m_ε and σ_ε have uniform prior distributions correspondingly in the intervals $[a,b]$ and $[c,d]$, the posterior density $\hbar\left(m_\varepsilon, \sigma_\varepsilon \mid \underset{\sim}{\varepsilon}\right)$ satisfies the relation

$$\hbar\left(m_\varepsilon, \sigma_\varepsilon \mid \underset{\sim}{\varepsilon}\right) \sim a_0(m_\varepsilon, \sigma_\varepsilon) = \frac{n}{\sigma_\varepsilon^n} \exp\left[-\frac{n}{2\sigma_\varepsilon^2}\left(v_2 - 2m_\varepsilon v_1 + m_\varepsilon^2\right)\right],$$

$$m_\varepsilon \in [a,b], \quad \sigma_\varepsilon \in [c,d]. \tag{10.81}$$

Using a quadratic loss function, we will find the pointwise posterior estimate of η in the form

$$\hat{\eta}^* = \frac{1}{\beta}\int_a^b \int_c^d \eta(m_\varepsilon, \sigma_\varepsilon) a_0(m_\varepsilon, \sigma_\varepsilon) dm_\varepsilon d\sigma_\varepsilon, \tag{10.82}$$

where

$$\beta = \int_a^b \int_c^d a_0(m_\varepsilon, \sigma_\varepsilon) dm_\varepsilon d\sigma_\varepsilon.$$

For the posterior variance we analogously have

$$\sigma_{\hat{\eta}^*}^2 = \frac{1}{\beta}\int_a^b \int_c^d \eta^2(m_\varepsilon, \sigma_\varepsilon) a_0(m_\varepsilon, \sigma_\varepsilon) dm_\varepsilon d\sigma_\varepsilon - \hat{\eta}^{*2}. \tag{10.83}$$

As some guaranteeing estimate of the safety coefficient, the upper confidence limit of the quantity η may be used, this is determined in accordance with the concept of the Bayes confidence estimation, from the equation

$$\iint_{\Theta\left(\bar{\eta}_\gamma^*\right)} a_0(m_\varepsilon, \sigma_\varepsilon) dm_\varepsilon d\sigma_\varepsilon = \gamma\beta \tag{10.84}$$

in which the unknown estimates lie in the integration domain. The last one appears to be the intersection of the rectangle $[a,b] \times [c,d]$ and the set of values of me and m_ε, determined by the inequality $\eta(m_\varepsilon, \sigma_\varepsilon) \leqslant \bar{\eta}_\gamma^*$.

The calculations from the relations (10.82)–(10.84) assume using numerical methods of double integration and solutions of transcendental equations.

10.4.6 *Numerical analysis of the obtained estimates*

In order to clarify the influence of different factors on the behavior of estimates of the safety coefficient, we have to carry out numerous calculations using formulas (10.82)–(10.84) for a wide range of values of initial data.

In Table 10.4 we represent calculated results with $v_Q = v_S = 0.05$, $s_\varepsilon = (v_2 - v_1^2)^{1/2} = 0.03$ and the following a priori information $m_\varepsilon \in [-0.10; 0.10]$, $\sigma_\varepsilon \in [0.01; 0.06]$. For each value of the variate parameter we have determined three estimates $\hat{\eta}^*$, $\sigma_{\hat{\eta}}$ and $\bar{\eta}_{0.9}^*$ represented in Table 10.4. As seen from Table 10.4, the increasing of the statistic v_1 implies decreasing of the safety coefficient. This tendency may be easily interpreted. That is, v_1 can be interpreted as the sample mean for the relative error ε. When $v_1 < 0$, it displays the preponderance of the negative values or ε_j in the experimental data $\underset{\sim}{\varepsilon}$. If such an experimental value is realized, the event $s_j^* < q_j$, i.e., the factual carrying capability s_j^*, is less than theoretical one q_j. In other words, from the experimental results it follows that theoretical model $Q = \phi(\mathbf{X})$ implies the overstating of representation about the carrying capability. In the alternative situation, when $v_1 > 0$, we meet the preponderance of the events $s_j^* > q_j$, that is, in this case the theoretical model understates in preference the factual carrying capability. It is clear that for compensation of model error in the first situation we need to choose a greater value of the safety coefficient.

The behavior of the estimate $\bar{\eta}_{0.9}^*$ in accordance with the change of the variation coefficient of the loading v_S is given in Fig. 10.4. The cause is the presence of the random scattering of the loading and factors of carrying capability is the second reason of introducing the safety coefficient. The random nature of the loading is well determined by the variation coefficient. Increasing of the loading implies increasing the safety coefficient. The quantitative nature of these circumstances is illustrated in Fig. 10.4.

Note one more peculiarity appearing in the calculating experiment. In the case when the empirical data, expressed by the statistics v_1 and s_ε, lie near the corresponding indeterminacy intervals $[a, b]$ and $[c, d]$. Increasing the length of these intervals doesn't give us an appreciable change in the estimates of the safety coefficient. Hence, we may conclude the following: we should not choose narrow intervals of prior uncertainty for the parameters of error for the theoretical working capacity model. Besides, based on this argument, we have more chances for not observing experimental results that contradict the prior information.

Table 10.4 Bayes estimates for the safety coefficient.

v_1	$R_{\text{req}} = 0.99$	$R_{\text{req}} = 0.999$	$R_{\text{req}} = 0.9999$
	1.2445	1.3412	1.4304
−0.09	0.0131	0.0202	0.0275
	1.2613	1.3670	1.4657
	1.2318	1.3231	1.4072
−0.06	0.0133	0.0203	0.0276
	1.2488	1.3490	1.4425
	1.2186	1.3043	1.3830
−0.03	0.0124	0.0187	0.0255
	1.2345	1.3283	1.4156
	1.2065	1.2872	1.3610
0	0.0115	0.0174	0.0236
	1.2213	1.3095	1.3911
	1.1955	1.2715	1.3409
0.03	0.0108	0.0163	0.0220
	1.2093	1.2923	1.3691
	1.1854	1.2573	1.3227
0.06	0.0098	0.0150	0.0202
	1.1980	1.2765	1.3485
	1.1763	1.2444	1.3061
0.09	0.0094	0.0141	0.0190
	1.1883	1.2624	1.3305

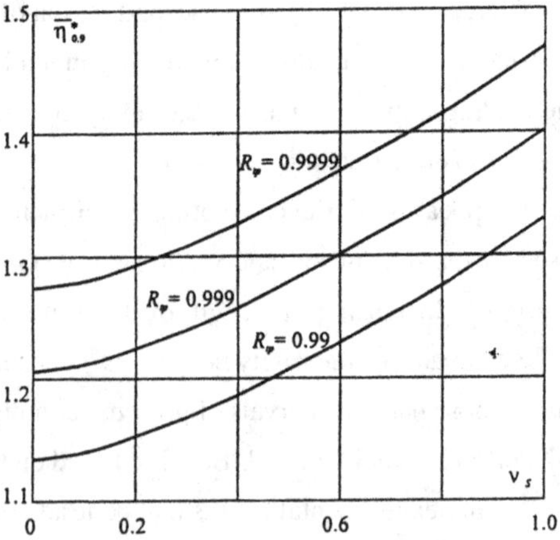

Fig. 10.5 The estimate for the safety coefficient as a function of the variance.

Bibliography

[1] J. Aitchison, *Two papers on the comparison of Bayesian and frequentist approaches to statistical problems of prediction,* Royal Stat. Soc., Ser. B., **26**, (1964), no. 2, 161–175.

[2] H. Akaike, *An objective use of Bayesian models,* Ann. Inst. Stat. Soc., Ser. B., **29**, (1977), 9–20.

[3] H. Akaike, *A New Look at the Bayes Procedure,* Biometrika, **65**, (1978), no. 6, 53–59.

[4] H. Akaike, *Likelihood and the Bayesian Procedure,* Trab. Estadist. y Invest. Oper., **21**, (1980), 143–166.

[5] A. Ando and G. M. Kaufman, *Bayesian Analysis of the Independent Multinormal Process-Neither Mean Nor Precision Known,* Amer. Statist. Assoc., **60**, (1965), no. 3, 345–358.

[6] R. A. Babillis and A. M. Smith, *Application of Bayesian statistics in reliability measurements,* in "Proc. Ann. R & M Conf.," vol. 4, 1965, pp. 357–365.

[7] H. S. Balaban, *Bayesian approach for designing component life tests,* in "Proc. 1967 Ann. Symp. Rel.," Washington, D.C., 1967, 59–74.

[8] G. A. Bancroft and I. R. Dunsmore, *Predictive distributions in life tests under competing causes of failure,* Biometrika, **63**, (1978), no. 2, 195–217.

[9] P. Barlow and F. Proshan, "Mathematical Reliability Theory," Soviet Radio, Moscow, 1969, 448 pgs. (Russian).

[10] P. Barlow and F. Proshan, "Statistical Reliability Theory and Failure–Free Testing," Science, Moscow, 1984, 328 pgs. (Russian).

[11] R. E. Barlow, *A Bayes explanation of an apparent failure rate paradox,* IEEE Transaction Reliab., **R-34**, (1985), no. 2, 107–108.

[12] D. Basu, *Randomization analysis of experimental data: the Fisher randomization,* Amer. Statist. Assoc., **75**, (1980), no. 371, 575–595.

[13] T. Bayes, *An essay towards solving a problem in the doctrine of chances,* (with a bibliographical note by G. A. Barnard), Biometrika, **45**, (1958), no. 2, 293–315.

[14] Ju. K. Belyaev, "Statistical Methods and Results of Reliability Testing," Znanie, Moscow, 1982, pp. 3–66. (Russian).

[15] Ju. K. Belyaev, *Multiple probability estimates of failure-free work,* Izv. AN SSSR, (1985), no. 4, 45–59.

[16] G. K. Bennett, *Basic concepts of empirical Bayes methods with some results for the Weibull distribution,* in "The Theory and Application of Realiability," vol. 1, Acad. Press, New York, 1981, pp. 181–202.

[17] G. K. Bennett and H. F. Martz, *A n empirical Bayes estimator for the scale parameter of the two-parameter Weibull distribution,* Nav. Res. Log. Quar., **20**, (1973), no. 4, 387–393.

[18] G. K. Bennett and H. F. Martz, *A continuous empirical Bayes smoothing technique,* Biometrika, **59**, (1972), 361–368.

[19] R. H. Berk, *Limited behavior of posterior distributions when the model is incorrect,* Ann.

Math. Statist., **37**, (1966), no. 1, 51–58.

[20] J. M. Bernardo, *Reference posterior distributions for Bayesian inference,* Royal Statist. Soc., Ser. B, **41**, (1979), no. 2, 113–147.

[21] J. Bernully, "On Large Numbers Law," Science, Moscow, 1986, 176 pgs. (Russian).

[22] S. K. Bhaltacharya, *Bayesian approach to the life testing and estimation,* Amer. Statist. Assoc., **62**, (1967), no. 1, 48–62.

[23] I. A. Birger, B. F. Shor and G. B. Iosilevich, "Reliabilty Estimation for Machine Details," Mashinostroenie, Moscow, 1979, 704 pgs. (Russian).

[24] P. J. Bickel and J. A. Yahow, *Asymptotically pointwise optimal procedures in sequential analysis,* Proc. Fifth Berkley Symp. Math. Statist. Prob. 1, (1965), 401–413.

[25] R. P. Bland, *On the definition of unbiasedness for estimating parameters which are random variables,* Commun. Statist. Simula. Computation, **B-I0**, (1981), no. 4, 435–436.

[26] V. V. Bolotin, "Probability and Reliabilty Methods in Equipment Design," Strojizdat, Moscow, 1982, 350 pgs. (Russian).

[27] G. Boole, "Studies in Logic and Probability," Walts, London, 1953.

[28] G. E. Box and G. C. Tico, *A further look at robustness via Bayes theorem,* Biometica, **49**, (1962), no. 4, 419–433.

[29] A. M. Breipohl, R. R. Priorie and W. J. Zimmer, *A consideration of the Bayesian approach in reliability evaluation,* IEEE Trans. Reliab., **R-14**, (1965), no. 1, 107–113.

[30] N. G. Bruevich and Yu. G. Milgram, "On the Question of Determining the Probabilty of Failure-Free Work of Equipments Based on Experience and Self-Learning," SOy. Radio, Moscow, 1975, pp. 7–26.

[31] K. V. Buers, R. W. S. Keith and M.D. Springer, *Bayesian confidence limits for the reliability of mixed cascade and parallel independent exponential subsystems,* IEEE Trans. Reliab., **R-23**, (1974), no. 1, 104–108.

[32] N. G. Bruevich and V. V. Sergeev, "The Basics of Non–Linear Device Reliabilty Theory," Science, Moscow, 1976, 136 pgs.

[33] K. V. Bury, *Bayesian decision analysis of the hazard rate for a twoparameter Weibull process,* IEEE Trans. Reliab., **R-21**, (1972), no. 2, 159–169.

[34] V. A. R. Camara and C. P. Tsokos, *The effect of loss functions on empirical Bayes reliability analysis,* Mathematical Problems in Engineering, **TMA**, (1999), to appear.

[35] V. A. R. Camara and C. P. Tsokos, *The effect of loss function on Bayesian reliability analysis,* in "Proceedings of the International Conference on Non-Linear Problems in Aviation and Aerospace," 1997, pp. 75–90.

[36] G. Cambell and M. Hollander, *Prediction intervals with Dirichlet process prior distribution,* Canad. J. Statist., **10**, (1982), no. 2, 103–111.

[37] G. C. Canavos, *Bayesian approach to parameter and reliability estimation in the Poisson distribution,* IEEE Trans. Reliab., **R-21**, (1972), no. 1, 52–56.

[38] G. C. Canavos, *An empirical Bayes approach for the Poisson life distribution,* IEEE Trans. Reliab., **R-22**, (1973), no. 1, 91–96.

[39] G. C. Canavos and C. P. Tsokos, *Bayesian estimation of life parameters in the Weibull distribution,* J. of Operations Research, **21**, (1973), no. 3, 755–763.

[40] G. C. Canavos and C. P. Tsokos, *Bayesian concepts for the estimation of reliability in the Wei bull life-testing model,* Ins. Stat. Ins. Rev., **40**, (1972), 153–160.

[41] E. Charatsis and C. P. Tsokos, *Sensitivity analysis of Bayesian reliability models,* in "Proc. IntI. Symposium of Measurement and Control," 1979.

[42] V. I. Cherneckij, "Analysis of Non–Linear Control Systems," Machinostroyeniye, Moscow, 1968, 246 pgs.

[43] A. A. Chervonyj, V. I. Lukjashenko and V. 1. Kotin, "Reliability of Composed Technical Systems," Machinostroyeniye, Moscow, 1976, 288 pgs. (Russian).

[44] P. V. Z. Cole, *A Bayesian reliability assessment of complex systems for binomial sampling,* IEEE Trans. Reliab., **R-24**, (1975), no. 1, 114–117.

[45] A. G. Colombo, D. Costantini and R. J. Jaarsma, *Bayes nonparametric estimation of time-dependent failure rate,* IEEE Trans. Reliab., **R-34**, (1985), no. 2, 109–113.

[46] P. G. Convert, *Entropie et theoreme de Bayes en theorie de l'estimation,* Rev. Techn. Thonson., **14**, (1967), no. 1, 5–17. (French).

[47] T. Cornfield, *The Bayesian outlook and its application,* Review Int. Stat. Inst., **35**, (1967), no. 1, 34–39.

[48] D. J. Couture and H. F. Martz, *Empirical Bayes estimation in the Weibull distribution,* IEEE Trans. Reliab., **R-21**, (1972), no. 1, 75–83.

[49] R. T. Cox, "The Algebra of Probable Inference," J. Hopkins Press, Baltimore, MD, 1961, 224 pgs.

[50] G. L. Crellin, *The philosophy and mathemamatics of Bayes equation,* IEEE Trans. Reliab., **R-21**, (1972), no. 3, 131–135.

[51] S. R. Dalal, *A note on adequacy of mixtures of Dirichlet processes,* Sankhya, A., **40**, (1978), no. 1, 185–191.

[52] S. R. Dalal and G. T. Hall, *On approximating parametric Bayes models,* Ann. Statist. 8 (1980), no. 5, 664–672.

[53] S. R. Dalal and E. C. Phadia, *Nonparametric Bayes inference for concordance in bivariate distributions,* Commun. Statist. Theor. Meth., **12**, (1983), no. 8, 947–963.

[54] A. P. Dawid, *On the limiting normality of posterior distributions,* Proc. Camb. Phil. Soc., **67**, (1970), no. 7, 625–633.

[55] A. P. Dawid and J. Guttman, *Conjugate Bayesian inference for structural models,* Commun. Statist., **A–I0**, (1981), no. 8, 739–748.

[56] A. P. Dawid, M. Stone and J. V. Zidek, *Marginalization paradoxes in Bayesian and statistical inference,* J. Royal Statist. Soc. B., **35**, (1974), no. 2, 189–223.

[57] C. H. Deans and C. P. Tsokos, *Bayesian estimation in the MakehamGompertz distribution,* METRON, **XXXVII**, (1980), nos. 3–4, 57–80.

[58] C. H. Deans and C. P. Tsokos, *Sensitivity of loss functions used to obtain Bayes estimates of survival,* Statistica (1981), 181–192.

[59] J. J. Deely and D. V. Lindley, *Bayes empirical Bayes,* Amer. Stat. Assoc., **76**, (1981), no. 376, 833–941.

[60] J. J. Deely, M. S. Tierney and W. J. Zimmer, *On the usefulness of the maximum entropy principle in the Bayesian estimation of reliability,* IEEE Trans. Reliab., **R-19**, (1970), no. 1, 110–115.

[61] B. De Finetti, *Bayesianism: its role for both the foundations and applications of statistics,* Internat. Statist. Rev., **42**, (1974), no. 1, 117–130.

[62] B. De Finetti, "Probability, Induction and Statistics," Wiley, London, 1972, 240 pgs.

[63] M. H. De Groot, "Optimal Statistical Solutions," Mir, Moscow, 1974, 492 pgs.

[64] M. H. De Groot and M. M. Rao, *Bayes estimation with convex loss,* Ann. Math. Statist., **34**, (1963), no. 6, 839–846.

[65] I. P. Devjatirenkov, *Rough Bayes estimates,* in "Proceedings of 4th All Union School on Additive Systems," Alma-Ata, 1978, pp. 70–75.

[66] T. Diaz, *Bayesian detection of the change of scale parameter in sequences of independent gamma random variables,* Econom., **19**, (1982), 23–29.

[67] K. Doksum, *Tailfree and neutral random probabilities and their posterior distributions,* Ann. Probability 2 (1974), 183–201.

[68] A. W. Drake, *Bayesian statistics for the reliability engineer,* in "Proc. Ann. Symp. Reliability," 1966, pp. 315–320.

[69] I. R. Dunsmore, *The Bayesian predictive distribution in life testing models,* Technometrics,

16, (1974), no. 3, 455–460.

[70] R. L. Dykstra and P. Loud, *A Bayesian nonparametric approach to reliability,* Ann. Statist. 9 (1981), no. 2, 356–367.

[71] R. G. Easterling, *A personal view of the Bayesian controversy on relability and statistics,* IEEE Trans. Reliab., **R-21**, (1972), no. 3, 186–194.

[72] A. W. E. Edwards, *Commentary on the arguments of Thomas Bayes,* Scand. J. Statist. 5 (1978), no. 2, 116–118.

[73] G. M. El–Sayyad, *Estimation of the parameter of an exponential distribution,* Royal Statist. Soc., Ser. B., **29**, (1967), no. 4, 525–532.

[74] R. A. Evans, *Prior knowledge: engineers versus statisticians,* IEEE Trans. Reliab., **R-18**, (1969), no. 2, p. 143.

[75] R. A. Evans, *The principle of minimum information,* IEEE Trans. Reliab., **R-18**, (1969), no. 1, 87–90.

[76] R. A. Evans, *Data we will never get,* IEEE Trans. Reliab., **R-20**, (1971), no. 1, p. 20.

[77] R. A. Evans, *Bayes: in theory and practice,* in "The Theory and Applications of Reliability," vol. 2, Acad. Press Inc., New York, 1977, pp. 50–54.

[78] I. G. Evans and A. M. Nigm, *Bayesian prediction for two-parameter Weibulllifetime models,* Commun. Statist. Theory Meth., **A-9**, (1980), no. 6, 649–658.

[79] B. Fellenberg and J. Pilz, *On the choice of prior distribution for Bayesian reliability analysis,* Freiberger Forsch, **D-170**, (1985), 49–68.

[80] T. S. Ferguson, *Bayesian analysis of some nonparametric problems,* Ann. Stat. 1 (1973), no. 2, 209–230.

[81] T. S. Ferguson, *Prior distribution on space of probability measures,* Ann. Statist. 2 (1974), no. 5, 615–629.

[82] T. S. Ferguson, *Sequential estimation with Dirichlet process priors,* in "Statistical Decision Theory and Related Topics," Acad. Press Inc., vol. 1, 1982, pp. 385–401.

[83] T. S. Ferguson and E. G. Phadia, *Bayesian nonparametric estimation based on censored data,* Ann. Statist. 1 (1979), no. 1, 163–186.

[84] R. A. Fisher, "Statistical Methods and Scientific Inference," Oliver I. Boyd, Edinburg, 1959.

[85] R. A. Fisher, *The logic of inductive inference* (with discussion), Royal Statist. Soc., **98**, (1935), no. 1, 39–82.

[86] J. Forsait, M. Malcolm and K. Mowler, "Machinery Methods of Mathematical Calculatons," Mir, Moscow, 1980, 279 pgs. (Russian).

[87] D. A. Freedman, *On the asymptotic behavior of Bayes' estimation in the discrete case,* Ann. Math. Statist., **34**, (1963), no. 12, 1386–1403.

[88] M. A. Girshick and L. G. Savage, *Bayes and minimax estimates for quadratic loss function,* in "Proc. Second Berkley Symp. Math. Statist. Prob.," vol. 1, 1951, pp. 53–74.

[89] V. F. Gladkij, "Probabilistic Method in Designing of Aircraft," Nauka, Moscow, 1982, 272 pgs. (Russian).

[90] B. V. Gnedenko, "Probability Theory," Nauka, Moscow, 1969, 400 pgs.

[91] B. V. Gnedenko, Ju. K. Belyaev and A. D. Solovijev, "Mathematical Methods in Reliability Theory," Nauka, Moscow, 1965, 524 pgs.

[92] I. J. Good, *The estimation of probabilities,* in "An Essay on Modern Bayesian Methods," Wiley, 1965, pp. 110.

[93] I. J. Good, "Probability and the Weighting of Evidence," Griffin, London, 1950, 168 pgs.

[94] I. J. Good, *Some history of the hierarchical Bayesian methodology,* Trab. Estadist. Invest. Oper., **31**, (1980), no. 1, 489–504.

[95] R. D. Guild, *Bayesian MFR life test sampling plans,* Quality Technology, 5 (1973), no. 1, 11–15.

[96] I. Guttman and G. C. Tiao, *A Bayesian approach to some best population problems,* Ann.

Math. Statist., **35**, (1964), no. 7, 825–835.

[97] C. W. Hamilton and J. E. Drenna, *Research towards a Bayesian procedure for calculating system reliability,* Aerospace Ann. of Rand M, (1964), 614–620.

[98] G. G. Haritonova, *Bayes probability estimation in the case of indetermined initial data,* Reliability and Quality Control (1986), no. 11, 24–26. (Russian).

[99] B. Harris, *A survey of statistical methods in systems reliability using Bernoulli sampling of components,* in "Proc. Conf. Theory and Appl. of Reliab. Emphasis Bayesian and Nonparametr. Meth.," PUBLISHER, New York, 1976, pp. 86–98.

[100] B. Harris and N. Singpurwalla, *Life distributions derived from stochastic hazard junctions,* IEEE Trans. Reliab., **R-17**, (1968), no. 1, 70–79.

[101] J. A. Hartigan, *Invariant prior distributions,* Ann. Math. Statist., **36**, (1964), 836–845.

[102] J. A. Hartigan, "Bayes Theory," Springer-Verlag, New York, 1983, 140 pgs.

[103] J. J. Higgins and C. P. Tsokos, *On the behavior of some quantities used in Bayesian reliability demonstration tests,* IEEE Trans. Reliab., **R-25**, (1976), no. 2, 261–264.

[104] J. J. Higgins and C. P. Tsokos, *Sensitivity of Bayes estimates of reciprocal MTBF and reliability to an incorrect failure model,* IEEE Trans. Reliab., **R-226**, (1977), no. 4, 286–289.

[105] J. J. Higgins and C. P. Tsokos, *Comparison of Bayesian estimates of failure intensity for fitted priors of life data,* in "Proceedings of the Conf. on the Theory and Applications of Reliability With Emphasis on Bayesian and Nonparametric Methods," vol. 1, Academic Press, New York, 1976, pp. 75–92.

[106] J. J. Higgins and C. P. Tsokos, *Comparison of Bayesian estimates of failure intensity for fitted priors of life data,* in "Proceedings of the Conf. on the Theory and Applications of Reliability," vol. 2, 1977, 75–92.

[107] J. J. Higgins and C. P. Tsokos, *Modified method-of-moments in empirical Bayes estimation,* IEEE Trans. Reliab., **R-28** (December 1979), no. 1, 27–31.

[108] J. J. Higgins and C. P. Tsokos, *A study of the effect of the loss function on Bayes estimation of failure intensity, MTBF, and reliability,* J. Applied Mathematics and Computation 6 (1980), 145–166.

[109] J. J. Higgins and C. P. Tsokos, *Pseudo Bayes estimation for the parameter of the Weibull process,* IEEE Transactions on Reliability? (1981), 111–117.

[110] J. J. Higgins and C. P. Tsokos, *A Quasi-Bayes estimate of the failure intensity of a reliability-growth model,* IEEE Transactions on Reliability, **R–30**, (1981), no. 5, 471–476.

[111] V. P. Iluhin, *An estimation of a priori distribution in statistical solution problems,* Mathematical Statistics and Applications 5 (1979), 114–162.

[112] K. A. Iudu, "Optimization of Automatic Devices With Reliability Criteria," Sov. Radio, Moscow, 1962, 194 pgs.

[113] E. T. Jaynes, *Prior probabilities,* IEEE Trans. Syst. Sci. Cybernetics **SSC–4**, (1968), no. 3, 227–241.

[114] H. Jeffreys, "Theory of Probability," Clarendon Press, Oxford, 1961, 240 pgs.

[115] H. Jeffreys, "Theory of Probability," Clarendon, Oxford, 1966, 428 pgs.

[116] A. M. Joglekar, *Reliability demonstration based on prior distributionsensitivity analysis and multi–sample plans,* in "Proc. 1975 Ann. Rel. and Maint. Symp.," PUBLISHER, Washington, DC, 1975, pp. 251–252.

[117] R. A. Johnson, *Asymptotic expansions associated with posterior distributions,* Ann. Math. Statist., **41**, (1970), no. 10, 851–864.

[118] J. D. Kalbflesch, *Non–parametric Bayesian analysis of survival time data,* Royal Stat. Soc. B., **40**, (1978), no. 2, 214–221.

[119] S. J. Kamat, *Bayesian estimation of system reliability for Weibull distribution using Monte Carlo simulation,* in "The Theory and Applications of Reliability with Emphasis on Bayesian and Nonparametric Methods," vol. 2, Academic Press, New York, 1977, pgs.

123–131.

[120] K. Kanur and L. Lamberson, "Reliability and System Design," Mir, Moscow, 1980, 604 pgs.

[121] E. L. Kaplan and P. Meier, *Nonparametric estimation from incomplete observations,* Amer. Statist. Assoc., **53**, (1958), 457–481.

[122] G. D. Kartashov, "Principles of Storage Use and Reliability Estimation," Znanie, Moscow, 1984, pp. 3–82.

[123] M. Kendall and A. Stuart, "Statistical Conclusions and Relations," Nauka, Moscow, 1973, 900 pgs.

[124] J. M. Keynes, "A Treatise on Probability," Harper and Row, New York, 1921.

[125] D. Koks and D. Hinkly, "Theoretical Statistics," Mir, Moscow, 1978, 560 pgs.

[126] B. O. Koopman, *The bases of probability,* Bull. Amer. Math. Soc., **46**, (1940), 763–774.

[127] S. P. Korolev, "Design Principles of Long–Range Ballistic Missiles," Nauka, Moscow, 1980, 208–290.

[128] R. Korwar and M. Hollander, *Empirical Bayes estimation of a distribution function,* Ann. Statist. 4 (1976), no. 3, 581–588.

[129] D. Koutras and C. P. Tsokos, *The alpha probability distribution as a failure model,* JournalofInter. Assoc. of Science and Technology, (1978), 1–5.

[130] D. Koutras and C. P. Tsokos, *Bayesian analysis of the alpha failure model,* Statistica **39**, (1979), no. 3, 399–412.

[131] B. A. Kozlov and 1. A. Ushakov, "Radioelectronics and Automatic Reliability Control Directory," Sov. Radio, Moscow, 1975, 472 pgs.

[132] G. Kramer, "Methods of Mathematical Statistics," Mir, Moscow, 1975, 648 pgs.

[133] G. Kramer and M. Lidbetter, "Stationary Random Processes," Mir, Moscow, 1969, 400 pgs.

[134] E. 1. Krineckij and V. A. Piskunov, "Reliability Control of Aircraft," MAl, Moscow, 1983, 78 pgs.

[135] A. A. Kuznecov, "Reliabilty of Ballistic Missile Construction," Mashinostroenie, Moscow, 1978, 256 pgs.

[136] L. Le Cam, *On some asymptotic properties of maximum likelihood estimates and related Bayes estimates,* Univ. Calif. Publ. Statist., 1, (1953), no. 11, 277–330.

[137] G. H. Lemon, *An empirical Bayes approach to reliability,* IEEE Trans. Reliab., **R-21**, (1972), 155–158.

[138] L. L. Levy and A. H. Moore, *A Monte–Carlo technique for obtaining system reliability confidence limits from component test data,* IEEE Trans. Reliab., **R-16**, (1967), no. 1, 69–72.

[139] B. P. Lientz, *Modified Bayesian procedures in reliability testing,* in "The theory and application of reliability with emphasis on Bayesian and nonparametric methods," vol. 2, Academic Press, New York, 1977, pp. 163–171.

[140] E. E. Limer, "Statistical Analysis of Non–Experimental Data," Financy i Statistika, Moscow, 1983, 381 pgs. (Russian).

[141] C. Y. Lin and G. L. Schick, *On–line (Console–Aided) assessment of prior distributions for reliability problems,* in "Proc. Ann. Rand M Conf.," vol. 9, 1970, pp. 13–19.

[142] D. V. Lindley, "Making Desisions," Wiley Interscience, London, 1971, 242 pgs.

[143] D. Y. Lindley, *The use of prior probability distributions in statistical inference and decisions,* in "Fourth Berkley Symp. Math. Statist. Prob.," vol. 1, 1961, pp. 453–468.

[144] D. Y. Lindley, "Bayesian Statistics: a Review," SIAM, Philadelphia, 1972, 68 pgs.

[145] D. Y. Lindley, *The future of statistics: a Bayesian 21st century,* Appl. Prob. 7 (1975), 106–115.

[146] D. Y. Lindley, *The Bayesian approach,* Scand. J. Statist. 5 (1978), no. 1, 1–26.

[147] K. D. Ling and C. Y. Leong, *Bayesian predictive distributions for samples from exponential distributions,* Tamkang J. Math. 8 (1977), no. 1, 11–16.

[148] G. S. Lingappaiah, *Bayesian approach to the prediction problem in the exponential population,* IEEE Trans. Reliab., **R-27**, (1978), no. 2, 222–225.

[149] G. S. Lingappaiah, *Bayesian approach to the prediction problem in complete and censored samples from the gamma and exponential population,* Commun. Statist. Theory Meth., **A-8**, (1979), no. 14, 1403–1423.

[150] B. Littlewood and J. L. Verrall, *A Bayesian reliability model with a stochastically monotone failure rate,* IEEE Trans. Reliab., **R-23**, (1974), no. 1, 108–114.

[151] V. T. Lizin and V. A. Pjatkin, "Design of Construction With a Thin Shell," Mashinostroenie, Moscow, 1985, 344 pgs. (Russian).

[152] D. Lloyd and M. Lipov, "Reliability," SOy. Radio, Moscow, 1964, 686 pgs. (Russian).

[153] R. H. Lochner and A. P. Basu, *Bayesian analysis of the two-sample problem with incomplete data,* Amer. Statist. Assoc., **67**, (1972), no. 3, 432–438.

[154] R. H. Lochner and A. P. Basu, *A generalized Dirichlet distribution in Bayesian life testing,* Royal Statist. Soc. B., **37**, (1975), no. 1, 103–113.

[155] R. H. Lochner and A. P. Basu, *A Bayesian approach for testing increasing failure rate,* in "The theory and application of reliability," vol. 1, Acad. Press, New York, 1977, pp. 67–83.

[156] M. Loev, "Probability Theory," International Literature, Moscow, 1962, 720 pgs.

[157] T. Lwin and N. Singh, *Bayesian analysis of the gamma distribution model in reliability estimation,* IEEE Trans. Reliab., **R-23**, (1974), no. 3, 314–319.

[158] N. R. Mann, *Computer–aided selection of prior distribution for generating Monte Carlo confidence bounds on system reliability,* Nav. Res. Log. Quart., **17**, (1970), 41–54.

[159] N. R. Mann and F. E. Grubbs, *Approximately optimum confidence bounds on series system reliability for exponential time to failure data,* Biometrka **59**, (1972), no. 2, 191–204.

[160] K. Mardia and P. Zemroch, "Tables of F-distributions and Related Ones," Science, Moscow, 1984, 256 pgs. (Russian).

[161] H. F. Martz, *Pooling life test data by means of the empirical Bayes method,* IEEE Trans. Reliab., **R-24**, (1975), 27–30.

[162] H. F. Martz and M. G. Lian, *Empirical Bayes estimation of the binomial parameter,* Biometrika, **62**, (1975), 517–523.

[163] H. F. Martz and M. G. Lian, *Bayes and empirical Bayes point and interval estimation of reliability for the Weibull model,* in "The Theory and Applications of Reliability with Emphasis on Bayesian and Nonparametric Methods," vol. 1, Academic Press, New York, 1977, pp. 203–233.

[164] G. Meeden and D. Isaacson, *Approximate behavior of the posterior distribution for a large observation,* Ann. Statist. 5 (1977), no. 5, 899–908.

[165] V. B. Mitrofanov, "On one multidimensional search algorithm," IPU AN SSSR, Moscow, 1974, 38 pgs.

[166] R. von Mizes, "Mathematical Theory of Probability and Statistics," Acad. Press, New York, 1964, 360 pgs.

[167] A. H. Moore and J. E. Bilikam, *Bayesian estimation of parameters of life distributions and reliability from type II censored samples,* IEEE Trans. Reliab., **R-27**, (1978), no. 1, 64–67.

[168] C. N. Morris, *Parametric empirical Bayes inference: theory and application,* Amer. Statist. Assoc., **78**, (1983), no. 381, 47–55.

[169] D. Neumann, "Two breakthroughs in the theory of statistical solutions search," vol. 8, no. 2, Mir, Moscow, 1964, pp. 113–140.

[170] W. G. Nichols and C. P. Tsokos, *Empirical Bayes point estimation in a family of probability distributions,* Intern. Stat. Inst., **40**, (1972), 146–161.

[171] W. G. Nichols and C. P. Tsokos, *An empirical Bayes approach to point estimation in adaptive control,* J. Information and Control, **20**, (1972), no. 3, 263–275.

[172] W. G. Nichols and C. P. Tsokos, *Empirical Bayes point estimation in a family of probability distributions,* Intl. Statistical Inst., **40**, (1972), no. 2, 147–151.

[173] D. D. Nikozakov, V. 1. Perlik and V. 1. Kukushkin, "Statistical Optimization of Aircraft Design," Mashinostroenie, Moscow, 1977, 240 pgs.

[174] T. O'Bryan and V. Susarla, *An empirical Bayes estimation problem with nonidentical componenets invoiving normal distributions,* Comm. Statist., 4 (1975), 1033–1042.

[175] W. J. Padgett and C. P. Tsokos, *Bayes estimation of reliability for the lognormal failure model,* in "The Theory and Applications of Reliability with Emphasis on Bayesian and Nonparametric Methods," vol. 2, Acad. Press, New York, 1977, 133–161.

[176] W. J. Padgett and C. P. Tsokos, *Bayesian reliability estimates of the binomial failure model,* Rep. Stat. Appl. Res., JUSE, **21**, (1974), no. 1, 9–26.

[177] W. J. Padgett and C. P. Tsokos, *Estimation of reliability for a class of life distributions with a stochastic parameter,* METRON, **34**, (1976), nos. 3-4, 333–360.

[178] W. J. Padgett and C. P. Tsokos, *Bayes estimation of reliability for the lognormal failure model,* in "Proceedings of the Conf. on the Theory and Appl. of Reliability With Emphasis on Bayesian and Nonparametric Methods," vol. 1, Academic Press, New York, 1976, pp. 131–161.

[179] W. J. Padgett and C. P. Tsokos, *Bayes estimation of reliability for the lognormal failure model,* in "Proceedings of the Conf. on the Theory and Appl. of Reliability," vol. 2, PUBLISHER, PUBADDR, 1977, pp. 133–161.

[180] W. J. Padgett and C. P. Tsokos, *On Bayes estimation for reliability for mixtures of life distributions,* SIAM J. Applied Math., **34**, (1978), no. 4, 692–703.

[181] W. J. Padgett and C. P. Tsokos, *Bayes estimation of reliability using an estimated prior distribution,* J. Operations Research, **27**, (1979), no. 6, 1143–1157.

[182] W. J. Padgett and L. J. Wei, *Bayesian lower bounds on reliability for the lognormal model,* IEEE Trans. Reliab., **R-27**, (1978), no. 2, 161–165.

[183] W. J. Padgett and L. J. Wei, *A Bayesian nonparametric estimator of survival probability assuming increasing failure rate,* Comm. Statist. Theor. Meth., **A-10**, (1981), no. 1, 49–63.

[184] A. S. Papadopoulos, *The Burr distribution as a failure model from a Bayesian approach,* IEEE Trans. Reliab., **R-27**, (1978), no. 3, 369–371.

[185] A. S. Papadopoulos and W. J. Padgett, *On Bayes estimation for mixture of two exponential-life-distribution from rate-censored samples,* IEEE Trans. Reliab., **R-35**, (1986), no. 1, 102–105.

[186] A. S. Papadopoulos and C. P. Tsokos, *Bayesian confidence bounds for the Weibull failure model,* IEEE Trans. Reliab., **R-24**, (1975), no. 1, 21–26.

[187] A. S. Papadopoulos and C. P. Tsokos, *Bayesian confidence bounds for the Wei bull failure model,* IEEE Transactions on Reliability, **R-24**, (April 1975), no. 1, 21–26.

[188] A. S. Papadopoulos and C. P. Tsokos, *Bayesian analysis of the Weibull failure model with unknown scale and shape parameters,* Statistica, **36**, (1976), no. 4, 547–560.

[189] A. S. Papadopoulos and A. N. V. Rao, *Bayesian confidence bounds for the Weibull failure model,* in "The theory and applications of reliability with emphasis on Bayesian and nonparametric methods," vol. 2, Academic Press, New York, 1977, pp. 107–121.

[190] J. B. Parker, *Bayesian prior distributions for multi-component systems,* Nav. Res. Log. Quatr., **19**, (1972), no. 3, 509–515.

[191] E. Parzen, *On the estimation of probability density function on mode,* Ann. Math. Statist., **33**, (1962), 1065–1075.

[192] M. Ja. Penskaja, *On A Priori Density Estimates,* in "Statistical Methods," Perm, 1982, pp. 115–124.

[193] V. I. Perlik, V. P. Savchuk and G. G. Haritonova, *Optimal probabilistic design of aircrajts,* no. 2, Aviacionnaja Tehnika (1984), no. 2, 59–63.

[194] E. G. Phadia, *A note on empirical Bayes estimation of a disribution function based on censored data, Ann.* Statist. 8 (1980), no. 1, 226–229.

[195] Ju. G. Polljak, "Probabilistic Design on Computer," SOy. Radio, Moscow, 1971, 360 pgs.
[196] A. M. Polovko, "The Basics of Reliability Theory," Science, Moscow, 1964, 342 pgs. (Russian).
[197] R. R. Prairie and W. J. Zimmer, *The role of the prior distributions in Bayesian decision making for the binomial situation,* Ann. Reliab. and Maint. 9 (1970), 2–12.
[198] F. Proschan and N. D. Singpurwalla, *Accelerated life testing-a pragmatic Bayesian approach,* in "Optimization in Statistics," J. Rustagi (ed.), Acad. Press, New York, 1979, pp. 78–90.
[199] F. Proschan and N. D. Singpurwalla, *A new approach to inference from accelerated life tests,* IEEE Trans. Reliab., **R-29**, (1980), no. 2, 98–102.
[200] V. S. Pugachev, "Random Function Theory," Fismatgiz, Moscow, 1971, 883 pgs.
[201] E. L. Pugh, *The best estimate of reliability in the exponential case,* Operation Research, **11**, (1963), 57–61.
[202] G. Raifa and R. Shleifer, "Applied Theory of Statistical Solutions," Statistics, Moscow, 1977, 360 pgs.
[203] F. P. Ramsey, "Truth and probability in the Foundations of Mathematics and Other Logical Essays," Kegan, London, 1926, 208 pgs.
[204] A. N. V. Rao and C. P. Tsokos, *Bayesian analysis of the Weibull failure model under stochastic variation of the shape and scale parameters,* METRON, **34**, (1976), nos. 3–4, 201–217.
[205] A. N. V. Rao and C. P. Tsokos, *Bayesian analysis of the extreme value distribution,* in "Proc. of Conf. on Theory and Application of Reliability," Academic Press, New York, 1976, pp. 171–186.
[206] A. N. V. Rao and C. P. Tsokos, *Robustness studies for Bayesian developments in reliability,* in "Decision Information," Academic Press, New York, 1979, pp. 239–258.
[207] A. N. V. Rao and C. P. Tsokos, *Estimation of failure intensity for the Weibull process,* Journal of Engineering Reliability and System Safety (1994), to appear.
[208] S. R. Rao, "Linear Statistical Methods and Their Applications," Science, Moscow, 1968, 548 pgs.
[209] K. Rai, V. Susarla and J. V. Ryzin, *Shrinkage estimation in nonparametric Bayesian survival analysis: a simulation study,* Commun. Statist. Simula. Compo, **B–9**, (1980), no. 3, 271–298.
[210] V. G. Repin and G. P. Tartakovski, "Statistical Synthesis With A Priori Indeterminancy and Adaptation of Informational Systems," Sov. Radio, Moscow, 1977, 432 pgs.
[211] H. Robbins, *Asymptotically subminimax solutions of compound statistical desision problems,* in "Proc. Second Berkley Symp. Math. Statist. and Reliab.," vol. ?, 1950, pp. 131–148.
[212] H. Robbins, *An empirical Bayes estimation problem,* in "Proc. National. Acad. Sci. USA," vol. 77, no. 12, 1980, pp. 6988–6989.
[213] H. Robbins, *An empirical bayes appoach to statistics,* in "Proc. 3rd Berkley Symp. Math. Statist. Probability," vol. 1, 1955, pp. 157–164.
[214] A. L. Rukhin, *Universal bayes estimator of real parameters,* Rend. Sem. Mat. Univers. Politechn. Torino, **35**, (1976-1977), 53–59.
[215] Y. S. Sathe and S. D. Yarde, *On minimum variance unbiased estimation of reliability,* Ann. Math. Statist., **40**, (1969), no. 7, 710–714.
[216] L. J. Savage, "The Foundations of Statistics," Wiley, New York, 1954, 308 pgs.
[217] V. P. Savchuk, *Bayes reliability estimate with linear failure intensity function,* Realiabilty and Quality Control, **11**, (1982), 19–25. (Russian).
[218] V. P. Savchuk, *Bayes probaility estimates of failure less work for articles with increasing intensivity function,* Realiabilty and Quality Control 9, (1983), 40–45. (Russian).
[219] V. P. Savchuk, *Approximate Bayesian estimation of failure–free work probability for the class of old distribution,* Izv. AN SSSR 6, (1985), 38–43.

[220] V. P. Savchuk, *Reliabilty estimation of non–recoverable devices with increasing intensivity function,* in "Reliability of machinery and equipment," no. 8, Nauk. Dumka, Kiev, 1985, pp. 35–43.

[221] V. P. Savchuk, *Bayes approach in the theory of reliabilty testing,* Reliability and Quality Control 2 (1985), 46–51.

[222] V. P. Savchuk, *Bayes reliability estimates for binomial testing in the case of partial a priori determinancy,* Reliability and Quality Control 1, (1986), 8–16.

[223] V. P. Savchuk, *Bayes reliability estimation of technical device based on workability model with error,* Izv. AN SSSR 1, (1986), 60–65.

[224] V. P. Savchuk, *Reliability definition for machinery details,* Reliability and Quality Control 5, (1986), 11–18.

[225] V. P. Savchuk, *Bayes mini–max estimates of technical systems reliability,* Automatics and Telemechanics 8 (1986), 156–162. (Russian).

[226] V. P. Savchuk, *Bayes probability estimates for bounded old distributions,* Izv. AN SSSR 6 (1987).

[227] V. P. Savchuk, *Approximate nonparametric empirical Bayes probability estimates for failure-free work,* Automatics and Telemechanics 2 (1988), ??–??

[228] R. F. Schafer and A. J. Feduccia, *Prior distributions fitted to observed reliability data,,* **IEEE** Trans. Reliab., **R-21**, (1972), no. 1, 55–67.

[229] G. J. Schick and T. M. Drnas, *Bayesian reliability demonstration,* Amer. Inst. Ind. Eng. 4 (1972), no. 4, 92–102.

[230] R. J. Schulhof and D. L. Lindstrom, *Application of Bayesian statistics in reliability,* Ann. Symp. Reliab. (1966), 684–695.

[231] L. Schwartz, *On Bayes procedures,* Wahrscheinlichkeitstheorie verw., **Bd**, 4 (1965), no. 1, 10–26.

[232] I. N. Shimi and C. P. Tsokos, *The Bayesian and nonparametric approach to reliability studies: a survey of recent work,* in "Proc. of the Conf. on the Theory and Applications of Reliability With Emphasis on Bayesian and Nonparametric Methods," vol. 1, Acad. Press, New York, 1977, pp. 5–47.

[233] "The Theory and Applications of Reliability With Emphasis on Bayesian and Nonparametric Methods," vol. I, I. Shimi and C. P. Tsokos (eds.), Academic Press, New York, 1976.

[234] D. R. Smith, *An analysis regarding the determination of Bayesian confidence limits for the reliability of distribution–free parallel subsystems,* in "The Theory and Applications of Reliability With Emphasis on Bayesian and Nonparametric Methods," vol. 1, Acad. Press, New York, 1977, pp. 93–106.

[235] J. Q. Smith, *Bayes estimates under bounded loss,* Biometrika, **67**, (1980), no. 3, 629–638.

[236] R. M. Soland, *Bayesian analysis of the Weibull process with unknown scale and shape parameters,* IEEE Trans. Reliab., **R-17**, (1968), no. 1, 84–90.

[237] R. M. Soland, *Bayesian analysis of the Weibull process with unknown scale and shape parameters,* IEEE Trans. ReHab., **R-18**, (1969), no. 2, 181–184.

[238] M. D. Springer and J. K. Byers, *Bayesian confidence limits for the reliability of mixed exponential and distribution–free cascade subsystems,* IEEE Trans. Reliab., **R-20**, (1971), no. 1, 24–28.

[239] M. D. Springer and W. E. Thompson, *Bayesian confidence limits for the product of N binormial parameters,* Biometrika, **53**, (1966), no. 3, 611–613.

[240] M. D. Springer and W. E. Thompson, *Bayesian confidence limits for the reliability of cascade exponential subsystems,* IEEE Trans. ReHab., **R-16**, (1967), no. 1, 86–89.

[241] M. D. Springer and W. E. Thompson, *Bayesian confidence limits for the reliability of redundent systems when tests are terminated at first failure,* Technometrics, **10**, (1968), no. 1, 29–36.

[242] H. Strasser, *Consistency of maximum likelihood and Bayes estimates,* Ann. Statist. 9 (1981), no. 5, 1107–1113.

[243] M. Stone and A. P. Dawid, *On Bayesian implications of improper Bayes inference in routine statistical problems,* Biometrika, **59**, (1972), no. 3, 369–373.

[244] R. S. Sudakov, *Nonparametric methods in system testing problems,* Reliability and Quality Control 1, (1983), no. 9, 12–21. (Russian).

[245] V. Susarla and J. Van Ryzin, *Nonparametric Bayesian estimation of survival curves from incomplete observation,* Amer. Statist. Assoc., **71**, (1976), no. 356, 897–902.

[246] V. Susarla and J. Van Ryzin, *Large sample theory for survival curve estimators under variable censoring,* in "Optimizing Methods in Statistics," Acad. Press, New York, 1979, pp. 16–32.

[247] O. I. Teskin, "Multidimensional Problems of Control and Planning of Reliability Testing With One Control Level," Znanie, Moscow, 1980, pp. 60–68. (Russian).

[248] W. E. Thompson and E. Y. Chang, *Bayes confidence limits for reliability of redundant systems,* Technometrics, **17**, (1975), no. 1, 89–93.

[249] F. A. Tillman, C. L. Hwang, W. Kuo and D. L. Grosh, *Bayesian reliability and availability-a review,* IEEE Trans. Reliab., **R-31**, (1982), no. 4, 362–372.

[250] M. Tribus, "Rational Descriptions, Decisions and Designs," Pergamon Press, New York, 1952, 120 pgs.

[251] C. P. Tsokos, *Bayesian approach to reliability using the Weibull distribution with unknown parameters with simulation,* JUSE, **19**, (1972), no. 4, 1–12.

[252] C. P. Tsokos, *Bayesian approach to reliability using the Weibull distribution with unknown parameters and its computer simulation,* JUSE, **19**, (1972), no. 4, 123–134.

[253] C. P. Tsokos, *Bayesian approach to reliability: theory and simulation,* in "Proc. of IEEE Symposium on Reliability," San Francisco, CA, January 1972, pp. 78–87.

[254] C. P. Tsokos, *Recent Advances in Life- Testing,* Chapter 17 in "Reliability Growth: Nonhomogeneous Poisson Process," CRC Press, Inc., CITY, 1995, pp. 319–334.

[255] V. M. R. Tummala and P. T. Sathe, *Minimum expected loss estimator of reliability and parameters of certain life time distributions,* IEEE Trans. Reliab., **R-27**, (1978), no. 4, 283–285.

[256] 1. A. Ushakov, "Methods of System Effectivity Calculation on the Design Stage," Znanie, Moscow, 1983, 92 pgs. (Russian).

[257] A. Vald, "Statistical Decision Functions: Position Games," Science, Moscow, 1976, pp. 300–522.

[258] S. D. Yarde, *Life testing and reliability estimation for the two parameter exponential distribution,* Amer. Statist. Assoc., **64**, (1969), 621–63l.

[259] J. A. Venn, "The Logic of Chance," Chelsea Publishing Co., London, 1962.

[260] L. 1. Volkov and A. M. Shishkevich, "Aircrafts Reliability," Vyshaja Shkola, Moscow, 1975, 293 pgs. (Russian).

[261] R. T. Wallenius, *Sequential reability assurance in finite lots,* Technometrics, **11**, (1969), no. 1, 61–74.

[262] A. M. Walker, *On the asymptotic behavior of posterior distributions,* Royal Statist. Soc. B., **31**, (1969), no. 1, pp. 80–88.

[263] H. Weiler, *The use of incomplete beta functions for prior distributions in binomial sampling,* Technometrics 7 (1965), no. 3, 335–347.

[264] R. L. W. Welch and C. P. Tsokos, *Robustness of Bayes optimal discriminal procedure with zero–one loss,* J. Appl. Math. and Compo 5, (1979), no. 2, 131–148.

[265] R. L. W. Welch and C. P. Tsokos, *Bayes discrimination with mean square error loss,* Pattern Recognition, **10**, (1978), 113–123.

[266] S. Wilks, "Mathematical Statistics," Science, Moscow, 1967, 632 pgs.